ADVANCES IN LONG-TERM CARE

Volume 2

ADVISORY BOARD

Advances in Long-Term Care

Advances in
LONG-TERM CARE

Volume 2

Paul R. Katz, MD
Robert L. Kane, MD
Mathy D. Mezey, RN, EdD

Editors

SPRINGER PUBLISHING COMPANY
New York

Springer Publishing Company, Inc.
536 Broadway
New York, NY 10012

93 94 95 96 97 / 5 4 3 2 1

ISBN 0-8261-6831-0
ISSN 1053-0606

Printed in the United States of America

Contents

v

Contributors

VOLUME EDITORS

Paul R. Katz, M.D., is Associate Professor of Medicine at the University of Rochester School of Medicine and Dentistry. He is currently Physician-in-Chief of Long-Term Care at Monroe Community Hospital and Director of the Geriatric Fellowship at the University of Rochester. His research interests have focused on physician practice patterns in long-term care and organizational correlates of quality and on medical education. He is coeditor of *Principles and Practice of Nursing Home Care* and *Practice of Geriatrics*. Dr. Katz is active in the American Medical Directors Association and the American Geriatrics Society and serves as chairman of an annual national conference in medical care in the nursing home.

Robert L. Kane, M.D., holds the Minnesota Endowed Chair in Long-Term Care and Aging at the University of Minnesota School of Public Health. He has studied and written widely in the areas of geriatrics and long-term care with special attention to issues of quality assurance, functional assessment, and international comparisons of care. Most recently he has coedited a volume on international perspectives on care of the elderly, *Improving the Health of Older Persons*, and, with Rosalie Kane, has written *Long-Term Care: Principles, Programs and Policies*. His coauthored text, *Essentials of Clinical Geriatrics*, will soon be issued in its third edition.

Mathy D. Mezey, R.N., Ed.D., F.A.A.N., is the Independence Foundation Professor of Nursing Education at New York University. She is past Director of the Robert Wood Johnson Foundation Teaching Nursing Home Program, a national initiative which sought to improve care to nursing home patients and to entice nurses to work in long-term care by linking schools of nursing and nursing homes. While a faculty member at the University of Pennsylvania, she was Associate Director of an ambulatory care facility for the elderly where she established interdisciplinary geriatric programs, including a nurse-managed urinary continence program. She has written widely on the role of nurse practitioners in improving health care to the elderly, on assessment and, more recently, on ethical decision-making concerning life-sustaining treatments. She is the coauthor of *Health Assessment of the Older Individual* which is in its second edition, *Nurses, Nurse Practitioners: The Evolution of Primary Care,* and *Nursing Homes and Nursing Care.*

VOLUME AUTHORS

Kyle R. Allen, D.O.
126 East 2nd Street Suite A
Chillicothe, Ohio 45601

Brenda Bergman, Ph.D., R.N.C.
University of Nebraska Medical Center
College of Nursing
600 South 42nd Street
Omaha, Nebraska 68198-5330

Warren H. Bock, Ph.D.
President and C.E.O. of Emeritus
Corp.
2550 University Ave W. #312N
St. Paul, MN 55114

Barbara J. Braden, Ph.D.
Professor, Creighton University School
of Nursing
2500 California
Omaha, NE 68178

Janet Cuddigan, M.S.N.
University of Nebraska Medical Center
College of Nursing
600 South 42nd Street
Omaha, Nebraska 68198-5330

Elizabeth Dean, Ph.D.
Associate Professor
School of Rehabilitation Medicine
University of British Columbia University Hospital, University Site
2211 Wesbrooke Mall
Vancouver, British Columbia

Linda Feins, B.SN, R.N., C.
Comprehensive Services on Aging
Institute for Alzheimer's Disease and
Related Disorders
UMDNJ, New Jersey's University of
the Health Sciences
667 Hoes Lane
Piscataway, NJ 08855-1392

Hilary Hanchuk, MD.
Clinical Assistant Professor of Psychiatry
Robert Wood Johnson Medical School
UMDNJ, New Jersey's University of
the Health Sciences
667 Hoes Lane
Piscataway, NJ 08855-1392

**Jeanie Schmit Kayser-Jones, R.N.,
Ph.D., FAAN**
Professor, Department of Physiological
Nursing
School of Nursing and Medical Anthropology Program
Department of Biostatistics and International Health
School of Medicine
University of California, San Francisco,
CA 94143

**Mary Knapp, M.S.N., R.N.,
G.N.P.C.**
John Whitman and Associates, Inc.
Philadelphia, PA

Steven A. Levenson, M.D.
Medical Director
Levindale Hebrew Geriatric Center
and Hospital
Belvedere and Greenspring Avenues
Baltimore, MD 21215-5299

Mildred G. Kemp, Ph.D., R.N., F.A.A.N.
Rush-Presbyterian—St. Luke's Medical
Center
Department of Operating Room and
Surgical Nursing
1653 West Congress Parkway
Chicago, IL 60612

Mark H. Overton, M.D.
Rush-Presbyterian—St. Luke's Medical
Center
Department of Internal Medicine,
Geriatric Section
1653 West Congress Parkway
Chicago, IL 60612

William E. Reichman, M.D.
Director, Division of Geriatric Psychiatry
Robert Wood Johnson Medical School
UMDNJ, New Jersey's University of
the Health Sciences
667 Hoes Lane
Piscataway, NJ 08855-1392

Gregg A. Warshaw, M.D.
Associate Professor of Family Medicine
Director, Office of Geriatric Medicine
University of Cincinnati Medical Center
231 Bethesda Avenue
Cincinnati, OH 45267-0504

Keren Brown Wilson, Ph.D.
President, Concepts in Community
Living, Inc.
5207 S.E. 80th Street
Portland, Oregon 97206

Preface

This volume of *Advances in Long-Term Care* continues the review of many of the current and oftentimes problematic issues confronting health care professionals engaged in long-term care while at the same time highlighting future trends in the field. Since long-term care encompasses such a wide array of issues, we have attempted to focus on a representative sample of thoughtful and thought-provoking reviews from a variety of disciplines. The success of the first installment in this series, including a book of the year award from the American Journal of Nursing, speaks to the need for a discourse of this kind. Educators and practitioners alike should find useful material in the chapters that follow.

In chapter 1 Elizabeth Dean examines recent advances in rehabilitation for older persons with cardiopulmonary dysfunction with special reference to the prescription of exercise programs. The negative effects of immobility are highlighted as well as the significance of gravitational stress and exercise stress on normal physiologic function. In the following chapter Barbara Braden and colleagues present an extremely practical and well rounded review of pressure sores, a problem impacting significantly on the morbidity and mortality of an increasingly frail long-term care population. Chapter 3 continues in the clinical vein with a problem-oriented treatise of disturbed behavior in the chronic care setting. Reichman, Hanchuk, and Feins provide order to what is often viewed as a problem with only one solution—chemical or physical restraint.

Issues specific to the nursing home are explored in chapters 4 through 6. Mezey and Knapp summarize the relationship between nurse staffing and quality of care in addition to factors currently impeding the increase of RN staffing in nursing facilities. Steve Levenson then reviews the evolving and often complex role of the nursing home medical director in light of ever changing regulations and expectations. Finally, Kayser-Jones explores the complex relationship between environment and falls in the nursing home while presenting a provocative conceptual model to guide practice and future research in this area.

In chapter 7 the focus shifts from the nursing home to other housing options for the chronically ill. Keren Brown Wilson looks specifically at the "assisted living" model and the underpinnings of its success in the State of Oregon. Drs. Allen and Warshaw's chapter follows with a discussion of how the basic tenets of health maintenance apply to the chronically disabled and frail older adult and the implications for health care in general. Warren Bock and Robert Kane close out the volume with a discussion of the computer management information systems, their applicability to the long-term care environment and to quality management.

Sincere appreciation and thanks are extended to the contributors of Volume 2 in addition to the Advisory Board for their continued counsel and the staff at Springer Publishing Company for their unwavering support.

Forthcoming

1
Advances in Rehabilitation for Older Persons with Cardiopulmonary Dysfunction

Elizabeth Dean

This chapter examines the advances in rehabilitation for older persons with special reference to the prescription of exercise programs for those with cardiopulmonary dysfunction. The literature on the benefits of exercise and the negative consequences of immobility is best synthesized in a quotation by Bland and Cooper (1984):

> The weakest and oldest among us can become some kind of athlete but only the strongest can survive as spectators, only the hardiest can withstand the perils of inertia, inactivity, and immobility. (p. 1)

Although the negative effects of immobility have been well documented during the past 50 years, this body of knowledge has not been fully integrated into clinical practice. This chapter briefly highlights this body of knowledge and the significance of gravitational stress and exercise stress on normal physiological function.

The number of studies on the exercise performance of older populations has been increasing; however, the validity of many studies is questionable because of inadequate attention to the quality control of exercise-testing methodology. Quality control and the validity of exercise testing can be severely compromised in older individuals. Compared with young persons, many older individuals may be unaccustomed to exercise; have musculoskeletal limitations, cardiopulmonary limitations, muscle weakness, and poor biomechanical efficiency; and may experience greater arousal particularly when a mouth piece and nose clip are used for respiratory gas analysis. The rationale for prescribing exercise programs for older persons who have cardiopulmonary dysfunction is described within the limitations of the existing literature.

In addition to the results of an exercise test, exercise prescription is based on a knowledge of the physiologic responses of older people to exercise, the superimposed effect of cardiopulmonary dysfunction, and other factors such as medical history and medications. Because many factors influence the exercise responses of older people, exercise needs to be prescribed as carefully as medications with particular attention to its indications, side effects and risks, contraindications, optimal therapeutic dosage, and anticipated effects.

Exercise testing and prescription is only one component of a comprehensive rehabilitation program that consists of several multidisciplinary components directed at all facets of an individual's life. Although the literature on the therapeutic efficacy and cost effectiveness of these programs is scant, there have been some reports on the benefits of some components. These are briefly described.

FACTORS CONTRIBUTING TO CARDIOPULMONARY DYSFUNCTION IN OLDER PERSONS

Cardiopulmonary dysfunction is a major contributor to reduced function in older persons (Epidemiology of Respiratory Diseases Task Force Report, 1980; Strasser, 1987). Factors responsible for this dysfunction include age-related changes in the cardiovascular and respiratory systems, reduced activity, and cardiopulmonary pathology.

Aging reduces the reserve capacity of the cardiovascular and respiratory systems, thereby reducing the efficiency of oxygen transport (Horvath & Borgia, 1984; Stamford, 1988). With respect to cardiovascular function, cardiac output and stroke volume are reduced (Horvath & Borgia, 1984; Mcelvaney et al., 1989). During vigorous exercise and comparable cardiac output, older subjects have lower heart rates compared with young people; this phenomenon has been associated with an increased stroke volume secondary to an increased end-diastolic volume (Lakatta, 1987; Rodeheffer et al., 1984). The extraction of oxygen by muscle has been reported to be diminished in older persons (Hossack & Bruce, 1982; Stamford, 1988). These changes reduce maximum oxygen consumption and functional work capacity (Buskirk & Hodgson, 1987; Hagberg et al., 1985; Hossack & Bruce, 1982). With respect to pulmonary function, residual volume increases with age, and vital capacity and maximal ventilation decline (Mahler et al., 1986; Robinson et al., 1973). Forced expiratory volume and peak flow rate also decline with age (Koenigsberg & Holden, 1989). The degree to which ventilatory limitation contributes to reduced work capacity in older persons is not known.

Few studies have examined the general activity levels of older people. The Framingham study showed that habitual daily activity is reduced with age (Kannel & Gordon, 1970). Compared with objective measures of their activity levels, older individuals tend to overestimate how active they are (Sidney & Shephard, 1977). Past and present physical activity patterns have been found to bear little relationship to fitness in older people (Sobolski et al., 1988). Reduced activity levels may contribute to reduced efficiency of the oxygen transport system, deconditioning (Bassey, 1978; Greenleaf & Kozlowski, 1982), and other multisystem consequences. Thus, optimal fitness levels do not simply reflect nonspecific levels of activity but exposure to a regular aerobic training stimulus as well as some genetic contribution.

Cardiac and pulmonary diseases are prevalent in older age groups (de Nicola & Tammaro, 1985a; Landin et al., 1985; Strasser, 1987). Common cardiovascular conditions include atherosclerosis, coronary artery disease, hypertension, cardiac dysrhythmias, congestive heart failure, and congenital heart defects. Atherosclerosis is the primary cause of peripheral vascular disease in older individuals. Common pulmonary conditions include obstructive lung diseases, such as chronic bronchitis and emphysema, and restrictive diseases associated with decreased lung compliance as in pulmonary fibrotic conditions and reduced chest wall compliance. In addition, dysfunction of either the heart or lungs invariably influences the other organ because of their close anatomical and physiological interdependence (Weber et al., 1983). If at rest the body is able to compensate adequately for dysfunction, no signs or symptoms are apparent. During exercise, however, the oxygen transport system is stressed, and the individual may become symptomatic because the ability to compensate is exceeded.

NEGATIVE EFFECTS OF IMMOBILITY

The perils of inactivity were documented in the medical literature 50 years ago (Dripps & Waters, 1941; Journal of the American Medical Association, 1944), and during the past 30 years, space physiology research has contributed significantly to our understanding of the effects of recumbency and inactivity on the human organism (Chase et al., 1966; Hyatt et al., 1969; Miller et al., 1964; Saltin et al., 1968). These have been central issues to space physiologists in that the conditions for optimal human function (i.e., being upright and moving in a gravitational field) are removed in space. Studies of bed rest, a model of a microgravity environment, have enhanced our understanding of the physiological effects of recumbency and inactivity as well as space travel.

A significant contribution of this literature to clinical science has been the finding that deconditioning resulting from recumbency is primarily due to the impairment of fluid volume regulating mechanisms rather than reduced activity (Chase et al., 1966; Convertino et al., 1982; Hahn Winslow, 1985). Recumbency results in the removal of the gravitational stimulus to the body fluids (Levine & Lown, 1952; Sandler, 1986; Sandler et al., 1988). Fluid is shifted centrally to the thorax from dependent areas. Plasma volume decreases (Sandler, 1986), and the work of the heart and breathing increases (Bydgeman & Wahren, 1974). Older individuals and those with cardiopulmonary dysfunction have particular difficulty compensating for this fluid shift when moving from supine to the erect position (Blomqvist & Stone, 1983; Bydgeman & Wahren, 1974). Even after only 24 hours of recumbency, cardiac underfilling and orthostatic hypotension can be observed.

There is only one means of countering position-induced fluid shift and its sequelae, and that is to assume a vertical upright position (Blomqvist & Stone, 1983; Hung et al., 1983; Wenger, 1982). Exercise in the recumbent position fails to prevent the consequences of recumbency even in young people exercising at high intensities (Chase et al., 1966). Thus, there is unequivocal physiological evidence to support maximizing the amount of time older individuals spend in the upright position.

Immobilization affects virtually every organ system in the body. These effects have been well documented (Klemic & Imle, 1989) and are summarized in Table 1.1. With respect to the cardiovascular system, resting and submaximal heart rates are increased (Deitrick et al., 1948), maximal oxygen consumption is reduced (Convertino et al., 1986; Saltin et al., 1968), total blood volume and plasma volume are reduced (Deitrick et al., 1948; Saltin et al., 1968), blood viscosity is increased along with the risk of thromboembolism (Lentz, 1981; Wenger, 1982). With respect to the respiratory system, recumbency results in reductions in total lung capacity, vital capacity, functional residual capacity, and residual volume (Craig et al., 1971; Svanberg, 1957). These changes lead to an increased potential for airway closure, and ventilation and perfusion mismatching (Risser, 1980). Forced expiratory volume is diminished (Craig et al., 1971; Svanberg, 1957). In addition, the alveolar-oxygen difference and the arterial-oxygen tension are reduced (Clauss et al., 1968; Ray et al., 1974). With respect to the musculoskeletal system, muscle mass and strength are reduced (Rice et al., 1989; Vandervoort et al., 1986) with associated mineral loss of the bone (Deitrick et al., 1948; Peacock, 1963; Sinaki, 1989). Inactivity can also be associated with joint contractures, skin lesions, and decubitus ulcers (Rubin, 1988). Effects of inactivity on the neurological system include slowed electrical activity in the brain, slowed reaction times, emotional and behavioral changes, sleep disturbance, and impaired psychomotor performance (Rubin, 1988; Ryback et al., 1971; Zubeck & MacNeill, 1966). Metabolic changes include increased calcium and nitrogen excretion (Deitrick et al., 1948; Hulley et al., 1971). Immunological changes have been reported—specifically, reduced antibody defense mechanisms and increased risk of infection (Ahlinder et al., 1970).

Cardiovascular and cardiopulmonary deterioration following immobilization occurs faster than musculoskeletal and other changes, and the rate of recovery has been reported to be slower than the rate of deconditioning (Kottke, 1966; Sandler et al., 1988). These effects can be expected to be accentuated in older people (Harper & Lyles, 1988), particularly those with cardiopulmonary dysfunction.

EXERCISE RESPONSES OF HEALTHY OLDER PERSONS

Exercise induces a hypermetabolic state wherein the activity of the cardiovascular and pulmonary systems are functionally coupled to meet the increased demand for oxygen and removal of carbon dioxide (Wasserman & Whipp, 1975). Oxygen transport depends on adequate ventilation of the lungs, diffusion of gas across the alveolar-capillary membrane, perfusion of the lungs, and transport of an adequate volume of oxygenated blood to the tissues (Wasserman & Whipp, 1975; Weber et al., 1983; West, 1990). Cardiac output and ventilation—hence, oxygen consumption—increase commensurate with work load. Cardiac output depends on stroke volume and the capacity to adjust heart rate. Ventilation depends on tidal volume (i.e., the volume of air per breath) and the capacity to increase breathing frequency. Oxygenated blood is transported to the working muscles, and the mitochondrial oxidative enzymes extract oxygen commensurate with physiologic demand.

Exercise training has been reported to reverse the effects of inactivity and improve physical work capacity in older as well as younger people, and potentially retard the aging process (Adams & de Vries, 1973; Aniansson et al., 1980; Clark et al., 1975; de Vries, 1970; de Vries, 1971; Kasch et al., 1988; Kent, 1982; Plowman et al., 1979; Stamford, 1972; Suominen et al., 1977; Thomas et al., 1985). Responses to aerobic exercise in older people include increased maximum aerobic capacity (Hodgson & Buskirk, 1977; Seals et al., 1984b), reduced resting and submaximal heart rate and blood pressure (Cooper et al., 1976; Stamford, 1988), increased maximal voluntary ventilation (Yeng et al., 1985), increased stroke volume and oxygen extraction by muscle (Hagberg et al., 1985), increased mineral content of bone (Smith et al., 1981), decreased body fat and increased lean body mass (Sidney et al., 1977), improved glucose tolerance (Saltin et al., 1979), increased high-density lipoproteins and decreased low-density lipoproteins (Seals et al., 1984a; Yano et al., 1986), improved flexibility (Frekany & Leslie, 1975), improved mental function, and greater ability to perform ADLs (Ingebretsen, 1982; Sidney & Shephard, 1976). The multisystem effects of

TABLE 1.1 Multisystem Consequences of Recumbency and Immobility

Cardiovascular effects of immobility
   ↓ Total blood volume
   ↓ Plasma volume
   ↓ Orthostatic tolerance
   ↑ Blood viscosity
   ↑ Venous stasis
   ↑ Risk of thromboembolism
   ↓ Hemoglobin
   ↑ Resting heart rate
   ↑ Submaximum heart rate
   ↓ Maximum heart rate
   ↑ Submaximum oxygen consumption owing to reduced mechanical efficiency
   ↓ Maximum oxygen consumption

Respiratory effects of recumbency
   ↓ Total lung capacity
   ↓ Vital capacity
   ↓ Functional residual capacity
   ↓ Residual volume
   ↓ Expiratory reserve volume
   ↓ Forced expiratory volume
   ↓ Peak flow rate
   ↓ Lung compliance
   ↓ Rib cage compliance
   ↑ Diaphragm-abdominal compliance
   ↑ Pulmonary vascular congestion
   ↑ Airway closure of dependent airways, and secondary ventilation and perfusion
     mismatch
   ↓ Anteroposterior diameter of chest wall or abdomen
   ↑ Lateral diameter of chest wall or abdomen
   ↓ Size of dependent alveoli
   ↓ Arterial oxygen pressure

Respiratory effects of immobility
   ↓ Arterial oxygen pressure
   ↓ Alveolar-arterial oxygen gradient
   ↑ Pulmonary arteriovenous shunt
   ↑ Functional residual capacity

Musculoskeletal effects of immobility
   ↑ Muscle atrophy
   ↑ Muscle shortening
   ↓ Muscle strength
   ↓ Muscle efficiency associated with ↑ oxygen demand
   ↑ Creatinine clearance
   ↑ Collagen production in connective tissue
   ↓ Bone density
   ↑ Joint contractures

TABLE 1.1 Continued

Metabolic effects of immobility
   ↑ Calcium excretion
   ↑ Nitrogen excretion
   ↑ Phosphorus excretion
   ↑ Magnesium excretion

Central nervous system effects of immobility
     Slowed brain-wave activity
     Emotional and behavioral changes
     Reduced psychomotor performance
     Secondary sensory deprivation
     Altered sleep patterns

Integumentary effects of immobility
     Skin lesions
     Decubitus ulcers

Gastrointestinal effects of immobility
     Impaired food processing
     Constipation
     Paralytic ileus

Genitourinary effects of immobility
     Renal stasis
     Risk of kidney or urethral stones

Immunological effects of immobility
     Depressed antibody defense mechanisms (?)

Sources. Adapted from Deitrick et al. (1948); Klemic and Imle (1989); Saltin et al. (1968); Svanberg (1957).

exercise training that have been reported in older people are summarized in Table 1.2.

Physiological adaptation to aerobic exercise can occur in old people with a minimum training intensity of 40% of maximum heart rate (de Vries, 1971), whereas in young people a minimum training intensity of 60% of the maximum heart rate is required (Karvonen et al., 1957). Despite this difference, physiological adaptation to exercise and the percentage increase in functional capacity are comparable across age groups (Stamford, 1988). Furthermore, exercise intensity is singularly important in effecting functional gains in older as well as in younger persons (Thomas et al., 1985).

Up to moderate levels of exercise, oxygen normally drives the biochemical reactions needed to meet these energy demands (aerobic metabolism). Anaerobic metabolism provides additional energy without oxygen; this system, however, is short term and results in the formation of lactic acid. Lactic acid normally accumulates at 55% of the healthy untrained person's maximum

TABLE 1.2 Beneficial Effects of Exercise in Older People

Cardiovascular effects
   ↑ Maximum aerobic capacity
   ↑ Stroke volume
   ↓ Vascular resistance
   ↓ Resting heart rate
   ↓ Resting blood pressure
   ↓ Submaximal heart rate
   ↓ Submaximal blood pressure
   ↓ Submaximal rate pressure product
   ↓ Submaximal exertion

Respiratory effects
   ↑ Maximum voluntary ventilation
   ↑ Arteriovenous oxygen difference secondary to improved muscle oxygen
     extraction
   ↑ Respiratory muscle strength and endurance

Musculoskeletal effects
   ↑ Muscle strength
   ↑ Muscle mass
   ↑ Bone mineral content
   ↓ Lean body mass
   ↓ Body fat
   ↑ Flexibility

Metabolic effects
   ↑ Glucose tolerance
   ↓ Low-density lipoproteins
   ↑ High-density lipoproteins

Psychological effects
   ↑ Mental function
   ↑ Ability to perform ADLs
   ↓ Quality of life

Source. Adapted from Adams and de Vries (1973); Hagberg et al. (1985); Hodgson and Buskirk (1977); Kent (1982); Seals et al. (1984b); Sidney and Shephard (1976); Stamford (1988); Thomas et al. (1985); Yano et al. (1986).

aerobic capacity (Davis et al., 1979). The precise interplay between aerobic and anaerobic metabolic processes are different for each individual and are determined by the type of activity and the fitness of the individual. With training, the blood lactate threshold (LT) occurs at a higher absolute value and at a higher percentage of aerobic capacity. Recently, Belman and Gaesser (1991) showed that sedentary older subjects (age range, 65–75 years) could increase maximum oxygen consumption ($\dot{V}_{O_2,MAX}$) and LT, and reduce cardiorespiratory responses to high-intensity exercise (i.e., training above the

LT), with only 8 weeks of training. These effects, however, were comparable to 8 weeks of low-intensity training below LT. This is not likely true for individuals with high aerobic capacities in which case higher training intensities would be necessary to enhance aerobic power further.

Several reports have established that muscle strengthening programs result in improved strength in older individuals including the frail elderly (Davies & White, 1983; Suominen et al., 1977). In addition to strength gains, Suominen et al. (1977) demonstrated connective tissue adaptation to training; Davies and White (1983) reported that exercise of high duration and intensity did not impair force-generating potential of muscle nor increase muscle fatiguability.

Despite the increasing number of reports on the benefits of exercise in older age groups, this work needs to be interpreted cautiously. Holloszy (1983) has argued that much of the evidence has been fragmentary and inconclusive, and that theories claiming exercise accelerates aging have not been adequately disproved. Longitudinal studies with adequate numbers of subjects are needed to examine in detail the role of exercise on health promotion and pathophysiological states in older age.

EXERCISE RESPONSES OF PERSONS WITH CARDIOPULMONARY DYSFUNCTION

The conventional categorization of either heart or lung disease may be too narrow in older persons whose cardiopulmonary dysfunction may refelect various underlying mechanisms. Practitioners involved with exercise testing and training such individuals need to be aware of these mechanisms and how each impacts on exercise capacity and function.

The principal mechanisms by which cardiopulmonary pathology interferes with oxygen transport are impaired ventilation of the lungs, impaired diffusion of gas across the alveolar capillary membrane, impaired lung perfusion, inadequate myocardial perfusion, inadequate cardiac output, inadequate transport of oxygenated blood from the heart to the peripheral tissues, and inadequate return of venous blood back to the heart (Goldring, 1984; Wasserman & Whipp, 1975). The precise mechanisms and severity of the underlying cardiopulmonary pathophysiology and the ability of an individual to compensate physiologically will determine both the degree of functional compromise and the degree to which training can enhance function.

Exercise testing and training in populations with cardiorespiratory dysfunction have been primarily directed at the assessment and enhancement of aerobic capacity. The interplay of aerobic and anaerobic metabolic processes in patients with cardiorespiratory dysfunction, and the ability of the anaerobic system to compensate for impaired oxygen transport are not well understood. Lactate production, the by-product of anaerobic metabolism, has been reported to be reduced, and LT increased following training in individuals with cardiopulmonary dysfunction (Fortini et al., 1991; Taniguchi et al., 1990; Woolf & Suero, 1969). Thus, the LT has been considered to be a significant indicator of the anaerobic threshold and functional impairment in these patients. Brown and Wasserman (1981) have reported, however, that the use of indices of the anaerobic threshold is limited in the assessment of individuals with severe cardiorespiratory compromise who reach their peak symptom-limited oxygen consumption before the anaerobic threshold. Considerable research is needed to elucidate the roles of aerobic and anaerobic therapeutic exercise prescription so that the metabolic reserves of a given individual can be exploited vis-à-vis optimizing potential function.

With respect to the effects of exercise on individuals with chronic lung disease, individuals with airway obstruction have been most frequently studied. The methodology and findings of a cross-section of frequently cited studies are summarized in Table 1.3. Individuals with chronic airflow limitation (e.g., chronic bronchitis and emphysema) can increase exercise endurance with training (Alpert et al., 1974; Chester et al., 1977; Christie, 1968; Mungall & Hainsworth, 1980; Niederman et al., 1991; Paez et al., 1967; Vyas et al., 1971; ZuWallack et al., 1991), and report less subjective distress on exertion (Belman & Wasserman, 1981; Cockcroft et al., 1981; Lertzman & Cherniack, 1976; McGavin et al., 1977; Mertens et al;., 1978; Sinclair & Ingram, 1980; Tydeman et al., 1984). Although many investigators have failed to observe significant improvements in pulmonary function and gas exchange in response to exercise training (Alpert et al., 1974; Chester et al., 1977; Cockcroft et al., 1981; Degre et al., 1974; Nicholas et al., 1970; Paez et al., 1967; Pierce et al., 1964; Ries et al., 1988; Tydeman et al., 1984), some investigators have reported some improvement (Mertens et al., 1978; Mungall & Hainsworth, 1980; Paez et al., 1967; Ries et al., 1988; Sinclair & Ingram, 1980). Because individuals with chronic lung disease may be unable to achieve sufficient exercise intensities to improve aerobic capacity, other mechanisms could explain the improvements observed (e.g., desensitization to dyspnea, increased motivation, improved movement efficiency, improved anaerobic exercise capacity, and improved ventilatory muscle endurance) (Belman & Kendregan, 1981; Belman & Kendregan, 1982; Horvath & Borgia, 1984).

Individuals with moderately severe restrictive patterns of lung disease respond to acute exercise with a rapid shallow breathing pattern, reduced cardiac output, arterial desaturation, increased pulmonary vascular resistance, and right ventricular work (Chung & Dean, 1989). The degree to which these individuals can adapt physiologically to a training stimulus has not been thoroughly investigated.

With respect to the effects of exercise on individuals with heart disease, individuals with coronary artery disease (CAD) and postcoronary artery bypass surgery (CABPS) have been most frequently studied. The methodology and findings of a cross-section of frequently cited studies are summarized in Table 1.4. Individuals with CAD can increase exercise tolerance, symptom-limited oxygen consumption, maximal heart rate and blood pressure, and their anginal threshold; and reduce their submaximal oxygen demands [Clausen & Trap-Jensen, 1976; Detry et al., 1971; Doba et al., 1990; Dressendorfer et al., 1982; Froehlicher et al., 1984; Hagberg et al., 1983; Laslett et al., 1985; May & Nagle, 1984; Rousseau et al., 1973; Taniguchi et al., 1990; Varnauskas et al., 1966; Williams et al., 1984). Similar beneficial effects have been reported for individuals who have undergone CABPS (Hedback et al., 1990; Kappagoda & Greenwood, 1984; Laslett et al., 1985). Training responses in individuals with CAD and post-CABPS have been reported to occur centrally (e.g., improved myocardial vascularity and coronary perfusion) (Eckstein, 1957; Kramsch et al., 1981) and peripherally (e.g., increased oxygen extraction within the muscle) (Detry et al., 1971; Hossack, 1987; Rousseau et al., 1973; Varnauskas et al., 1966).

Evidence to date supports a role for exercise testing and training individuals with chronic cardiopulmonary failure. Maximum testing can be performed safely in these individuals with appropriate medical supervision and monitoring facilities. Exercise testing is used to assess the functional manifestations of the underflying pathophysiology and treatment interventions. With respect to the management of ventilatory failure, Holten et al. (1972) studied the training responses of patients with long-standing severe disease to a 4-week program of cycle ergometry. An interrupted protocol was used in which patients cycled for two 3-minute bouts with a 3-minute rest between; the protocol was repeated twice daily. All patients used supplemental oxygen. Patients demonstrated aerobic training effects including an improved sense of well-being. With respect to the management of cardiac failure, exercise testing has become an important adjunct in the assessment of the disease (Wasserman, 1990; Wilson, 1987). Because left-ventricular performance and exercise capacity are poorly related in patients with failure secondary to coronary artery disease, the exercise capacity of these patients is extremely heterogeneous (Williams, 1985). The training exercise intensity for these patients is maintained below the threshold for myocardial ischemia, increased pulmonary vascular congestion, exertional hypotension, or sustained ventricular dysrhythmias (Williams, 1985). Patients who have demonstrable cardiac decompensation, manifested by vascular congestion at rest that is refractory to pharmacological therapy, are not considered candidates for exercise training. Within these guidelines, individuals with ventricular ejection fractions of 40% or less can increase their work capacities in response to training (Lee et al., 1979; Williams et al., 1981). These studies support that selected patients with severe ventricular dysfunction can show

TABLE 1.3 Cross-Section of Studies Evaluating Effect of Exercise on Patients with Chronic Lung Disease

Investigators	Research Design	Subjects	Smoking	Medications	Pretesting & Posttesting Preparation	Pretesting & Posttesting Procedures
Alpert et al. (1974)	Single-group pre-training & posttraining design	12 pts with COPD (?) & emphysema; all pts experienced dyspnea during self-paced walking on level, or on washing & dressing	All had smoked at least 1 ppd for 20 yr, but had quit prior to study	Not reported	None	S-S cycle erg test, resp gas analysis; 30-min baseline, then 6 min of S-S ex at max wkld tolerated
Chester et al. (1977)	Controlled pretraining & posttraining design	21 pts with COPD; all at least partially disabled with SOB (could walk on TM at 2 mph with 0% grade for 6 min); E grp: mean age = 51 ± 6 yrs, C grp: mean age = ?	Not reported	Meds & resp therapy withheld 12 hr before testing	None, other than ex performed in postabsorptive state	(a) 2 mph with 0% grade for at least 6 min (b) erg test at 150 or 300 kgm/min for 6 min
Christie (1968)	Single-group pre-training & posttraining design	10 pts with clinically stable COAD with marked dec ex tolerance; pts unable to walk at own pace for 15 min or 0.5 mi; 2 pts could not keep pace with others; mean age, 59.8 yr	Not reported	Generally unchanged; occasional short course of antibiotics given	None	Step test with resp gas analysis; 5–6 step exs (4 min) of inc'g wklds performed consecutively with 20-min rest between; peak wkld = wkld pt can maintain for ≥ 3 min

Training Duration	Exercise Training Procedures	Dropouts & Complications	Adherence	Reported Results
15 wk	Initially pts cycled at moderate resistance that permitted them to ex 5–7 min before tiring; at home, pts worked up to 20 min 3×/day, pts then inc resis & repeated the above process; wk 1 supervised & thereafter home erg ex on own	None reported	Not reported	Subj change inc ex tolerance Dec dyspnea Obj change No change PFTs Mod dec specific & static lung compliance No change dynamic compliance Dec V_{O_2REST} ($p < .05$) Dec $V_{O_2SUBMAX}$ ($p < .05$) Dec HR_{SUBMAX} ($p < .05$) No change C0, L, & R ht pressures, resistances, & ventricular stroke work Dec systemic a-v O_2 diff in ex ($p < .01$)
4 wk	Daily walking at inc'g speeds & grades, & other activities; mean TM walking dur'n = 15 min daily; daily program lasted 1–2 hr; pts also exercised with rowing machines, erg, & pulley wts to tolerance; training HR = 125 ± 18 bpm (approx 70% HRmax, HRmax not defined)	None reported	Not reported	No change pulmonary function (i.e., spirometry, lung volumes, ABGs) No change hemodynamic function (i.e., HR, CI, SI, PVR, a-v O_2 diff) Inc PAWP at rest & during ex Dec $V_{O_2SUBMAX}$ & VE_{SUBMAX} Inc total work performed
Mean duration = 9.7 wk, range 6–17 wk	Outpt training; 15 min ex, walking 0.5–1 mi/day 4 exs—int & freq inc'd on ind'l basis 5-min step ex, up/down self-paced encouragement for pt to integrate ex into ADLs	1 pt died (unrelated to ex prog)	Not reported	Subj changes Inc ex tolerance Inc well-being Inc physical work capacity Obj changes Inc V_{O_2MAX} & VE_{MAX} ($p < .01$) Inc max work ($p < .01$) Dec VE_{SUBMAX} No change $V_{O_2SUBMAX}$

TABLE 1.3 Continued

Investi-gators	Research Design	Subjects	Smoking	Medica-tions	Pretesting & Posttest-ing Prepa-ration	Pretesting & Posttesting Procedures
Cockcroft et al. (1981)	Random-ized pre-training & posttraining design with a delayed treatment control grp	39 pts with chronic respira-tory disability, varying degrees of restrictive disease & COAD, all pts breathless on exertion First 20 pts randomly assigned to grps, remaining 19 assigned by "minimization" process to spread out ex-traneous varia-tion eg age effects, smok-ing, 12 MWD	"Minimiza-tion" proc-ess used to assign smokers across grps	Not re-ported	None, other than mean for 2 repeated 12 MWD tests performed same day A.M. & P.M.	Tested initially, 2 & 4 mo; test included 12 MWD (mean of 2 repeated tests) & pro-gressive TM test (3 kph with 1.5% grade inc'ts/min; endpoint = at 10 min or sooner if pt could not con-tinue
Degre et al. (1974)	Controlled pretraining & post-training de-sign	16 pts with stable moderate to severe CAO (mean age, 50 ± 7 yr), E grp = 11, C grp = 5	Not re-ported	Pts re-ceived 3–4 L O$_2$ nasal-ly during ex	?	Initial 6-wk observation period pre-ceded & fol-lowed evalua-tion with a SLV02 max (progressively inc'g wklds of 10W/min) & submax erg test, submax test day after max test at 40, 70, & if possi-ble, 100 W for 6 min at S-S
McGavin et al. (1977)	Controlled pretraining & post-training de-sign	24 pts with stable chronic bronchitis, pt not included if FEV1 inc'd > 30% with bdtor; random assignment to the E & C grps; E grp = 12 pts (mean age 61.4 ± 5.6 yr; range 53–69 yr), C grp = 12 pt (mean age 57.2 ± 7.9 yr; range 40–69 yr)	Both grps advised not to smoke (no data)	Not re-ported, other than no pt on steroids	12 MWD tests repe-ated on 2 diff days; first test discarded	12 MWD tests & erg test with resp gas analy-sis (performed 20 min after walk test), ini-tial wkld 17 W for 2 min then inc'd 17 W/min; severe pts initial & inc'l wklds of 8.5 W/min Endpoint: pt could not go further or ex-cessive HR

Training Duration	Exercise Training Procedures	Dropouts & Complications	Adherence	Reported Results

6 wk	C grp: delayed training for 4 mo with no special advice, then 6 wk of rehab'n prog consisting of erg, rowing machine, swimming, water exs, & walking 2×/day over inc'g distances of up to 2 mi, then home prog of stair climbing & level walking
	
	E grp: 6 wks of rehab'n prog, then 6 wks home ex
		C grp = 4 dropouts
		E grp = 1 dropout
			Not reported	Subj change
				  C grp: no subjective improvement
				  E grp: improvement in well-being & walking ability, 50% dec breathlessness, 50% dec cough, 30% dec sputum
				
				Obj change
				  E grp: inc 12 MWD ($p <$ .05)
				  Little change TM ex performance
				  No change PFTs
				  Inc V_{0_2MAX}
				  Maintained improvement 7 mo after study
				
				Delayed treatment C grp: overall improvement greater than the E grp

6 wk	E grp: 6 wk training prog & br ex prog; ex prog was 25 min 3×/wk consisting of 5-min warm-up at 25–40 W, 25 min at 75% max wkld, 5 min warm-down C grp: br ex prog only	Most (?) controls did not complete	Not reported	C grp: no improvement on SLV_{0_2MAX} test E grp: no change $C0_{MAX}$, SV_{MAX} Inc Pa_{0_2} at rest (suggested improved V/Q ratio) Inc mean PAP at rest No change lung vols & diffusing capacity

3 mo	E grp: unsupervised home prog including progressive stair climbing exs, pt to climb up/down given no steps for given no mins at least 1×/day at least 5×/wk; goal: to be able to climb 10 steps for at least 10 min daily
	
	C grp: no ex instruction but attended monthly clinic
		4 of original 28 dropouts; following illness retraining commenced; more illness in E grp	Not reported	C grp
				  No changes
				
				E grp
				  Dec breathlessness ($p <$ .01)
				  Inc well-being ($p <$ .07)
				  Inc ex tolerance
				  No change ADL ability
				  Dec cough ($p <$ .02)
				  Dec sputum ($p <$ .07)
				  Inc mean stride length in walking
				  No change body wt, PFTs, or ex HR

TABLE 1.3 Continued

Investigators	Research Design	Subjects	Smoking	Medications	Pretesting & Posttesting Preparation	Pretesting & Posttesting Procedures
Mertens et al. (1978)	Single-group pretraining & posttraining design	13 pts with stable mild or moderate COLD (6 with emphysema or emphysema/chronic bronchitis, 7 with chronic bronchitis only); emphysema pts more disabled than emphysema/chronic bronchitis pts; all pts limited in effort tolerance; all < 15% improvement of FEV1 postbdtor, all sedentary lifestyles	Not reported	Not reported	None	2 erg tests repeated on same day pretraining, 6 & 12 mo; also 6 pts had repeated tests at 18 & 24 mo Test 1: pedaling 6 min at 60 rpm; wkld adjusted to develop 75% of pt's V_{O_2MAX} Test 2: erg test at same wkld for C0 determination
Mungall & Hainsworth (1980)	Single-group pretraining & posttraining design	10 pts with COAD (chronic bronchitis & emphysema) (mean age, 56.7 yr; range 50–64 yr; all pts < 20% improvement of FEV1 postbdtor	Noted at each attendance (no data)	Checked regularly as part of ongoing medical management (?)	None	Retests every 2 wk over 3–12-wk period (i.e., before, during, & after training period); tests included 12 MWD (mean of 4 repeated tests) & ex test at 2 TM wklds based on each pt
Nicholas et al. (1970)	Controlled pretraining & posttraining design; prolonged notraining control baseline (3 mo) followed by training prog (6 mo)	15 pts with COPD, prolonged Hx of exertional dyspnea, (mean age, 59.5 ± 6.6 yr; range, 43–71 yr)	All pts had been heavy smokers; all but one had quit before to study, this one had quit after the initial evaluation	Some pts had been treated with digitalis, current med regimens (?)	None	In baseline period ex tolerance repeatedly measured; pts given chance to become familiar with TM walking; control period: 2 ex tests repeated; best one used for baseline Pts permitted to hold hand rail

16

Training Duration	Exercise Training Procedures	Dropouts & Complications	Adherence	Reported Results
1 yr, 6 pts cont'd for 2nd yr	Supervised end training prog, 1×/wk & continued home prog the remaining days of week	Difficult to maintain pt motivation; interruptions made training discontinuous	3 pts who showed little/no improvement had failed to ex regularly	Subj change 8 pts noted symptomatic improvement Obj change 5 showed no improvement/ deterioration (3 had failed to ex regularly) Dec HR_{SUBMAX} Inc aerobic power (8% in emphysema pts, 15% chronic bronchitic pts) Inc muscle end (bronchitics > emphysema pts) Small dec O_2 debt Dec air trapping & CO_2 retention (emphysema pts) Cessation dec lung vols (bronchitic pts) 20% inc in tolerance to submax wklds.
3 mo	Period 1: no change Period 2: supervised ex training; 11–12 min of activity/ day in PT dept or home, Canadian Air Force prog for women Period 3: cessation of prog, return to pretraining activity levels	Pts instructed not to attend prog during exacerbation of illness	Not reported	Inc 12 MWD ($n = 7$), dec 12 MWD ($n = 1$), no change 12 MWD ($n = 2$) Inc FEV1, dec TLC, inc DLC0, dec A-a O_2 diff at end of training Inc 12 MWD, inc DLCo & O_2 tension diff maintained at rest after period 3
6 mo	Control period: for standardization all pts instructed in PD & br exs; 1 session of 2 TM walks/wk Exp'l period: 3×/wk, 3 TM walks/session, int = 1.7 mph with 0% grade; or 3 mph with 10% grade; set of Master's two-steps to climb at home 10 min daily; encourage to walk as much as possible & inc phys activity	7 dropouts; interruptions owing to vacations or illness; 3 pts required 12 mo to complete 9-mo study	Not reported	Considerable inc in ex tolerance in 4 of 8 who completed Other 4 showed little or no improvement No change PFTs No change gas exchange Most change occurred in first 6 wk

TABLE 1.3 Continued

Investi-gators	Research Design	Subjects	Smoking	Medica-tions	Pretesting & Posttest-ing Prepa-ration	Pretesting & Posttesting Procedures
Niederman et al. (1991)	Single-group pre-training & posttraining design	33 outpts with stable CLD (emphysema, chronic bron-chitis, asthma, pulmonary fib-rosis); all pts had limited ex capacity (mean FEV1, 1.2 ± 0.8 L; mean age, 65.8 ± 8.1 yr; range, 50–82 yr)	No pt was current smoker; 26 pts had previously smoked	Stable med regimens, 13 required steroid therapy	None	12 MWD & multistage erg test with ramp-ing protocol (10–25 W/min) & resp gas analysis; end-point: symp-tomatic en-dpoint, max pred HR or $SaO_2 < 85\%$
Paez et al. (1967)	Single group pre-training & posttraining design	8 pts with stable severe emphysema (i.e., walk ≤ 3 min without ex intolerance); no wt change over study; pts assigned ran-domly to air or O_2 breathing grps (age range, 49-69 yr)	Not re-ported	Some pts maintained on dose of digitalis	None	Submax erg GXT with resp gas analysis; all pts on room air; submax erg test, constant wkld (range, 120–198 kgm/min) 5 min. TM test: on first & last day of training
Pierce et al. (1964)	Single-group pre-training & posttraining design	9 pts with se-vere emphysema, generalized physical debil-ity (mean FVC = 72% pred, FEV1 = 30% FVC, MVV = 26% pred)	Not re-ported	Not re-ported	2–3 days familiariza-tion with TM & apparatus; on test days pts re-ceived bdtor Tx & bronchial toilet fol-lowed by a light break-fast, & 60-min rest interval be-fore testing	Highest speed pts could walk for 2.5 min was individually de-termined; resp gas analysis

Training Duration	Exercise Training Procedures	Dropouts & Complications	Adherence	Reported Results
9 wk	2.5-hr session, 3×/wk 1 hr—support grp, educational lectures on physiology, disease, meds, nutrition, relax'n, stress management, breathing retraining 1.5-hr ex session—20-min rotation between erg (int = 50% max Watts for 20 min), TM, U/E erg & wts; exercise to same RPE Ex prescription revised weekly; inc wklds 15% when pt can sustain prescribed wkld for 20 min	None reported	Not reported	Subj change Dec depression Dec sense of disability Inc knowledge on health education info Incorporated education into ADL Dec dyspnea Obj change Inc sustained submax performance on erg ($p < .01$) Inc 12 MWD ($p < .01$) Dec VE/V_{O_2MAX} Little improvement max ex performance on graded erg test Magnitude of change in physiological & psychological parameters not directly related to lung function
21 days	TM walking, 5–10-min sessions/day; at least 30 min between sessions; int prog'd according to tolerance 4 pts trained breathing compressed room air & 4 pts trained on O_2; all pts breathed air or O_2 with face mask at same flow rates	1 pt developed bronchospasm on retest	Not reported	Inc walking capacity Inc stride length Dec HR_{SUBMAX} Inc walking speed of O_2 breathers Dec HR_{REST} Dec RBC vol O_2 breathers Inc RBC vol air breathers No change $V_{O_2SUBMAX}$ & RQ No change VE_{SUBMAX} or $VE/V_{O_2SUBMAX}$ Inc PAO_2 at end of ex Dec A-a O_2 diff usually during ex No change pH & $PACO_2$ during ex Dec CO_{SUBMAX} Inc a-v O_2 diff No change lactate production & O_2 debt
	Regular physical training, other routine therapy unchanged 2.5-min walks with 0% grade, 5–10×/day, at speeds usually slower than pt's max attainable Walks separated by rests so vital signs returned to baseline Pts encouraged to be active	No ill effects noted	Not reported	No change PFTs 24% dec submax HR, 40% dec submax RR, 40% dec submax VE, 23% dec V_{O_2} & VC_{O_2} Inc wk tolerated Facilitation of ADL

TABLE 1.3 Continued

Investigators	Research Design	Subjects	Smoking	Medications	Pretesting & Posttesting Preparation	Pretesting & Posttesting Procedures
Ries et al (1988)	Single-group pretraining & posttraining design	45 pts with stable COPD; random assignment to 3 grps (1 C grp & 2 E grps); C grp: no U/E training, E grp 1: U/E wt training, & E grp 2: U/E PNF exs	Not reported	Hypoxemic pts tested with O_2	None	S-S TM walking test max isokinetic U/E erg test, incremental protocol, endpoint = symptom limitation After 20-min rest, end erg test wkld one stage below max; if maintained for > 12 min, test repeated at higher load
Sinclair & Ingram (1980)	Controlled pretraining & posttraining design	33 pts with chronic bronchitis; E grp: pts living close by, C grp: pts living away from city	All had been smokers & had symptoms of chronic bronchitis; both grps advised to quit; more E pts than C pts quit	As much as possible meds not changed	Familiarization with ex regimens following acute exacerbation in hospital	12 MWD (1 trial as pts previously familiarized), erg GXT

Training Duration	Exercise Training Procedures	Dropouts & Complications	Adherence	Reported Results
6 wk	All pts particpated in rehab prog including walking ex education: instruction in PT & OT, & psychological support 2 E grps: isokinetic erg 15 min/wk; wkld inc'd when wkld in end test sustained for 15 min E grp 1: gravity resisted strengthening exs, 5 low resis-high reps ex, 1×/day for 1 wk & then 2×/day E grp 2: PNF ex, low freq, resistraining with wts 4 ex with same wt; 3 sets of 4–10 reps of each ex (initial wt = max wt pt could complete 6 reps of first ex, range 1–5 lbs pt trained alternate days for 1 wk & then 1×/day Prog'n: pt moved to next wt when could complete 3 sets of at least 6 reps of each ex	17 drop-outs	90%	Inc no lifts on U/E performance test & end time on isokinetic arm erg ($p < .05$) Inc max wkld on erg ($p < .05$) Inc TM speed Dec V_{O_2}, VE, HR in all grps ($p < .05$) Dec RPE & fatigue in all grps ($p < .05$) Dec RV, FRC, RV/TLC, FVC ($p < .05$) No change FEV1, FEV1/FVC, FEF25%–75% No change in U/E erg performance, ventilatory muscle endurance, or simulated ADL performance
Mean period between tests for E grp 10.3 mo	E grp: supervised training prog, 12 min walk 1×/day, stair climbing, stepping up/down 2 steps for 1.5–2 min 2×/day; prog'n based on pts C grp: did not perform prog & were not reviewed	E grp: 2 dropouts, 1 died (unrelated to prog); pts restarted prog after bronchitis bout; C grp: 2 died resp failure, 1 had MI; 10 readmissions affected 7 pts	Not reported	Subj change Dec dyspnea ($p < .02$) Inc well-being ($p < .02$) Inc daily activity ($p < .02$) Obj change C grp: no change E grp: inc FVC (suggested dec air trapping) 24% inc walking distance (range 12%–83%) Dec cadence (i.e., inc stride length) Gradual improvement; most improvement between 8–12 mo

TABLE 1.3 Continued

Investigators	Research Design	Subjects	Smoking	Medications	Pretesting & Posttesting Preparation	Pretesting & Posttesting Procedures
Tydeman et al. (1984)	Randomized pretraining & posttraining design	24 pts with CAO, mean age 56–69 yrs; no pt > 30% improvement of FEV1 past bdtor; pts randomly assigned to grps, grp 1: initially supervised prog in hospital & then ex'd at home, grp 2: ex'd only at home	All pts ex smokers	All drug therapy aside from antibiotics was unchanged	12 min walk test repeated 3× with 20-min rest between, mean of tests 2 & 3 averaged	12 MWD test
Vyas et al. (1971)	Single-group pretraining & posttraining design	14 pts with stable moderately severe to severe CAO (mean age, 61 yr; range, 41–68 yr)	Not reported	Not reported	Morning testing ranging from 1.5–3 hr after breakfast; no practice	Symptom-limited multistage erg test with resp gas analysis 5 min warmup, 60 kgm/min; wkld then inc'd in approx equal steps so pt reaches limit in 3–4 min Posttest: repeated pretest, included progressive wklds until max reached

22

Training Duration	Exercise Training Procedures	Dropouts & Complications	Adherence	Reported Results

Mean 36 wk, range 26–51 wk	PT class: 15-min rest before ex step ex, int = stepping on/off until SOB (rate constant) Walking ex—self-paced rate until feel SOB Chair ex—standing/sitting until feel SOB (rate constant)
	
	Home ex: exs cont'd at home on daily basis
		In illness, ex discont'd; when well, instructed to strive for past performance immediately but responding to SOB
		
		8 dropouts owing to thoracic/lumbar pain, repeated illness, 1 death
			Not reported	Subj change
				  Improved well-being, ADL performance, confidence, & relaxation in most pts
				
				Obj change
				  Inc walking distance (mean inc of 42%, peak inc between 26–51 wk)
				  No change FEV1, FVC, PEF, or HR recovery from ex
				  All pts could walk 1600 m in own time without stopping (distance consistent with performing most normal social activities)
				  Pts improved at home & in PT prog with exception of walking ex (i.e., peak performance at home lower & occurred sooner)

Mean 10 wk; range 6–26 wk	Outpts: 20–30 min/day on erg; inpts: 20 min 2×/day 5-min warm-up at 0 load, 1–2 min at 90% max wkld & 2 min at 30% max wkld, 5-min rest & protocol repeated Prog'n: when pt completed 3–4 sessions easily, int & dur'n inc'd	3 dropouts	Not reported	Inc max wk rate, total work done, V_{O_2MAX}, total V_{O_2} ($p < .01$) 10% inc V_{O_2MAX}, degree of improvement not related disease severity or efficiency of work performance, but to change in PA_{O_2} on ex in combination with $\dot{V}C$ or Hb Dec VE_{SUBMAX} Inc PA_{O_2} (possibly owing to improved V/Q matching)

TABLE 1.3 Continued

Investi-gators	Research Design	Subjects	Smoking	Medica-tions	Pretesting & Posttest-ing Prepa-ration	Pretesting & Posttesting Procedures
Woolf & Suero (1969)	Single-group pre-training & posttraining design	14 pts with stable advanced COLD (mean age, 59 yr; range, 48–72 yr)	Not re-ported	All pts on stable reg-imens (e.g., bdtors, steroids, digitalis, diuretics)	None	No ex test, but lung mechanics & gas exchange measures
Zu Wallack et al. (1991)	Single-group pre-training & posttraining design	50 ambulatory pts with CLD & significant resp symptoms; pts included 40 with COPD, 3 asthmatics, 3 with pulmonary fibrosis, 2 with chest wall de-formity, 1 with bronchiectasis	Not re-ported	13 pts on low flow 0_2 during ex; 3 pts ste-roid-treated asthmatics	None	(a) 12 MWD (b) multistage GXT (n = 44), protocol not specified; resp gas analysis (n = 34); end-point = fatigue or dyspnea, max HR = 79.4 ± 9.8% pred; tests re-peated before, during, & after 6 wk

Training Duration	Exercise Training Procedures	Dropouts & Complications	Adherence	Reported Results
Grp 1: 1 mo; grp 2: 2 mo	Goal: 30 min of continuous walking breathing room air Grp 1 ($n = 6$): TM walking, 1 mph with 4% grade, pts breathed room air, inc walking dur'n by 1 min/session up to 30 min Grp 2 ($n = 9$): TM walking, 2 mph with 8% grade; 8 pts reached 4 min, then req'd approx 60% O_2 to inc to 30 min walking; O_2 withdrawn & pt returned to room air, walking dur'n only 5 min, training cont'd until pt able to walk easily for 30 min breathing room air all pts trained 2×/day, 5×/week, & encouraged to walk freq'ly	None reported	Not reported	Slower deeper breathing Inc V/Q relationship suggested by dec A-a O_2 Diff & improved venous admixture, & shorter 90% desat time Inc dynamic compliance Dec work of breathing Dec blood lactate levels (suggests dec anaerobic metabolism) Trend toward dec V_{O_2} Improved general muscle function
6 wk	12 3-hr sessions 50% – education, breathing retraining, control of dyspnea, nutrition, energy conservation, work simplification, stress management, relaxation 50% – inspiratory resistive loading TM & cycle erg Supervised stair climbing Upper-body & limb strengthening Br exs Ex protocol: to produce moderate dyspnea or HR between 70%–85% max Prog'n: dur'n & int inc'd small (?) amts Pts encouraged to ex at home	6 pts not given physician approval for TM GXT before training	1 pt missed first 2 sessions	28% inc 12 MWD No relationship between inc 12 MWD & age, sex, O_2 req't, ABGs, PFTs Pos relationship between inc 12 MWD & vent reserve Greater % improvement in 12 MWD in pts with low peak O_2 & O_2 pulse

TABLE 1.4 Cross-Section of Studies Evaluating Effect of Exercise on Patients with Heart Disease

Investi-gators	Research Design	Subjects	Smoking	Medica-tions	Pretesting & Posttest-ing Prepa-ration	Pretesting & Posttesting Procedures
Clausen & Trap-Jensen (1976)	Single-group pre-training & posttraining design	29 pts with ex-ertional angina (mean age, 55 yr; range, 44–66 yr)	Not re-ported	1 pt on di-gitalis & diuretics, 4 pts on β blockers for several mo; other pts on anti-anginal meds prn	None, other than testing per-formed in A.M. in fasting state	Erg GXT at 3–4 diff wklds; lowest wkld det'd which provoked an-gina between 3–5 min after ex onset, & highest load sustainable for at least 1 min before angina onset

12 pts per-formed 2 arm erg ex periods 17 pts repeated 1 leg load 2× on erg; nitro given at start of last ex per-iod; between ex periods, pts rested 5–10 min after cessa-tion pain |
| Detry et al. (1971) | Single group pre-training & posttraining design | 12 pts with CAD (8 in Seattle, 4 in Belgium) (mean age, 47.8 yr; range, 34–48 yr), $n = 6$ with angina, $n = 6$ prior MI with-out angina | Not re-ported | 2 pts on β-blockers; schedules unchanged | None re-ported | Seattle: multi-stage TM test, V_{0_2MAX} test with resp gas analysis; Bel-gium: multi-stage erg test (initial wkld 10 W & suc-cessive inc of 10 W/min); endpoint: max tolerable fa-tigue, dyspnea, leg wkness, or angina |

Training Duration	Exercise Training Procedures	Dropouts/ Complications	Adherence	Reported Results
3 mo	1 hr daily or 3×/wk; prog averaged 38 training sessions in 3 mo; included ergometer ex, ex periods normally 5 min with approx equal rests, 4–6 ex periods/ex session Wklds set so chest pain occurred at end of 5-min period Prog'n: wklds inc'd with inc'd ex tolerance to maintain same work int	4 dropouts; no reasons given	Not reported other than pts attended ave of 38 training sessions in 3 mo	100% inc total work before angina Improvement in ex tolerance with training approx same as improvement with nitro 10% dec HR_{SUBMAX} No change SBP Angina onset independence of wkld & occurred at fairly constant value of RPP, HR, & SBP for each pt Pain t'holds for RPP, HR, & SBP higher in arm ex than leg ex
3 mo	45 min 3×/wk Seattle: 6 graded levels of walking, jogging, running & 12 calisthenics scaled from 5-15 reps; int adjusted to pt Belgium: walking, calisthenics, jogging, rowing, cycling at 5 graded levels; int adjusted to pt	None reported	Not reported	Subj change All pts reported improvement Obj change 23% inc V_{O_2MAX} ($p < .0001$) Inc HR max angina pts; not in pts without angina Dec submax HR, MAP, CO No change SV Inc a-v O_2 diff Dec RPP & LV work

TABLE 1.4 Continued

Investigators	Research Design	Subjects	Smoking	Medications	Pretesting & Posttesting Preparation	Pretesting & Posttesting Procedures
Doba et al. (1990)	Single group pretraining & posttraining design	81 pts with stable CAD; n = 41 with single, n = 20 with double & n = 9 with tripple vessel disease, n = 11 CABG (mean age, 53 ± 10 yr, 57 ± 7 yr, 57 ± 6 yr, & 55 ± 9 yr, respectively)	Not reported	Pts stabilized with long-acting nitrates & Ca antagonists	None	SL_{MAX} TM GXT; Bruce protocol
Dressendorfer et al. (1982)	Single group pretraining & posttraining design	8 pts with CAD (mean age, 52 yr, range, 37–64 yrs); all physically active but none in formal ex prog	Not reported	2 pts on β-blockers daily	None	(a) SL_{MAX} graded TM test (fatigue limited) (b) single-stage S-S test with 0% grade (pt walked for 10 min at speed that provoked 0.1-mV flat ST seg depression from baseline at rest) TM walking with handrail support
Froelicher et al. (1984)	Randomized controlled pretraining & posttraining	146 pts with stable CAD (E grp = 72, C grp = 74) (mean age, 53 ± 8 yr; range, 35–65 yr)	Not reported	Some pts on digoxin & β-blockers; inclusion criterion: pts could be discont'd for 3 days before testing; other meds included long-acting nitrates, antidysrhythmics, & antihypertensives	None, other than pts in fasting state	3 entry level ex tests done on separate days within 2 wk performed initially & 1 yr later, included TM GXT with modified Balke-Ware protocol, Thallium scintigraphy; all tests symptom or sign limited max effort

Training Duration	Exercise Training Procedures	Dropouts/Complications	Adherence	Reported Results
12 wk	1 hr/wk; int 70%–85% symptom-limited HR max, circuit training, ex modalities sequentially performed for 3-min intervals—warm-up 5 min, followed by randomly assigned ex for 8 min each including stepping (Master's step), rowing, cycle erg, walking/jogging on TM, & cool-down 5 min Home prog: walking/jogging at same int 20–30 min 2×/wk	None reported	> 85% attendance at institutional sessions	Inc TMT for all grps ($p <$ .05) Inc V_{O_2MAX} all grps ($p <$ .05) Inc HR max for SVD & CABG grps ($p <$ .05) Inc RPP for SVD grp ($p <$ .01) Dec EDI in all grps ($p <$ .01) Dec FAI in all grps ($p <$ .01) Dec CRI for SVD & CABG grps ($p <$ .01) Dec MRI for SVD grp ($p <$ .01) Dec PCI for SVD & DVD grps ($p <$ .001)
Mean 16 wk; range, 14–20 wk	40 min, 3×/wk, walking speeds on level ranged from 3.4–4 mph (mean, 3.9 mph); ex HR based on each pt's ischemic t'hold i.e., 0.1 mV ST seg depression in pretraining submax test Mean training HRs ranged from 74%–83% max (corresponds 56%–78% V_{O_2MAX})	None reported	80% of scheduled ex sessions attended	No change V_{O_2MAX} 16% dec submax HR, SBP, & 16% dec RPP ($p <$ .05) No pts had ischemic ECG changes posttraining 10% dec V_{O_2} (suggests improved external work efficiency) Inc ex t'hold for myocardial ischemia
1 yr	E grp: supervised ex prog including arm, leg, or arm & leg erg, 45 min 3×/wk, initially int set at minimum of 60% estimated V_{O_2MAX} from initial TM test Prog'n: int progressively inc'd to 85% of estimated V_{O_2MAX} by wk 8 of training After 8 wk, pt assigned to gym prog or outdoor walk-run prog C grp—low int walking prog	C grp: 5 medical dropouts E grp: 6 medical dropouts 7 quit owing to conflicts, lack of motivation; repeat testing performed on 59 of 72 pts of E grp & 69 of 74 pts of C grp No episodes of cardiac arrest or other major complications	Mean attendance 76% ± 18%; range, 23%–97%	Improved aerobic capacity Improved thallium ischemia scores Improved ventricular function Modest improvement in myocardial perfusion in some pts

TABLE 1.4 Continued

Investigators	Research Design	Subjects	Smoking	Medications	Pretesting & Posttesting Preparation	Pretesting & Posttesting Procedures
Hagberg et al. (1983)	Controlled pretraining & posttraining design	E grp: 11 pts with stable CAD (9 with single previous MI & 2 with significant 1 & 3 vessel disease) (mean age, 52 ± 7 yr; range 42–62 yr) C grp: 6 additional pts with comparable ex tolerance as E grp (mean age, 43 ± 5 yr; range 38–51 yr)	Not reported	E grp: 6 pts on propranolol, 7 pts on long-acting nitrates, 3 pts on digoxin, 1 pt on quinidine; 7 pts had changes in meds during prog C grp: 4 pts on propranolol, 1 pt on long-acting nitrates	None, other than testing done after light meal & 3 hr after meds	Pretests & posttests performed over 3 wks; TM V_{O_2MAX} test, Bruce protocol, resp gas analysis; endpoint: exhaustion or angina 9 asymptomatic pts attained true V_{O_2MAX} (leveling off criterion) & 2 pts with angina attained SL V_{O_2MAX}
Hedback et al. (1990)	Controlled pretraining & posttraining design	E grp: 43 pts post-CABG 2 C grps: from list of 1-yr survivors; matched for age, gender, yrs post-CABG, max wkld, CABG Hx, occupation, employment	Discouraged; same proportion smokers in C & E grps	Pts on β-blockers analyzed separately; C grp had high proportion of pts on long-acting nitrates & diuretics	None	SL erg test at 6 wk, 4 & 12 mo post-CABG protocol started at 30 W with 10 W/min inc in wkld

Training Duration	Exercise Training Procedures	Dropouts/ Complications	Adherence	Reported Results
12 mo	10 min of walking & stretching; period of end ex either jogging or cycle erg; prog'n: dur'n, int & freq progressively inc'd (?) After approx 6 mos, pts performing 50–60 min end ex at 70%–90% V_{O_2MAX}, 4–6×/wk; in last 6 mo, pts averaged 5×/wk; in last 3 mo, pts running 20–25 mi/wk or performing equivalent amounts of erg ex	9 pts developed MI, serious ventricular arrhythmias, or cardiac arrest	Not reported	C grp No changes in submax HR, CO, SV, SBP, DBP, MAP, LVSW, SVR E grp Dec body wt ($p < .01$) 39% inc V_{O_2MAX} 18% inc ex SV 18% inc LVSW ($p < .01$)
3 mo	E grp: high int dynamic interval training prog, 30–40 min 2×/wk, included warm-up on erg, 5-min high int & 3-min low int alternated; high int: target HR = max HR during SL_{MAX} ex test 6 wk post-CABG, low int: 30% below high int HR Initially hi-int periods performed on erg, after 3–4 wk, 2 of these periods were replaced by jogging & calisthenics or gymnastics, plus pts had home prog 3–5×/wk; after 3 mo pts transferred to community prog Education—risk factor control, cessation of smoking, & nutrition counseling C grp: no organized physical training prog	No cardiac complications or other adverse effects	80% training sessions attended	Less inc RPP ($p < .05$) Dec freq angina during ex tes ($p < .01$) Dec resting SBP & DBP ($p < .01$) Fewer smokers ($p < .05$) Fewer pts on long-acting nitrates ($p < .05$)

TABLE 1.4 Continued

Investigators	Research Design	Subjects	Smoking	Medications	Pretesting & Posttesting Preparation	Pretesting & Posttesting Procedures
Kappagoda & Greenwood (1984)	Controlled pretraining & posttraining design	30 pts post-CABPS NYHA-grp-II); E grp = 15 pts who lived close by (mean age, 50.1 ± 2.2 yr); C grp = 15 pts who lived farther away (mean age, 52.3 ± 2.2 yr)	Not reported	Anturan 3×/day all pts	None	Cycle erg GXT; initial wkld 200 kpm/min, inc'd by 100 kpm/min every 3 min; testing performed before, 8–10 wk after & 9 mo after surgery; endpoints: net depolarization > 0.01 mV in the ST seg 80 msec after QRS, HR of 80% age-predicted max & severe angina
Laslett et al. (1985)	Single-group pretraining & posttraining design	10 pts with CAD including pts post-CABPS, catheterization-documented CAD & classic angina (mean age, 56.2 yr; range, 27–71 yr)	Not reported	Pts excluded if cardiac meds inc'd during study or if pts req'd digoxin during testing	None	SL_{MAX} test, Balke TM protocol; endpoint: highest SL wkld attained
May & Nagle (1984)	Controlled pretraining & posttraining design	121 pts with CAD; E grp = 71 pts with MIs or severe myocardial ischemia (mean age, 50.7 ± 7 yr); C grp 1 = 26 pts with MI or severe myocardial ischemia (mean age, 57.5 ± 8.1 yr); C grp 2 = 24 pts with neg tests, ECG changes & blood enzyme levels (mean age, 48.6 ± 5.9 yrs)	Not reported	No pts on meds to control HR or BP	None	SL_{MAX} test, Balke TM protocol; endpoint = exhuastion, angina, severe dysrhythmia or HR_{MAX} Mean times for retests: E grp = 9.6 ± 1.2 mo, C grp 1 = 12.9 ± 4.3 mo, C grp 2 = 18.8 ± 11.8 mo

Training Duration	Exercise Training Procedures	Dropouts/Complications	Adherence	Reported Results
6–7 mo (?)	E grp: training began between tests 2 & 3; 3×/wk for first 2 wk (hospital visits) & after 2 wk pt ex'd at home; Canadian Air Force 5BX prog (modified for outpt use) wk 1 — 1st level, wk 2 — 2nd level, subsequent levels performed at home, 11 min each session C grp: self-administered activity prog based on symptoms	No unusual responses to ex tests E grp: 3 dropouts	Not reported	Surgery improved effort tolerance RPP training further inc'd wk capacity & peak RPP ($p < .05$)
6 mo	20 min 3×/wk, int = 70% HR_{MAX}, activities included walking, jogging, running, cycling, or rowing depending on pt	None reported	Not reported	1.6 MET inc functional wk capacity (range, 0.5–2.5 METs ($p < .001$) Inc mean HR at which ECG evidence of ischemia ($p < .05$) Inc RPP ($p < .05$)
10–12 mo (?)	E grp: aerobic ex (?), 30 min/day or 50 min 3×/wk or 75 min 2×/wk; training wkld = (60 + max METs)/100 × max METs, training HR = [(HR max − HRrest) × (60 + max METs)/100] + HR rest; prog'n: wkld inc'd to maintain training HR C grp 1 & C grp 2: no regular ex	None reported	Not reported	C grps: no sig change V_{0_2MAX}, RPP_{MAX}, RPP_{SUBMAX} E grp Inc est'd V_{0_2MAX} ($p < .01$) Inc RPP_{MAX} ($p < .01$) Dec RPP_{SUBMAX} ($p < .01$)

TABLE 1.4 Continued

Investi-gators	Research Design	Subjects	Smoking	Medica-tions	Pretesting & Posttesting Prepa-ration	Pretesting & Posttesting Procedures
Rousseau et al. (1973)	Controlled pretraining & post-training design	14 pts with healed MI (no angina); C grp: $n = 7$ (studied for 2 mo before study, E grp: $n = 7$ (studied for 3–31 mo prior)	Not re-ported	Pts on β-blockers excluded	None	Multistage max erg test with resp gas analy-sis; initial wkld 50 W for 1 min, int inc'd 10 or 25 W/min; pedaling rate 50 rpm; endpoint = subj exhaustion
Taniguchi et al. (1990)	Single-group pre-training & posttraining design	17 acute MI pts ($n = 10$ with anterior MIs, $n = 7$ with inferior MIs) (mean age, 60 ± 11 yr); 2 wk post-acute MI; all pts could walk safely on flat surface > 200 m	Not re-ported	Not re-ported	2 days be-fore ex test, pts walked on TM for 3–5 min at 2 kph with 0% grade	Pretest repeat-ed after wk 1 & 2 (a) Ramp ex test (AT de-termination) with resp gas analysis (b)One stage S-S ex test (tar-get HR de-termination = 90% of HR at AT)
Varnauskas et al (1966)	Single-group pre-training & posttraining design	9 pts with CAD (age range, 43–59 yr); pts gener-ally active in professions & in recreational & other physical activi-ties	Not re-ported	4 pts on nitrates occasionally	None, other than investigated in A.M. be-fore break-fast	SL TM GXT & SL erg test done 2–3 days before training & repeated 4–6 wk after train-ing, ex pro-tocols (?), peak erg wklds be-tween 150–500 kpm/min
Williams et al. (1984)	Single-group pre-training & posttraining design	53 pts with CAD including prior MI or pos angiogra-phy ($n = 25$ with angina, $n = 21$ with an-gina &/or ECG ischemic changes) (me-dian age, 52 yr; range 36–68 yr; local resi-dents has su-pervised prog, nonlocal resi-dents had un-supervised prog	Not re-ported	Prescribed as in-dicated, but were with-drawn for testing β-Blockers tapered off 7–10 days before test-ing & stop-ped for at least 48 hr before; all other drugs stopped at least 12 hr before	None	SL erg GXT, protocol = ?. peak ex wkld attained ranged between 300–1200 kpm/min; SL TM GXT, protocol = ?; endpoints: fatigue/angina

Training Duration	Exercise Training Procedures	Dropouts/ Complications	Adherence	Reported Results
13.5 mo	Individually graded exs (?), 45 min 3×/wk, int = approx 70%–80% V_{O_2MAX}	None reported	Not reported	Inc V_{O_2MAX}, HR_{MAX}, CO_{MAX} Inc a-v O_2 diff Dec SV at V_{O_2MAX} in both E & C grps
2 wk	Predischarge pts walked on flat surface, 20–30 min 2×/day at target HR based on AT; pts discharged with new target HR	6 pts discont'd owing to angina with ST seg depression, pain & unsteadiness of legs, cerebral embolism & drug hepatitis	Not reported	Dec HR_{REST}, warming-up & AT ($p < .05$) No change peak HR Inc O_2 pulse at AT & endpoint ($p < .05$) Inc AT & peak V_{O_2} ($p < .05$)
4–6 wk	Cycle erg training Initial baseline wkld selected for each pt; inc'd by 50 W/1–3 min at intervals of 5 min wk 1 daily ex, following wks ex on alt days (except Sun)	Illness ($n = 3$), technical problems, 1 pt VT but ex not discont'd, 1 pt heel cord problem & off 1 wk; 5 pts had chest pain on ex at least ×1	Not reported	No wt loss Inc work capacity Inc exertion req'd to elicit angina/breathlessness No change HR No change V_{O_2}, VE Dec CO & SV Inc a-v O_2 diff Dec BP posttraining Dec LV work Dec blood lactate Inc Hb
6–12 mo	3–5×/wk, 30–60 min using a combination of cycle erg, stair climbing, walking & jogging; int = training HR between 65%–86% HRR	None reported	Not reported	Inc peak wkld ($p < .0001$) Inc total work performed ($p < .0001$) Inc total METs ($p < .0001$) Dec HR at max pretraining wkld ($p < .002$) Inc HR at peak effort ($p < .009$) Inc $LVEF_{REST}$ ($p < .075$) Inc LVEF at max pretraining wkld ($p < .002$) No change LVEF at peak

objective improvements in work performance following training without deleterious effects on ventricular function or unusual incidence of morbidity or mortality. Most studies have examined individuals with cardiac failure secondary to coronary artery disease; the role of exercise in the management of individuals with cardiac myopathies is less clear.

Several other conditions that commonly occur in older people affect functional capacity but may be attenuated by regular physical exercise. These include peripheral vascular disease (Skinner & Strandness, 1967), hypertension (Pickering, 1987), diabetes (Jette, 1984; Leon, 1989), hyperlipoproteinemia (Superko & Haskell, 1987) and obesity (Lampman & Schteingart, 1989). Thus, judiciously prescribed exercise may have a significant role in attenuating the effects of multisystem disease as well as maintaining function and reducing the negative sequelae of immobility.

EXERCISE TEST: BASIS FOR TRAINING

The indications for exercise prescription in older populations are based on the individual's history, physical examination, and the results of the exercise test (Smith & Gilligan, 1983). The most common complaints of individuals who have cardiopulmonary dysfunction are dyspnea, reduced endurance (Leblanc et al., 1986; Pardy et al., 1984), fatigue (Weber et al., 1988), and chest pain (Pollack & Pels, 1984). Thus, mitigating these complaints are reasonable goals for the exercise program. An exercise test can objectively assess work performance and the degree to which subjective complaints compromise performance. Basing the exercise prescription on the results of an exercise test ensures that the prescription is associated with maximal benefit and minimal risk for the individual.

The validity, reliability, and safety of exercise testing are maximized when performed by qualified and experienced practitioners (Shephard, 1991). Practice and familiarization with the exercise testing modality and testing procedures have been shown to be significant factors in maximizing test validity [Davies et al., 1970; Dean et al., 1989; Wall & Charteris, 1981]. Activity and substances ingested before the test can also affect exercise performance and thus need to be standardized (e.g., the avoidance of any unusual or strenuous exercise for 24 hours before the test; and the avoidance of smoking, drinking caffeinated or alcoholic beverages or ingesting a heavy meal within 3 hours of testing).

Types of Exercise Tests

There are several types of exercise tests that are clinically useful; these are classified according to their endpoints. Common tests include the maximal test, the symptom or sign-limited test, the submaximal exercise test, and the anaerobic threshold test.

The $\dot{V}_{O_2MAX}$ exercise test is the gold standard for determining functional work capacity. The hallmark of the maximal test is the plateau of oxygen consumption with further increases in work load [McArdle et al., 1986]. Symptom or sign-limited exercise tests are terminated by symptoms such as dyspnea, chest pain, or muscle fatigue; or by signs such as cardiac dysrhythmias and abnormal changes in heart rate or blood pressure (Blair et al., 1988, pp. 155–235; Jones, 1988, pp. 135–144). Submaximal exercise tests are terminated when predetermined criteria are reached (e.g., a submaximal work rate, oxygen consumption, heart rate, blood pressure, or perceived exertion level) (Braun et al., 1982; Miyashita et al., 1985). Submaximal exercise responses can be used to predict $\dot{V}_{O_2MAX}$ (Shephard et al., 1968; Siconolfi et al., 1982).

Before any exercise test, the absolute or relative contraindications for being tested are reviewed on an individual basis (American College of Sports Medicine, 1991, pp. 121–159; Jones, 1988, pp. 135–144). These are summarized in Table 1.5. Also, the criteria for terminating the exercise test are determined beforehand. These criteria are based on the individual's history, indications for the exercise test, and its objectives. General criteria for prematurely terminating an exercise test in the event of unusual exercise responses appear in Table 1.6.

The simplest exercise test is a time-based walk test and includes monitoring of heart rate, blood pressure, breathing frequency, arterial saturation, perceived exertion, and breathlessness [McGavin et al., 1976]. Tests such as the 12-minute walk test and its modifications (3- and 6-minute walk tests) have several advantages in testing older or debilitated persons (Guyatt et al., 1985). They are easy to perform, can be performed in a variety of settings, and are easy to administer (Swerts et al., 1990). The individual walks as far as possible in the specified time, slowing down or stopping if necessary. Because of a significant practice effect, the walk test needs to be repeated on at least two different days. The results of the second test are used. Disadvantages of this test include the risk of an individual performing a maximal test without the benefit of detailed monitoring. The use of the test is therefore limited in severely compromised or high-risk individuals.

Complex, more sophisticated tests involve respiratory gas analysis performed during incremental treadmill or ergometer protocols (e.g., Balke and Bruce protocols) (Balke & Ware, 1959; Bruce & Horsten, 1969). Respiratory gas analysis is performed in tests requiring detailed analysis of the energetics of exercise (e.g., $\dot{V}_{O_2MAX}$ tests, symptom-limited $\dot{V}_{O_2MAX}$ tests, and anaerobic tests). The individual wears a nose clip and breathes through a mouth piece connected to a one-way valve system. The expired gas is analyzed for its oxygen and carbon dioxide content. Often, ventilation, tidal volume, and

TABLE 1.5 Relative and Absolute Contraindications to Exercise Testing an Individual with Cardiopulmonary Dysfunction

Absolute contraindications
    Congestive heart failure
    Acute EKG changes of myocardial ischemia
    Unstable angina
    Ventricular or dissecting aneurysm
    Ventricular tachycardia
    Multifocal ectopic beats
    Repetitive ventricular ectopic activity
    Untreated or refractory tachycardia
    Supraventricular dysrhythmia
    Recent thromboembolic event (pulmonary or other)
    Uncontrolled asthma
    Uncontrolled heart failure
    Pulmonary edema
    Uncontrolled hypertension (above 250 mm Hg systolic, 120 mm Hg diastolic)
    Acute infections

Relative contraindications
    Recent myocardial infarction [less than 4 weeks ago]
    Aortic valve disease
    Severe cardiomegaly
    Pulmonary hypertension
    Resting tachycardia
    Resting EKG abnormalities
    Poorly controlled diabetes
    Severe electrolyte disturbance
    Severe systemic hypertension
    Significant conduction disturbance
    Complete atrioventricular block
    Fixed rate pacemakers
    Acute cerebrovascular disease
    Respiratory failure
    Left ventricular failure
    Epilepsy

Source. Adapted from Jones (1988), and Kellermann (1977).

breathing frequency are also measured. These detailed studies are particularly useful if the metabolic characteristics of exercise are of interest or if the contribution of cardiac to pulmonary compromise in exercise needs to be examined (Wasserman & Whipp, 1975). In addition, oxygen consumption for a given work load gives an index of movement economy. Improved movement economy may be an important determinant of improved work performance with training in some individuals with cardiopulmonary compromise (Belman & Wasserman, 1981). Practice and familiarization with the procedures are as important in these complex tests to maximize test va-

TABLE 1.6 Criteria for Prematurely Terminating an Exercise Test

Miscellaneous
  Wish of individual for any reason
  Failure of monitoring equipment

General signs and symptoms
  Fatigue
  Lightheadedness, confusion, ataxia, pallor, cyanosis, dyspnea, nausea, or peripheral
    vascular insufficiency
  Onset of angina

Electrocardiographic signs
  Symptomatic supraventricular tachycardia
  ST displacement (3 mm) horizontal or downsploping from rest
  Ventricular tachycardia
  Exercise-induced left bundle branch block
  Onset of second- or third-degree atrioventricular block
  R on T premature ventricular contractions (one)
  Frequent multifocal premature ventricular contractions (frequent runs of three or
    more)
  Atrial fibrillation when absent at rest
  Appearance of a Q wave

Cardiovascular signs
  Any fall in blood pressure below the resting level
  Exercise hypotension (> 20 mm Hg drop in systolic blood pressure)
  Excessive blood pressure increase (systolic $\geq$ 220 or diastolic $\geq$ 110 mm Hg)
  Inappropriate bradycardia (drop in heart rate greater than 10 beats/min with
    increase or no change in work load)

Source. Adapted from American College of Sports Medicine (1991); Jones (1988).

lidity as in less complicated tests. These factors may be even more important in older debilitated people who are less accustomed to activity and who may experience greater arousal in novel situations compared with younger people. The steady-state exercise test examines an individual's exercise responses to one or more submaximal work rates, each maintained for several minutes until a physiological steady state in achieved. The results of a submaximal exercise test may be used to estimate $\dot{V}_{O_2MAX}$ and functional work capacity (Shephard et al., 1968; Siconolfi et al., 1982). This test has also been used for the noninvasive determination of cardiac output during exercise (Mcelvaney et al., 1989). Less emphasis, however, has been placed on serially comparing steady-state exercise responses and monitoring responses over time, or before and after interventions (Dean & Ross, 1988). In older or disabled persons, responses to steady-state exercise could be used to assess endurance during a moderate level of physical exertion, which may be of great functional significance in these populations.

The anaerobic threshold (AT) is measured using respiratory gas analysis during an incremental maximum stress test. Based on ventilatory parameters, the AT is defined as the ($\dot{V}_{O_2}$) at which the linear relationship between ventilation and $\dot{V}_{O_2}$ is lost, whereas the relationship between ventilation and carbon dioxide production is unchanged (Wasserman et al., 1987). Fortini et al. (1991) have reported that the AT can be determined in a high proportion of patients with exercise-induced angina. They suggest that determining the AT can be a useful index of functional impairment, and that it is not affected if the test is prematurely stopped by exhaustion or dyspnea. The AT cannot be determined, however, if the patient's performance is symptom limited below the level at which the AT occurs (Belman & Wasserman, 1981). The relationship of the anaerobic and lactate thresholds has been the subject of intense debate during the past decade.

The treadmill and the cycle ergometer are commonly used exercise-testing modalities and offer different advantages. Walking on a treadmill represents a familiar functional activity and provides a higher estimate of $\dot{V}_{O_2MAX}$ than the cycle ergometer (Astrand, 1976). The individual needs to be able to walk with minimal, if any, handrail support, however, (Zeimetz et al., 1979). This requirement may exclude individuals who are unsteady or poorly coordinated. Cycle ergometry may be more appropriate for these individuals; however, ergometer tests are often terminated because of leg fatigue or discomfort from the ergometer seat, and thus may preclude the individual reaching $\dot{V}_{O_2MAX}$. For maximal test validity and reliability, the height of the seat and handle bars are standardized according the person's height and leg length (Jones, 1988, pp. 135–144).

Upper-extremity cycle ergometry has been reported to have some application in determining aerobic capacity in some individuals such as those with spinal cord injuries. Upper-extremity work, however, is associated with greater cardiovascular demands (e.g., increased blood pressure and heart rate for the same work load in the lower extremities) (Astrand & Saltin, 1961; Franklin, 1985). Despite this caveat, Ries et al. (1988) have reported that moderate upper-extremity exercise can be beneficial in the rehabilitation of individuals with chronic obstructive lung disease (i.e., exercise-test performance improved, and breathlessness and fatigue decreased). Research is needed to examine the full potential of upper-extremity work in the rehabilitation of older individuals with cardiopulmonary compromise.

Protocols

Numerous exercise-test protocols have been described for the individual who has cardiopulmonary dysfunction (Balke & Ware, 1959; Bruce & Horsten, 1969; Chung, 1983; Ellestad et al., 1969; Guyatt et al., 1985; McGavin et al., 1976; McHenry et al., 1972). These protocols typically begin at low intensities and increase in graded increments every 2 to 3 minutes. These increments are usually no more than 1 MET (3.5 ml/kg of body weight/ minute or equivalent to a step increment of the oxygen consumption at rest). In disabled and older persons increments of 0.5 MET or less is more desirable (Smith & Gilligan, 1983). Once the individual has reached the test termination criterion, the cool-down begins (i.e., the work loads are decreased gradually every few minutes until vital signs approach resting values). The individual continues to be monitored during the postexercise recovery period, for 10 to 15 minutes, to minimize the possibility of delayed abnormal responses (Pollack & Pels, 1984). The metabolic cost of the work rates for some common exercise-test protocols are shown in Figure 1.1. These can be compared with the metabolic cost of some common activities shown in Table 1.7. Note, however, that these values are approximate and that these will be inflated in cases in which the work of breathing is increased.

Because maximum $\dot{V}_{O_2}$—hence, MET level—declines significantly with advancing age, exercise-test protocols used for older persons, particularly those with compromised functional capacity, need to start at very low work loads. Compared with the average healthy 60-year-old who has an average $\dot{V}_{O_2 MAX}$ of 7 to 8 METs and the 75-year-old who has an average $\dot{V}_{O_2 MAX}$ of 5 to 6 METs, the 75-year-old who lives in a nursing home has a maximum MET level of only 2 to 4 (Smith, 1981). In addition, older persons require a longer period to reach an exercise steady state; therefore, they may require at least 3 minutes at each work load (Skinner, 1987). Premature test termination is more common in older than in younger populations. Exercise tests of individuals with cardiopulmonary dysfunction are more likely to be terminated because of signs of abnormal exercise responses (e.g., abnormal heart rate or rhythm, abnormal change in blood pressure, arterial saturation less than 85%, pallor, or excessive sweating) or exercise-induced symptoms (e.g., dyspnea, chest pain, leg pain, leg fatigue, or discomfort) (Jones, 1988, pp. 135–144).

Interrupted exercise protocols have been advocated for individuals with extremely low functional work capacity (Astrand 1960; Sheffield & Roitman, 1977; Zadai, 1985). These protocols alternate bouts of exercise with rest; the duration of exercise is often followed by a comparable duration of rest. Interrupted exercise protocols may result in greater total energy expenditure than a single bout of uninterrupted exercise. In addition, they may increase the individual's exercise duration and total work output imposing excessive physiological demands or undue risk.

Monitoring

Heart rate, electrocardiogram (EKG), blood pressure, breathing frequency, and arterial saturation are fundamental measures recorded during an exercise test of an individual with cardiopulmonary dysfunction. Mean arterial pres-

FIGURE 1.1 Oxygen Cost of Work Stages of Some Commonly Used Exercise Test Protocols

Source. Froehlicher, V. F. (1987). *Exercise and the heart* (ed. 2, p. 15). Chicago: Year Book Medical. Reprinted with permission.

TREADMILL PROTOCOLS

Functional Class	Clinical Status	O_2 Cost ML/KG/MIN	METS	Bicycle Ergometer 1 WATT = 60 KPDS FOR 70 KG BODY WEIGHT (KPDS)	Bruce 3 MIN STAGES MPH	Bruce %GR	Kattus MPH	Kattus %GR	Balke Ware % GRAD AT 3.3 MPH 1-MIN STAGES	Ellestad 3/2-3 MIN STAGES MPH	Ellestad %GR	USAFSAM 2 OR 3 MIN STAGES MPH	USAFSAM %GR	"SLOW" USAFSAM MPH	"SLOW" USAFSAM %GR	McHenry MPH	McHenry %GR	Stanford % GRADE AT 3 MPH	Stanford % GRADE AT 2 MPH	METS
NORMAL AND I (HEALTHY DEPENDENT ON AGE ACTIVITY)		56.0	16		5.5	20			26, 25, 24, 23, 22, 21, 20, 19, 18, 17, 16, 15, 14, 13, 12, 11, 10, 9, 8, 7, 6, 5, 4, 3, 2, 1											16
		52.5	15		5.0	18				6	15									15
		49.0	14.									3.3	25			3.3	21			14
		45.5	13	1500						5	15									13
		42.0	12	1350	4.2	16	4	22				3.3	20			3.3	18			12
	SEDENTARY HEALTHY	38.5	11	1200												3.3	15	22.5		11
		35.0	10	1050			4	18		5	10	3.3	15			3.3	12	20.0		10
		31.5	9	900	3.4	14	4	14						2	25	3.3	9	17.5		9
		28.0	8	750			4	10		4	10	3.3	10	2	20			15.0		8
II	LIMITED	24.5	7	600	2.5	12	3	10		3	10			2	15	3.3	6	12.5		7
		21.0	6	450			2	10		1.7	10	3.3	5	2	10			10.0	17.5	6
		17.5	5		1.7	10								2	5			7.5	14	5
III		14.0	4	300								3.3	0	2	0	2.0	3	5.0	10.5	4
		10.5	3	150	1.7	5						2.0	0					2.5	7	3
IV	SYMPTOMATIC	7.0	2		1.7	0												0.0	3.5	2
		3.5	1																	1

sure and rate pressure product can be derived from heart rate and blood pressure. Mean arterial pressure, the average pressure within the arterial system, is equal to diastolic pressure plus one third (systolic pressure minus diastolic pressure). The rate pressure product that is highly correlated with myocardial oxygen demand and the work of the heart (de Nicola & Tammaro, 1985b) is the product of heart rate and systolic blood pressure. At maximal levels of exercise, the rate pressure product increases three- to five-fold from rest. Cardiac dysrhythmias and asymptomatic ischemic heart disease are common in older persons with cardiopulmonary dysfunction (Stamford, 1988). Therefore, EKG monitoring needs to be used more routinely in exercise testing for older individuals—even those without overt cardiopulmonary disease. Arterial saturation monitored noninvasively with a pulse oximeter has been shown to produce valid measures provided the device is calibrated and applied appropriately. Although pulse oximetry has been reported to be less valid at high work rates (Hanson & Casaburi, 1987), this limitation is not a concern in exercise testing for individuals with low functional work capacities. Saturation is not usually permitted to fall below 85% preferably remaining within a couple of percentage points of the resting value.

Given that exercise is largely limited by subjective complaints in individuals with impaired functional capacity, assessment of the subjective experience of exercise is clinically relevant. Subjective scales of perceived exertion (Borg, 1982) and modified scales to assess breathlessness (Killian, 1985) and angina (American College of Sports Medicine, 1991, pp. 55–91) have been developed. Compared with objective measures of exercise response, however, subjective measures have received relatively little attention. Further development and refinement of subjective exercise responses is therefore warranted to enhance clinical exercise testing and training procedures.

EXERCISE PRESCRIPTION

The exercise prescription is based on the results of the exercise test and quantifies the exercise dose needed to effect the desired training response (Hanson et al., 1980). Although the exercise prescription for older persons with cardiopulmonary dysfunction is comparable with that for healthy people, each component of the prescription can be modified to meet the needs of the individual. Specifically, the following are addressed including the indications for an exercise program, the parameters of the exercise program, the means of monitoring the individual's responses to exercise, and exercise progression and follow-up.

TABLE 1.7 Oxygen Cost of Some Common Activities

Intensity (70-kg Person)	Endurance Promoting	Occupational	Recreational
1½–2 METs 4–7 ml/kg/min 2–2½ kcal/min	Two low in energy level	Desk work, driving auto, electric calculating machine operation, light housework, polishing furniture, washing clothes	Standing, strolling (1 mph), flying, motorcycling, playing cards, sewing, knitting
2–3 METs 7–11 ml/kg/min 2½–4 kcal/min	Too low in energy level unless capacity is very low	Auto repair, radio and television repair, janitorial work, bartending, riding lawn mower, light woodworking	Level walking (2 mph), level bicycling (5 mph), billiards, bowling, skeet shooting, shuffleboard, powerboat driving, golfing with power cart, canoeing, horseback riding at a walk
3–4 METs 11–14 ml/kg/min 4–5 kcal/min	Yes, if continuous and if target heart rate is reached	Brick laying, plastering, wheelbarrow (100-lb load), machine assembly, welding (moderate load), cleaning windows, mopping floors, vacuuming, pushing light power mower	Walking (3 mph), bicycling (6 mph), horseshoe pitching, volleyball (6-person, noncompetitive), golfing (pulling bag cart), archery, sailing (handling small boat), fly fishing (standing in waders), horseback riding (trotting), badminton (social doubles)
4–5 METs 14–18 ml/kg/min	Recreational activities promote endurance. Occupational activities must be continuous, lasting longer than 2 min	Painting, masonry, paperhanging, light carpentry, scrubbing floors, raking leaves, hoeing	Walking (3⅓ mph), bicycling (8 mph), table tennis, golfing (carrying clubs), dancing (foxtrot), badminton (singles), tennis (doubles), many calisthenics, ballet
5–6 METs 18–21 ml/kg/min	Yes	Digging garden, shoveling light earth	Walking (4 mph), bicycling (10 mph), canoeing (4 mph), horseback riding (post-

			ing to trotting), stream fishing (walking in light current in waders), ice or roller skating (9 mph)
6–7 METs 21–25 ml/kg/min 7–8 kcal/min	Yes	Shoveling 10 times/min (4½ kg or 10 lb), splitting wood, snow shoveling, hand lawn mowing	Walking (5 mph), bicycling (11 mph), competitive badminton, tennis (singles), folk and square dancing, light downhill skiing, ski touring (2½ mph), water skiing, swimming (20 yards/min)
7–8 METs 25–28 ml/kg/min 8–10 kcal/min	Yes	Digging ditches, carrying 36 kg or 80 lb, sawing hardwood	Jogging (5 mph), bicycling (12 mph), horseback riding (gallop), vigorous downhill skiing, basketball, mountain climbing, ice hockey, canoeing (5 mph), touch football, paddleball
8–9 METs 28–32 ml/kg/min 10–11 kcal/min	Yes	Shoveling 10 times/min (5½ kg or 14 lb)	Running (5½ mph), bicycling (13 mph), ski touring (4 mph), squash (social), hadball (social), fencing, basketball (vigorous), swimming (30 yards/min), rope skipping
10 + METs 32 + ml/kg/min 11 + kcal/min	Yes	Shoveling 10 times/min (7½ kg or 16 lb)	Running (6 mph = 10 METs, 7 mph = 11½ METs, 8 mph = 13½ METs, 9 mph = 15 METs, 10 mph = 17 METs), ski touring (5+ mph), handball (competitive), squash (competitive), swimming (greater than 40 yards/min)

Source. From Fox, S. M., Naughton, J. P., & Gorman, P. A. (1972). Physical activity and cardiovascular health: 3. The exercise prescription: Frequency and type of activity. *Modern Concepts of Cardiovascular Disease, 41*, 25–30. Reprinted with permission.

Parameters

The parameters of an exercise prescription include the type of exercise; its intensity, duration, and frequency; and the course of the exercise program (Blair et al., 1988, pp. 239–262). A typical exercise session includes a warm-up, a period of steady-state aerobic exercise at the required intensity for the specified duration, and a cool-down and recovery period (Figure 1.2). The warm-up consists of several minutes of exercising at increasing intensities to prepare the individual for the training exercise intensity. The cool-down is the reverse (i.e., it consists of several minutes of decreasing exercise intensities to return the individual's vital signs gradually to baseline resting values).

The optimal aerobic training stimulus consists of rhythmic continuous exercise of a large muscle group, usually the quadriceps. Walking is an ideal activity for older persons as it enhances mobility and independence (Porcari et al., 1987). Cycle ergometry for the lower extremities may be beneficial for some individuals who may be unable to physically support themselves safely walking and who are free from orthopedic problems in the lower extremities.

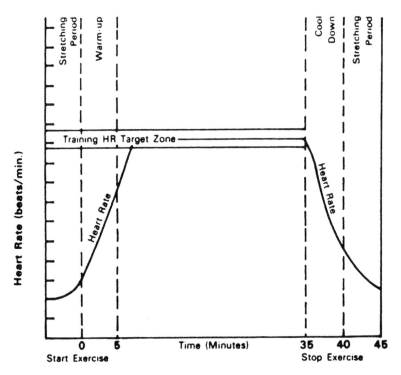

FIGURE 1.2 Components of Exercise Training Session

Upper-extremity training using an arm ergometer may have less application in the rehabilitation of the older adult because of the greater myocardial demands associated with it (Astrand & Saltin, 1961). Swimming and aquatic exercise may be beneficial for individuals who have orthopedic problems in that biomechanical stress through the weight-bearing joints is minimized. Although water exercise can be an effective means of eliciting cardiorespiratory training responses, cardiovascular responses have been reported to be significantly greater in the water than on land for comparable work rates (Whitley & Schoene, 1987). Thus, the parameters of the exercise prescription in the water have to be adjusted accordingly.

O'Hara et al. (1984) and O'Hara et al. (1987) attempted to examine the effect of anaerobic training, characterized by high-intensity short-duration exercise, in individuals with cardiopulmonary dysfunction given that these individuals are often unable to achieve an aerobic training intensity (Belman & Wasserman, 1981). Following a training program of upper-extremity weight training and back packing, these investigators reported that maximal work capacity was significantly improved, probably as a result of a 16% reduction in ventilation. Whether the subjects in this study were actually performing anaerobic work was not verified, however.

If the effects of training are to be assessed in a valid manner, the activity or modality used in training should be the same as that used in pretraining exercise testing (Sharkey, 1988). Moreover, maximal transfer of training will be achieved if the training activity is comparable with activities the individual routinely performs (Vandervoort et al., 1986).

To achieve an optimal aerobic training response, it is currently held that a healthy person needs to perform aerobic exercise for 30 minutes 3 times a week at a heart rate that is 70% to 85% of that individual's maximum heart rate (i.e., at an $\dot{V}_{O_2}$ of 60% to 75% of maximum (American College of Sports Medicine, 1991, pp. 93–119). Individuals with cardiopulmonary dysfunction can demonstrate a training effect when they train at lower intensities (Ward et al., 1987). For these individuals, the exercise intensity may be set at 50% to 75% of the peak heart rate achieved in a symptom- or sign-limited exercise test (Hanson et al., 1980; Shephard, 1976). If an individual has particularly low functional work capacity, the intensity based on heart rate can be set at the resting heart rate plus 50% to 80% of the heart rate reserve (i.e., peak heart rate minus resting heart rate) (de Vries, 1971; Karvonen et al., 1957). As the exercise program proceeds, the intensity may be increased from the lower to the higher end of the training range (American College of Sports Medicine, 1991, pp. 93–119; Smith & Gilligan, 1983).

Sidney & Shephard (1978) examined the effects of exercise frequency and intensity on the exercise responses of 60- to 83-year-old healthy subjects. Specifically, they studied the effect of high frequency (HF) and low frequency

(LF) of exercise in combination with either high intensity (HI) or low intensity (LI). HF and LF were defined as more or less than two 1-hour exercise sessions a week; and high and low intensity referred to training at 120 to 130 beats per minute and 140 to 150 beats per minute, respectively. They reported that subjects in the HF-HI exhibited higher predicted $\dot{V}_{O_2MAX}$ (29%) compared with the other groups. The LF-HI group showed more modest gains followed by small but significant gains made by HF-LI group. The LF-LI group showed no change. A secondary finding was that the HF-HI group reached maximal gains by 7 weeks, whereas the LF-HI and HF-LI groups showed progressive increases over 14 weeks. Thus, although HI regimens were more effective in producing a cardiopulmonary training effect, a LI regimen could induce a training effect in conjunction with a high-training frequency.

Exercise intensity can be defined on the basis of subjective parameters that have particular application for disabled and older persons whose exercise tolerance is frequently limited by their symptoms. Comparable with an exercise intensity based on heart rate from the results of the pretraining exercise test, so too can training intensity be defined on the basis of subjective measures. Perceived exertion or breathlessness can be specified on the Borg scale, which ranges from 0 (nothing at all) to 10 (maximal exertion or breathlessness) (Borg, 1982). The training intensity is set at a range of severity for a given symptom (e.g., training based on perceived exertion may range between moderate and heavy on the Borg scale). The use of subjective parameters to define training intensity may be particularly important in the individual with chronic airflow limitation who may be expending considerable energy to breathe (Pardy et al., 1984) or whose condition fluctuates from day to day. In this case, the subjective experience is maintained constant while the power output varies [Myles & Maclean, 1986], thereby increasing the duration of exercise that can be tolerated.

The duration of the exercise session primarily depends on the severity of the individual's cardiopulmonary compromise. Duration may range from only a few minutes in the severely compromised individual to between 20 to 40 minutes for the mildly impaired individual. As a rule, individuals who need to train at low intensities are likely to train for a shorter duration, more frequently, to achieve a training response (Samsoe, 1984). For example, an individual may train for 15 minutes twice a day, whereas an individual who trains for 30 minutes will likely train every other day. Individuals with extremely low functional capacities may need to train several times within 1 day to elicit an optimal training response. Pierce et al. (1964) reported a training response in patients who walked for 2.5 minutes 5 to 10 times daily. Given that older people detrain rapidly when an exercise stimulus or a gravitational stimulus is removed provides physiological support for incorporating short, frequent bouts of exercise in exercise prescriptions for older people.

Given the heterogeneity of an older population with respect to general health status, cardiopulmonary dysfunction, medications, and so forth, exercise prescription for this group constitutes a relatively greater challenge than for a younger population. The diversity among older individuals will inevitably lead to greater diversity among the exercise programs prescribed for them.

Monitoring

The indications for training on a given exercise day are comparable with those for exercise testing—specifically, the individual feels well, has been free of any infection for several days, and exhibits none of the contraindications to exercise (see Table 1.5). The individual will likely benefit more from the training session if the individual feels energetic, and if training does not immediately follow meals or compete with other activities.

Objective parameters (e.g., heart rate, blood pressure, and arterial saturation) and subjective parameters (e.g., perceived exertion, breathlessness, and angina) are monitored before, during, and after exercise. Resting baseline measures are taken after 15 minutes of sitting quietly. During the exercise session, these parameters can be recorded every couple of minutes or less frequently once the target exercise parameters have stabilized. Following the training session, the exercise responses continue to be recorded for 10 to 15 minutes until they approach resting values, and the individual exhibits no aftereffects of the exercise. Continuous EKG monitoring is indicated for those individuals who showed irregularities in the exercise test. Indications for prematurely terminating an exercise training session are comparable with those for terminating an exercise test (see Table 1.6).

Exercise recovery data yield important information about an individual's cardiovascular status. Compared with individuals who are conditioned, deconditioned individuals exhibit longer time courses for recovery of their vital signs to resting levels. In individuals with coronary artery disease, an interesting relationship has been reported between the severity of their disease and the recovery of blood pressure following exercise. The proportion that recovery systolic blood pressure is to peak systolic blood pressure at 1, 2, and 3 minutes postexercise has been reported to be more sensitive than EKG and angina in detecting coronary artery disease (Amon et al., 1984; Nelson et al., 1989). Abnormal proportions have been defined as greater than 1.0, 0.9, and 0.8 at 1, 2, and 3 minutes postexercise, respectively. This information can be used for ongoing functional assessment of an individual's coronary artery disease.

Exercise Progression and Follow-Up

Over the course of training, the individual exercises at increasing intensities until consistently training within the middle to high end of the range (American College of Sports Medicine, 1991, pp. 93–119; Smith & Gilligan, 1983). The exercise intensity in not increased above the upper limit of this range without another exercise test being performed. In the retest, if the individual is able to exercise to a higher limit before symptoms occur, then the training range of objective and subjective symptoms can be justifiably increased.

The course of adaptation to training is gradual for older persons with different time courses for different organ systems (Bassey, 1978; Moritani & de Vries, 1981; Orlander et al., 1980). Musculoskeletal adaptation to exercise is generally slower than cardiopulmonary adaptation, and in older persons age-related changes in joints and connective tissue likely slow the rate of this adaptation further. Prolonged periods of warm-up and cool-down are advocated to augment this adaptation and avert potential problems (Hanson et al., 1980; Landin et al., 1985; Pollack & Pels, 1984). The anticipated time course for adaptation in an individual who has cardiopulmonary dysfunction and the mechanisms of that adaptation depend on the type and severity of cardiopulmonary dysfunction.

After completion of the exercise program, which may range from several weeks to months, a retest is scheduled so that the effect of training can be evaluated. The retest, a repeat of the preexercise test, will establish whether the training intensity needs to be changed or whether a maintenance program is indicated. The effectiveness of the exercise program can be gauged by the maximal and submaximal exercise responses for comparable work rates in the pretraining and posttraining tests. Such changes may include reaching a higher level of maximal exercise and, thus, greater maximum exercise responses as well as reductions in heart rate, blood pressure, rate pressure product, perceived exertion and breathlessness at submaximal work loads, and the maintenance of adequate arterial saturation.

FACTORS LIMITING TRAINING EFFICACY

In an older population with underlying cardiopulmonary disease, many factors can disrupt a training program. These factors need to be considered so that disruptions and detraining can be minimized. In addition to cardiopulmonary dysfunction, older individuals may have osteoarthritis, postural defects, musculoskeletal abnormalities, foot problems, glucose intolerance, thyroid problems, hearing and visual disturbances, hypertension, coronary artery disease, malnourishment, obesity, fluid and electrolyte imbalance, and balance problems (Feigenbaum, 1985). Changes in medication schedules can influence exercise performance and thus need to be monitored. Visual and hearing deficits can interfere with communication and limit the validity of subjective reports. Intercurrent illnesses and constitutional problems are more likely to disrupt the exercise programs of older compared with younger people (Naso et al., 1990). The exercise test and training program can be modified to consider these factors for an individual and thereby improve the efficacy of these procedures.

The effectiveness of an exercise program is highly dependent on motivation across all age groups (Belman & Wasserman, 1981). Motivation may be enhanced if the individual understands the benefits of the training program and is actively involved in planning the program so that it is designed to meet the individual's needs and interests. Exercise that is social and carried out with others may provide an additional incentive to adhere to an exercise program (Smith & Gilligan, 1983). In addition, exercise that is habitual and accommodated within the individual's daily activities may also improve adherence particularly for those who are less inclined to exercise.

Avoidance of detraining in older individuals may be as important a priority as exercise training itself. Naso et al. (1990) reported a small but significant benefit from endurance training program in individuals between 66 and 97 years of age. The limited magnitude of the training effect was explained by the LI of training, functional limitations in the legs, and intercurrent illness. The investigators proposed that prevention of the sequelae of detraining is a high priority in an older population, considering that any benefit of training is quickly lost with inactivity and bed rest. Research is needed to elucidate the role of frequent short bouts of exercise in older populations as a means of averting detraining effects when exercise training is interrupted. Further, the role of exercise during bouts of acute illness, and the degree to which modified exercise during illness could offset some of the effects of detraining, remain to be elucidated.

OTHER COMPONENTS OF COMPREHENSIVE REHABILITATION PROGRAM

The definition of pulmonary rehabilitation published by the American College of Chest Physicians (Petty, 1975) can be extended to individuals with cardiopulmonary dysfunction.

> Cardiopulmonary rehabilitation may be defined as an art of health care practice wherein individually tailored multidisciplinary programs are formulated which through accurate diagnosis, therapy, emotional support, and education stabilizes or reverses both the physio- and psychopathology of cardiopulmonary diseases and attempts to return individuals to their highest possible functional capacity allowed by their cardiopulmonary dysfunction and overall life situation.

To complete this definition, rehabilitation is also directed at health promotion and prevention of further disability. Thus, in addition to the exercise training component of the rehabilitation program, the focus of this chapter, several other components have been reported to have beneficial effects and are briefly discussed. These components include promotion and maintenance of good health, optimal medications, respiratory support, physical therapy, occupational therapy; and sexual, psychosocial, and vocational rehabilitation (see Table 1.8) (American Thoracic Society, 1981; Hodgkin et al., 1983; Holle et al., 1988; Make, 1986; Vallbona & Baker, 1984). The role of exercise classes and fall prevention is also discussed. The comprehensive rehabilitation program is a multidisciplinary effort designed to meet the specific needs of each individual.

Health Promotion and Maintenance

Without fundamental good health habits, an individual is not likely to derive maximal benefit from a rehabilitation program (Lampman, 1987; Make, 1986). The basic tenets of healthy living are common to all age groups and provide the focus for patient education (Gilmartin, 1986); specifically, these include good nutrition and weight control, adequate hydration, avoidance of smoking, avoidance of infections, good sleeping habits, a comfortable ambient environment, a safe barrier-free environment, and a healthy social environment. Health promotion and maintenance may be especially important in an older age group.

Medications

Individuals with cardiopulmonary dysfunction are frequently on short- or long-term medication regimens. In addition to understanding the purpose of the medications and their side effects, the individual needs to know the time course of these agents, and their maximal or minimal potencies depending on their positive or negative effects on exercise performance (American Heart Association, 1975; Haas et al., 1979). Some medications are taken in conjunction with aerosol therapy; thus, it is important that the individual's skill in administering these agents is satisfactory. Some individuals require supplemental oxygen during exercise. The dose may need to be increased immediately before, during, and immediately after exercise. (This adjustment is made by an appropriately qualified health care practitioner.) The adequacy of oxygen delivery can be ensured by continuous arterial saturation monitoring (Hanson & Casaburi, 1987).

TABLE 1.8 Components of the Comprehensive Rehabilitation Program

Health promotion and maintenance
  Good general health care
  Balanced diet
  Adequate hydration
  Weight control
  Avoidance of smoking and second-hand smoke
  Air quality
  Avoidance of infections
  Good sleeping habits
  Comfortable ambient environment
  Safe barrier-free environment
  Social support

Medications
  Cardiac inotropic agents
  Cardiac chronotropic agents
  Digitalis
  Diuretics
  Corticosteroids
  Bronchodilators
  Mucolytic agents
  Psychopharmacological agents
  Avoidance of drug toxicity and interactions

Respiratory support
  Oxygen therapy
  Aerosol therapy
  Mechanical ventilatory support

Physical therapy
  Exercise testing
  Exercise training
  Muscle strengthening
  Breathing control
  Relaxation procedures
  Activity pacing/and energy conservation
  Airway clearance

Occupational therapy
  Work simplification including ADLs
  Energy conservation

Sexual rehabilitation

Psychosocial rehabilitation

Vocational rehabilitation

Physical Therapy and Occupational Therapy

Physical therapy is often the primary focus of the rehabilitation program and frequently involves a training program. In addition, muscle strengthening regimens may be prescribed even for frail older people with beneficial results (Fisher et al., 1991; Frontera et al., 1988). Exercise or activities that involve straining, isometric contractions, or are discontinuous or arrhythmic, however, may be detrimental as these are associated with increased cardiopulmonary stress (Hanson & Nagle, 1987) and are not associated with improved endurance and function. Breathing control and airway clearance procedures such as postural drainage or postural drainage in conjunction with chest percussion may be indicated for some individuals with chronic lung diseases. In recent years, however, the efficacy of these procedures has been questioned (Faling, 1986; Kirilloff et al., 1985; Ross & Dean, 1989). These procedures may not be indicated if exercise alone is effective as an airway clearance procedure (International Journal of Sports Medicine, 1988; Wolff et al., 1977). Some individuals with severe chronic lung disease may require an assessment of their respiratory muscle strength and endurance (Hudson, 1984), and the contribution of respiratory muscle weakness versus fatigue. This distinction is critical in prescribing treatment in that weak muscles may require strength or endurance training (Pardy et al., 1981), and fatigued muscles are likely to benefit from judicious rest (Braun & Marino, 1984). Ventilatory muscle training consists of inspiring at a given flow rate through a hand-held device that can provide variable resistance; the nose is clipped during the training session, which ranges from 15 to 30 minutes. Although ventilatory muscle training can improve exercise tolerance (Belman & Mittman, 1980), the reverse may be also true (Keens et al., 1977); further, exercise may be a more practical and functional means of improving ventilatory muscle function (Belman et al., 1984). Relaxation procedures and body positioning may also have a role in reducing excessive energy expenditure in the individual with significantly increased work of breathing or of the heart (Cox et al., 1988). The interrelationship of the individual's functional capacity and ability to perform ADLs can be determined by the physical therapist. Such an examination can shed light on ways in which the individual might conserve energy during daily activities.

Occupational therapy may have a role in identifying alternative means of accomplishing daily tasks and work simplification. Although such energy conservation strategies are commonly used, little is known about their efficacy. Research is needed to investigate the role of energy conservation strategies in the rehabilitation of individuals with cardiopulmonary dysfunction so that these interventions can be prescribed on a rational basis.

Group Exercise

Exercise classes have become increasingly common in residential homes for the elderly, extended care units and community seniors' programs. These classes are often conducted 2 or 3 times a week, and include stretching and range-of-motion exercises, a warm-up routine, several minutes of aerobic exercise, and a cool-down. Individuals are not typically screened for participation in these classes, nor are they exercise tested or monitored during exercise. This practice needs to be examined given that it may expose participants to undue risk (Gutman et al., 1977).

Relatively few studies have examined the efficacy of exercise classes. One study, however, by Sidney & Shephard (1977) showed that healthy individuals older than age 60 benefited from a 1-hour class of endurance activity 4 times a week. These individuals demonstrated improved aerobic power and body composition, and improved ability to carry out ADLs. Whether the benefits of the program were augmented by the class format is not known. It can be argued that for older persons with cardiopulmonary dysfunction exercise classes have a limited role in enhancing physical function, in that older persons require prescribed exercise to ensure that exercise is both beneficial and not deleterious. Because exercise testing and monitoring are not usually performed, there is no means of predicting who is exercising above or below the optimal therapeutic range. Permitting an individual to exercise outside this range does not constitute therapeutic, safe, or cost-effective practice (Baruch & Mossberg, 1983; Gutman et al., 1977; Stamford, 1988).

A growing number of shopping malls across the United States and Canada are open outside working hours to provide a year-round walking circuit for the public. The social aspects of walking in a public place may improve adherence to an exercise program that has been problematic in some studies (Smith & Gilligan, 1983). This potentially rich data base has not been exploited by researchers; thus, there is negligible information available on the benefits of mall walking. Malls provide conditions that are ideal for scientific investigations (e.g., there is easy access; the air quality, temperature, and humidity are relatively constant; and the walking surface is even, slip proofed, and obstacle free). In addition, distances can be objectively measured and recorded.

Prevention of Falls

Falls are a major hazard for older persons and are associated with high rates of morbidity and mortality (Danish Medical Bulletin, 1987; Rubenstein et al., 1991). Programs directed at older persons need to assess an individual's potential risk for falling and implement means of minimizing this risk (Wolf-Klein et al., 1988). Those individuals who are in walking programs not involving a treadmill need to ensure that the walking surface is even, free of obstructions, and free of sudden inclines and declines. Walkways and corridors with railings are invaluable in providing an older person with additional confidence and mobility independence. Walking aids such as canes and walkers may be indicated; however, they are frequently misused and may constitute a hazard (Jebsen, 1967). Wheeled walkers may be a preferable alternative in that they may be safer and preserve movement continuity. Individuals with chronic airway obstruction may benefit from a high-wheeled walker so they can lean forward to facilitate breathing during exercise.

Sexual Rehabilitation

Of the components of a rehabilitation program, sexual rehabilitation has been relatively neglected. Because of the physical demands of sexual activity, older individuals with cardiopulmonary dysfunction have unique concerns. The threat of attacks of shortness of breath or chest pain can be extremely anxiety provoking to individuals and their partners. In addition, these apprehensions can be compounded by concerns about performing sexually and pleasing one's partner (Haas et al., 1979).

The physical demands of sexual activity at home with a long-term partner are relatively low for older adults (American Heart Association, 1975) compared with younger adults (Bartlett & Bohr, 1956). Oxygen cost has been reported to be equivalent to a brisk walk or climbing two flights of stairs. The American Heart Association guideline (1975) specifies that sexual activity can likely be tolerated if the individual with heart disease can maintain a steady-state exercise intensity of 6 to 8 calories per minute on a treadmill or 600 kilopond-meters on the cycle ergometer. This is only a rough guideline; however, the precise energy cost of sexual activity in older persons with various cardiopulmonary pathologies needs to be studied in detail so that recommendations can be made on a rational basis.

Although empirical data are lacking, several recommendations can be made to enhance sexual performance in older individuals who have cardiopulmomary dysfunction (American Heart Association, 1975; Haas et al., 1979). Comparable with other types of physical activity, medications can improve sexual performance (e.g., β-blockers, coronary artery vasodilators, and bronchodilators) or impair it (e.g., tranquilizers and antidepressants). Therefore an individual may benefit from adjusting medications whenever possible. Sexual performance may also be enhanced in the absence of alcohol and a few hours after a heavy meal (Selecky, 1987). Less physically demanding positions during intercourse (e.g., the individual does not have to support the weight of the partner, and sitting or standing positions) may reduce energy cost and anxiety (Selecky, 1987). Sexual encounters can be coordinated with peak energy periods during the day rather than restricting intercourse to bedtime when the individual can be expected to be fatigued. The role of exercise training to enhance sexual performance has not been studied in detail. One study by Stein (1977) reported that following a 16-week ergometer training program, the mean maximal heart rate during sexual intercourse was lower than for a control group. This result suggests that the physical demands of intercourse may be reduced with improved exercise tolerance; thus, improved tolerance may help reduce potential risk associated with this activity.

Psychosocial and Vocational Rehabilitation

Psychosocial and vocational counseling are commonly included in the comprehensive rehabilitation program to assist its participants adjust to changing functional status and deal with reactions such as fear, depression, and anxiety (Dudley et al., 1980a; Dudley et al., 1980b; Dudley et al., 1980c; Hudson, 1984; Sandu, 1986). The demand for vocational counseling in older age groups may become more significant with the prospect of nonmandatory retirement. The ability to work can be predicted on the basis of an exercise stress test. The guidelines of the American Thoracic Society (1987) specify that if the $\dot{V}_{O_2}$ required in a given occupation exceeds 40% of the individual's $\dot{V}_{O_2MAX}$ in the stress test, that individual would not be able to tolerate working at that occupation. Exercise testing has a significant role in estimating an individual's potential to perform various tasks including ADLs and types of employment. The application of exercise testing to predicting work capacity in older individuals with cardiopulmonary dysfunction warrants further refinement.

The occupational environment and the quality of the ambient air can have a significant effect on pulmonary function both acutely and over the long term, which can predispose an individual to chronic obstructive disease, restrictive disease, or both. An individual's sensitivity to the air quality may rule out potential employment options. If individuals are working in these environments, appropriate education and physical protection are important in minimizing any hazard (Kanner, 1987).

CONCLUSION

Although the evidence during the past 50 years has been unequivocal regarding the critical role of both gravity and exercise in normal physiological function, this literature has not been fully integrated into current health care practice. The removal of a significant gravitational stimulus and exercise stimulus during recumbency and reduced activity significantly complicate the management of older people with underlying pathology. This literature therefore constitutes the basis for this chapter on advances in rehabilitation for older persons with cardiopulmonary dysfunction.

Exercise testing and training older individuals with cardiopulmonary compromise is a specialized area of exercise physiology. Older persons are diverse with respect to general health, medications, musculoskeletal status, and conditioning levels; therefore, exercise tests and prescriptions have to be appropriately modified to meet the specific needs of each individual. Even with such modifications exercise tests can yield valuable information regarding the cardiopulmonary status of an individual, the degree to which it compromises function, and the parameters for a training program. Despite the advances that have been made, many questions remain regarding optimal testing and training procedures for older persons with cardiopulmonary dysfunction. These need to be addressed in controlled clinical trials.

The comprehensive rehabilitation program is a multidisciplinary health care effort of which the exercise test and training program is one component. Other components that have been reported to have some benefit include health promotion and maintenance, teaching the individual about medications, various physical therapy and occupational therapy interventions; and sexual, psychosocial, and vocational rehabilitation. The literature examining the role of rehabilitation programs is scant. Each of the individual components warrants detailed study with respect to its efficacy and cost effectiveness.

To paraphrase the quotation by Bland and Cooper (1984) that opened this chapter, the weakest and oldest can be trained, but only the very strongest can endure the perils of immobility. This quotation synthesizes literature from the past 50 years that has unequivocally established that the human organism is designed to be bipedal, upright, and moving in a gravitational field, and that the removal of gravitational stress and exercise stress constitutes a death knell for the older person. This literature needs to be exploited in current health care practice; at the same time, health care workers need to examine their attitudes regarding immobility and recumbency in older people so that the mobility potential of individuals assigned to their care can be maximized.

REFERENCES

Adams, G. M., & de Vries, H. A. (1973). Physiological effects of an exercise training regimen upon women aged 52 to 79. *Journal of Gerontology, 28,* 50–55.
Ahlinder, S., Birke, G., Norberg, R., Plantin, L. O., & Reizenstein, P. (1970). Metabolism and distribution of IgG in patients confined to prolonged strict bed rest. *Acta Medica Scandinavica, 187,* 267–270.

Alpert, J. S., Bass, H., Szucs, M. M., Banas, J. S., Dalen, J. E., & Dexter, L. (1974). Effects of physical training on hemodynamics and pulmonary function at rest and during exercise in patients with chronic obstructive pulmonary disease. *Chest, 66,* 647–651.

American Heart Association, Committee on Exercise (1975). Recommendations concerning sexual activity in post-coronary patients. In *Exercise testing and training of individuals with heart disease or at high risk for its debelopment: A handbook for physicians* (pp. 57–58).

American College of Sports Medicine (1991). Guidelines for exercise testing and prescription (4th ed.). Philadelphia: Lea & Febiger.

American Thoracic Society (1981). Pulmonary rehabilitation. *American Review of Respiratory Diseases, 124,* 663–666.

American Thoracic Society (1987). Evaluation of impairment/disability secondary to respiratory disorders. *American Review Respiratory Diseases, 130,* 1205–1209.

Amon, K. W., Richardsm K. L., & Crawford, M. H. (1984). Usefulness of the postexercise response of systolic blood pressure in the diagnosis of coronary artery disease. *Circulation, 70,* 951–956.

Aniansson, A., Grimby, G., Rundgren, A., Svanborg, A., & Orlander, J. (1980). Physical training in older men, *Age and Ageing, 9,* 186–187.

Astrand, I. (1960). Aerobic work capacity in men and women with special reference to age. Acta Physiologica Scandinavica, 169(Suppl.), 1–92.

Astrand, P. O. (1976). Quantification of exercise capability and evaluation of physical capacity in man. *Progress in Cardiovascular Diseases, 19,* 51–59.

Astrand, P. O., & Saltin, B. (1961). Maximal oxygen uptake and heart rate in various types of muscle activity. *Journal of Applied Physiology, 16,* 977–983.

Balke, B., & Ware, R. W. (1959). An experimental study of physical fitness of air force personnel. *U.S. Armed Forces Medical Journal, 10,* 675–688.

Bartlett, R. G., & Bohr, V. C. (1956). Physiologic responses during coitus in the human. *Federation Proceedings, 15,* 10.

Baruch, I. M., & Mossberg, K. A. (1983). Heart-rate response of elderly women to nonweight-bearing ambulation with a walker. *Physical Therapy, 63,* 1782–1787.

Bassey, E. J. (1978). Age, inactivity and some physiological responses to exercise. *Gerontology, 24,* 66–77.

Belman, M. J., & Gaesser, G. A. (1991). Exercise training below and above the lactate threshold in the elderly. *Medicine and Science in Sports and Exercise, 23,* 562–568.

Belman, M. J., & Kendregan, B. A. (1981). Exercise training fails to increase skeletal muscle enzymes in patients with chronic obstructive pulmonary disease. *American Review of Respiratory Diseases, 123,* 256–261.

Belman, M. J., & Kendregan, B. A. (1982). Physical training fails to improve ventilatory muscle endurance in patients with chronic obstructive pulmonary disease. *Chest, 81,* 440–443.

Beman, M. J., & Mittman, C. (1980). Ventilatory muscle training improves exercise capacity in chronic obstructive pulmonary disease patients. *American Review of Respiratory Diseases, 121,* 273–280.

Belman, M. J., Sieck, G., & Mazar, A. (1984). Ventilatory muscle training and pulmonary rehabilitation. Chest (Suppl.), 83S.

Belman, M. J., & Wasserman, K. (1981). Exercise training and testing in patients with chronic obstructive pulmonary disease. *Basics of Respiratory Disease, 10,* 1–6.

Blair, S. N., Painter, P., Pate, R. R., Smith, L. K., & Taylor, C. B. (Eds.). (1988). *Resource manual for guidelines for exercise testing and prescription.* Philadelphia: Lea & Febiger.

Bland, J. H., & Cooper S. M. (1984). Osteoarthritis: A review of the cell biology involved and evidence for reversibility. Management rationally related to known genersis and pathophysiology. *Seminars in Arthritis and Rheumatism, 14*, 106–133.

Blomqvist, C. G., & Stone H. L. (1983). Cardiovascular adjustments to gravitational stress. In J. T. Shepherd & F. M. Abboud (Eds.), *Handbook of physiology. Section 2: Circulation* (Vol. 2, pp. 1025–1063). Bethesda: American Physiological Society.

Borg, G. A. V. (1982). Psychophysiological bases of perceived exertion. *Medicine and Science in Sports and Exercise, 14*, 377–381.

Braun, N., & Marino, W. D. (1984). The effect of daily intermittent rest of respiratory muscles in patients with severe chronic airflow limitation. *Chest* (Suppl.), 59S.

Braun, S. R., Fregosi, R., & Reddan, W. G. (1982). Exercise training in patients with chronic obstructive lung disease. *Postgraduate Medicine, 71*, 163–173.

Brown, H. V., & Wasserman, K. (1981). Exercise performance in chronic obstructive pulmonary disease. *Medical Clinics of North America, 65*, 525–547.

Bruce, R. A., & Hornsten, T. R. (1969). Exercise stress testing in evaluation of patients with ischemic heart disease. *Progress in Cardiovascular Disease, 11*, 371–390.

Buskirk, E. R., & Hodgson, J. L. (1987). Age and aerobic power: The rate of change in men and women. *Federation Proceedings, 46*, 1824–1829.

Bydgeman, S., & Wahren, J. (1974). Influence of body position on the anginal threshold during leg exercise. *European Journal of Clinical Investigation, 4*, 201–206.

Chase, G. A., Grave, C., & Rowell, L. B. (1966). Independence of changes in functional and performance capacities attending prolonged bed rest. *Aerospace Medicine, 37*, 1232–1237.

Chester, E. H., Belman, M. J., Bahler, R. C., Baum, G. L., Schey, G., & Buch, P. (1977). Multidisciplinary treatment of chronic pulmonary insufficiency: 3. The effect of physical training on cardiopulmonary performance in patients with chronic obstructive pulmonary disease. *Chest, 72*, 695–702.

Christie, D. (1968). Physical training in chronic obstructive lung disease. *British Medical Journal, 2*, 150–151.

Chung, E. K. (1983). Protocols for the Exercise ECG Test. In E. K. Chung (Ed.), *Exercise electrocardiography: Practical Approach* (2nd ed., pp. 119–131). Baltimore: Williams & Wilkins.

Chung, F., & Dean, E. (1989). Pathophysiology and cardiorespiratory consequences of interstitial lung disease. *Physical Therapy, 69*, 956–966.

Clark, B. A., Wade, M. G., Massey, B. H., & Van Dyke, R. (1975). Response of institutionalized geriatric mental patients to a twelve-week program of regular physical activity. *Journal of Gerontology, 30*, 565–573.

Clausen, J. P., & Trap-Jensen, J. (1976). Heart rate and arterial blood pressure during exercise in patients with angina pectoris. *Circulation, 53*, 436–442.

Clauss, R. H., Scalabrini, B. Y., Ray, J. F., & Reed, G. E. (1968). Effects of changing body positions upon improved ventilation-perfusion relationships. *Circulation, 37*(Suppl. 2), 214–218.

Cockcroft, A. E., Saunders, M. J., & Berry, G. (1981). Randomised controlled trial of rehabilitation in chronic respiratory disability. *Thorax, 36*, 200–203.

Convertino, V. A., Goldwater, D. J., & Sandler, H. (1986). Bedrest-induced peak VO_2 reduction associated with age, gender, and aerobic capacity. *Aviation, Space and Environmental Medicine, 57*, 17–22.

Convertino, V. A., Hung, J., Goldwater, D., & DeBusk, R. F. (1982). Cardiovascular

responses to exercise in middle-aged men after 10 days of bedrest. *Circulation, 65,* 134–140.
Cooper, K. H., Pollock, M. L., Martin, R. P., White, S. R., Linnerud, A. C., & Jackson, A. (1976). Physical fitness levels vs. selected coronary risk factors. *Journal of the American Medical Association, 236,* 116–119.
Cox, N. J. M., van Herwaarden, C. L. A., Folgering, H., & Binkhorst, R. A. (1988). Exercise and training in patients with chronic obstructive lung disease. *Sports Medicine, 6,* 180–192.
Craig, D. B., Wahba, W. M., & Don, H. (1971). "Closing volume" and its relationship to gas exchange in the seated and supine positions. *Journal of Applied Physiology, 31,* 717–721.
Danish Medical Bulletin (1987). The prevention of falls in later life. *Gerontology.* 4(Suppl.).
Davies, C. T. M., Tuxworth, W., & Young, J. M. (1970). Physiological effects of repeated exercise. *Clinical Science, 39,* 247–258.
Davies, C. T. M., & White, M. J. (1983). Effects of dynamic exercise on muscle function in elderly men, aged 70 years. *Gerontology, 29,* 26–31.
Davis, J. A., Frank, M. H., & Whipp, B. J. (1979). Anaerobic threshold alterations caused by endurance training in middle-aged men. *Journal of Applied Physiology, 46,* 1039–1046.
Dean, E., & Ross, J. (1988). Effect of walking program on patients with postpolio syndrome symptoms. *Archives of Physical Medicine and Rehabilitation, 69,* 1033–1038.
Dean, E., Ross, J., Bartz, J., & Purves, S. (1989). Improving the validity of exercise testing: the effect of practice on performance. *Archives of Physical Medicine and Rehabilitation, 70,* 599–604.
Degre, S., Sergysels, R., Messin, R., Vandermoten, P., Salhadin, P., Denolin, H., & De Coster, A. (1974). Hemodynamic responses to physical training in patients with chronic lung disease. *American Review of Respiratory Disease, 110,* 395–402.
Deitrick, J. E., Whedon, G. D., Shorr, E., Toscani, V., & Davis, V. B. (1948). Effects of immobilization upon various metabolic and physiologic functions of normal men. *American Journal of Medicine, 4,* 3–36.
de Nicola, P., & Tammaro, A. E. (1985a). Coronary heart disease. In *Cardiology in the aged* (pp. 107–119). New York: Schattauer.
de Nicola, P., & Tammaro, A. E. (1985b). Cardiologic semeiology in the aged. In *Cardiology in the aged* (pp. 23–57). New York: Schattauer.
Detry, J. R., Rousseau, M., Vandenbroucke, G., Kusumi, F., Brasseur, L. A., & Bruce, R. A. (1971). Increased arteriovenous oxygen difference after physical training in coronary heart disease. *Circulation, 44,* 109–118.
de Vries, H. A. (1970). Physiological effects of an exercise training regimen upon men aged 52 to 88. *Journal of Gerontology, 25,* 325–336.
de Vries, H. A. (1971). Exercise intensity threshold for improvement of cardiovascular-respiratory function in older men. *Geriatrics, 26,* 94–101.
Doba, N., Shukuya, M., Yoshida, H., Inagaki, M., Inaji, J., & Hinohara, S. (1990). Physical training of patients with coronary heart disease: Noninvasive strategies for the evaluation of its effects on the oxygen transport system and myocardial ischemia. *Japanese Circulation Journal, 54,* 1409–1418.
Dressendorfer, R. H., Smith, J. L., Amsterdam, E. A., & Mason, D. T. (1982). Reduction of submaximal exercise myocardial oxygen demand post-walk training program in coronary patients due to improved physical work efficiency. *American Heart Journal, 103,* 358–362.

Dripps, R. D., & Waters, R. M. (1941). Nursing care of surgical patients: 1. The "stir-up." *American Journal of Nursing, 41,* 530–534.

Dudley, D. L., Glaser, E. M., Jorgenson, E. M., & Logan, D. L. (1980a). Psychosocial concomitants to rehabilitation in chronic obstructive pulmonary disease: 1. Psychological and psychosocial considerations. *Chest, 77,* 413–420.

Dudley, D. L., Glaser, E. M., Jorgenson, E. M., & Logan, D. L. (1980b). Psychosocial concomitants to rehabilitation in chronic obstructive pulmonary disease: 2. Psychosocial treatment. *Chest, 77,* 544–551.

Dudley, D. L., Glaser, E. M., Jorgenson, E. M., & Logan, D. L. (1980c). Psychosocial concomitants to rehabilitation in chronic obstructive pulmonary disease: 3. Dealing with the psychiatric diseases (as distinguished from psychosocial or psychophysiologic problems). *Chest, 77,* 677–684.

Eckstein, R. W. (1957). Effect of exercise and coronary artery narrowing on coronary collateral circulation. *Circulation Research, 5,* 230–235.

Ellestad, M. H., Allen, W., & Wan, M. C. K. (1969). Maximal treadmill stress testing for cardiovascular evaluation. *Circulation, 39,* 517–522.

Epidemiology of Respiratory Diseases Task Force Report. (1980). *State of knowledge, problems and needs* (Publication No. 81-2019, p. 84). Bethesda: U.S. Department of Health and Human Services, National Heart, Lung, and Blood Institute.

Faling, L. J. (1986). Pulmonary rehabilitation-physical modalities. *Clinics in Chest Medicine, 7,* 599–618.

Feigenbaum, L. Z. (1985). Geriatric medicine and the elderly patient. In M. A. Krupp (Ed.), *Current medical diagnosis and treatment* (pp. 19–26). Los Altos: Lange Medical Productions.

Fisher, N. M., Pendergast, D. R., & Calkins, E. (1991). Muscle rehabilitation in impaired elderly nursing home residents. *Archives of Physical Medicine and Rehabilitation, 72,* 181–185.

Fortini, A., Bonechi, F., Taddei, T., Gensini, G. F., Malfanti, P. L., & Serneri, G. G. N. (1991). Anaerobic threshold in patients with exercise-induced myocardial ischemia. *Circulation* 83(Suppl. 3), 50–53.

Fox, S. M., Naughton, J. P., & Gorman, P. A. (1972). Physical activity and cardiovascular health: 3. The exercise prescription: Frequency and type of activity. *Modern Concepts of Cardiovascular Disease, 41,* 25–30.

Franklin, B. A. (1985). Exercise testing, training and arm ergometry. *Sports Medicine, 2,* 100–119.

Frekany, G. A., & Leslie, D. K. (1975). Effects of an exercise program on selected flexibility measurements of senior citizens. *Gerontology, 15,* 182–183.

Froelicher, V. F. (1987). *Exercise and the heart.* (ed. 2, p. 15). Chicago: Year Book Medical.

Froelicher, V., Jensen, D., Genter, F., Sullivan, M., McKirnan, M. D., Witztum, K., Scharf, J., Strong, M. L., & Ashburn, W. (1984). A randomized trial of exercise training in patients with coronary heart disease. *Journal of the American Medical Association, 252,* 1291–1297.

Frontera, W. R., Meredith, C. N., O'Reilly, K. P., Knuttgen, H. G., & Evans, W. J. (1988). Strength conditioning in older men: Skeletal muscle hypertrophy and improved function. *Journal of Applied Physiology, 64,* 1038–1044.

Gilmartin, M. E. (1986). Patient and family education. *Clinics in Chest Medicine, 7,* 619–627.

Goldring, R. M. (1984). Specific defects in cardiopulmonary gas transport. *American Review of Respiratory Disease, 129*(Suppl.), S57–S59.

Greenleaf, J. E., & Kozlowski, S. (1982). Physiological consequences of reduced physical activity during bed rest. *Exercise and Sports Sciences Reviews, 10,* 84–119.

Gutman, G. M., Herbert, C. P., & Brown, S. R. (1977)/ Feldenkrais versus conventional exercise for the elderly. *Journal of Gerontology, 32,* 562–572.

Guyatt, G. H., Sullivan, M. J., Thompson, P. J., Fallen, E. L., Pugsley, S. O., Taylor, D. W., & Berman, L. B. (1985). The 6-minute walk: A new measure of exercise capacity in patients with chronic heart failure. *Candian Medical Association Journal, 132,* 919–923.

Haas, A., Pineda, H., Haas, F., & Axen, K. (1979). Sexual aspects of the COPD patient. In *Pulmonary therapy and rehabilitation* (pp. 158–163). Baltimore: Williams & Wilkins.

Hagberg, J. M., Allen, W. K., Seals, D. R., Hurley, B. F., Ehsani, A. A., & Holloszy, J. O. (1985). A hemodynamic comparison of young and older endurance athletes during exercise. *Journal of Applied Physiology, 58,* 2041–2046.

Hagberg, J. M., Ehsani, A. A., & Holloszy, J. O. (1983). Effect of 12 months of intense exercise training on stroke volume in patients with coronary artery disease. *Circulation, 67,* 1194–1199.

Hahn Winslow, E. (1985). Cardiovascular consequences of bed rest. *Heart and Lung, 14,* 236–246.

Hansen, J. E., & Casaburi, R. (1987). Validity of ear oximetry in clinical exercise testing. *Chest, 91,* 333–337.

Hanson, P. G., Giese, M. D., & Corliss, R. J. (1980). Clinical guidelines for exercise training. *Postgraduate Medicine, 67,* 120–138.

Hanson, P., & Nagle, F. (1987). Isometric exercise: Cardiovascular responses in normal and cardiac populations. In P. Hansen (Ed.), *Exercise and the heart* (pp. 157–170). Philadelphia: W. B. Saunders.

Harper, C. M., & Lyles, Y. M. (1988). Physiology and complications of bed rest. *Journal of the American Geriatrics Society, 36,* 1047–1054.

Hedback, E. L., Perk, J., Engvall, J., & Areskog, N. (1990). Cardiac rehabilitation after coronary artery bypass grafting: Effects on exercise performance and risk factors. *Archives of Physical Medicine and Rehabilitation, 71,* 1069–1073.

Hodgkin, J. E., Gray, L. S., & Connors G. A. (Eds.). (1983). Pulmonary rehabilitation and continuing care [Special issue]. *Respiratory Care, 28,* 1419–1528.

Hodgson, J. L., & Buskirk, E. R. (1977). Physical fitness and age, with emphasis on cardiovascular function in the elderly. *Journal of the American Geriatric Society, 25,* 385–392.

Holle, R. H. O., Williams, D. V., Vandree, J. C., Starks, G. L., & Schoene, R. B. (1988). Increased muscle efficiency and sustained benefits in an outpatient community hospital-based pulmonary rehabilitation program. *Chest, 94,* 1161–1168.

Holloszy, J. O. (1983). Exercise, health, and aging: A need for more information. *Medicine and Science in Sports and Exercise, 15,* 1–5.

Holten, K. (1972). Training effect in patients with severe ventilatory failure. *Scandinavian Journal of Respiratory Disease, 53,* 65–76.

Horvath, S. M., & Borgia, J. F. (1984). Cardiopulmonary gas transport and aging. *American Review of Respiratory Diseases, 129*(Suppl.), S68–S71.

Hossack, K. F. (1987). Cardiovascular responses to dynamic exercise. In P. Hanson (Ed.), Exercise and the heart (pp. 147–156). Philadelphia: W. B. Saunders.

Hossack, K. F.; & Bruce, R. A. (1982). Maximal cardiac function in sedentary normal men and women: Comparison of age-related changes. *Journal of Applied Physiology, 53,* 799–804.

Hudson, L. D. (1984). Management of COPD. *Chest, 84,* 76S–81S.

Hulley, S. B., Vogel, J. M., Donaldson, C. L., Bayers, J. H., Friedman, R. J., & Rosen, S. N. (1971). The effect of supplemental oral phosphate on the bone mineral changes during prolonged bedrest. *Journal of Clinical Investigations, 50,* 2506–2518.

Hung, J., Goldwater, D., Convertino, V. A., McKillop, J. H., Goris, M. L., & DeBusk, R. F. (1983). Mechanisms for decreased exercise capacity after bed rest in normal middle-aged men. *American Journal of Cardiology, 51,* 344–348.

Hyatt, K. H., Kamenetsky, L. G., & Smith, W. M. (1969). Extravascular dehydration as an etiologic factor in post-recumbency orthostatism. *Aerospace Medicine, 40,* 644–650.

Ingebretsen, R. (1982). The relationship between physical activity and mental factors in the elderly. *Scandinavian Journal of Social Medicine, 29,* 153–159.

(1988). Cystic fibrosis and physical activity. *International Journal of Sports Medicine, 9*[Suppl. 1], 1–64.

Jebson, R. H. (1967). Use and abuse of ambulation aids. *Journal of the American Medical Association, 199,* 63–68.

Jette, D. U. (1984). Physiological effects of exercise in the diabetic. *Physical Therapy, 64,* 339–342.

Jones, N. L. (1988). *Clinical exercise testing* (3rd ed.). Philadelphia: W. B. Saunders.

(1944). [Special issue on the effects of bed rest]. *Journal of the American Medical Association, 125.*

Kannel, W. B., & Gordon, T. (1970). *The Framingham study: An epidemiological investigation of cardiovascular disease* (Section 24, Publication No. 0-409-080). Washington, DC: U.S. Government Printing Office.

Kanner, R. E. (1987). Impairment and disability evaluation and vocational rehabilitation. In Hodgkin, J. E. & Petty, T. L. (Eds.), (pp. 173–182). *Chronic obstructive pulmonary disease: Current concepts* Philadelphia: W. B. Saunders.

Kappagoda, C. T., & Greenwood, P. V. (1984). Physical training with minimal hospital supervision of patients after coronary artery bypass surgery. *Archives of Physical Medicine and Rehabilitation, 65,* 57–60.

Karvonen, M. J., Kentala, E., & Mustala, O. (1957). The effects of training on heart rate: A longitudinal study. *Annals of Experimental Medicine and Biology* [Fenn], *35,* 307–315.

Kasch, F. W., Wallace, J. P., Van Camp, S. P., & Verity, L. (1988). A longitudinal study of cardiovascular stability in active men aged 45 to 65 years. *The Physician and Sportsmedicine, 16,* 117–124.

Keens, T. C., Krastins, R. B., Wannamaker, E. M., Levison, H., Crozier, D. N., & Bryan, A. C. (1977). Ventilatory muscle endurance training in normal subjects and patients with cystic fibrosis. *American Review of Respiratory Diseases, 116,* 853–860.

Kellermann, J. J. (1977). Rehabilitation of patients with coronary heart disease. In E. H. Sonnenblick & M. Lesch (Eds.), *Exercise and heart disease* (pp. 183–208). New York: Grune & Stratton.

Kent, S. (1982). Exercise and aging. *Geriatrics, 37,* 132–135.

Killian, K. J. (1985). The objective measurement of breathlessness. *Chest, 88,* 84S–90S.

Kirilloff, L. H., Owens, G. R., Rogers, R. M., & Mazzocco, M. C. (1985). Does chest physical therapy work? *Chest, 88,* 436–444.

Klemic, N., & Imle, P. C. (1989). Changes with immobility and methods of mobilization. In C. F. Mackenzie (Ed.), *Chest physiotherapy in the intensive care unit* (2 ed., pp. 188–214). Baltimore: Williams & Wilkins.

Koenigsberg, M. R., & Holden, D. M. (1989). Peak expiratory flow rates in the elderly. *The Journal of Family Practice, 29,* 503–506.

Kottke, F. J. (1966). The effects of limitation of activity upon the human body. *Journal of the American Medical Association, 196,* 825–830.

Kramsch, D. M., Aspen, A. J., Abramowitz, B. M., Kreimendahl, T., & Hood, W. B. (1981). Reduction of coronary atherosclerosis in moderate conditioning exercise in monkeys on an atherogenic diet. *New England Journal of Medicine, 305,* 1483–1489.

Lakatta, E. G. (1987). Catecholamines and cardiovascular function in aging. *Endocrinology and Metabolism Clinics, 16,* 877–891.

Lampman, R. M. (1987). Evaluating and prescribing exercise for elderly patients. *Geriatrics, 42,* 63–76.

Lampman, R. M., & Schteingart, D. E. (1989). Moderate and extreme obesity. In B. A. Franklin, S. Gordon, & G. C. Timmers (Eds.), *Exercise in modern medicine* (pp. 156–178). Baltimore: Williams & Wilkins.

Landin, R. J., Linnemeier, T. J., Rothbaum, D. A., Chappelear, J., & Noble, R. J. (1985). Exercise testing and training of the elderly patient. In N. K. Wenger (Ed.), *Exercise and the heart* (2nd ed., pp. 201–218). Philadelphia: F. A. Davis.

Laslett, L. J., Paumer, L., & Amsterdam, E. A. (1985). Increase in myocardial oxygen consumption indexes by exercise training at onset of ischemia in patients with coronary artery disease. *Circulation, 71,* 958–962.

Laslett, L., Paumer, L., & Amsterdam, E. (1987). Exercise training in coronary artery disease. In P. Hanson (Ed.), *Exercise and the heart* (pp. 211–226). Philadelphia: W. B. Saunders.

Leblanc, P., Bowie, D. M., Summers, E., Jones, N. L., & Killian, K. J. (1986). Breathlessness and exercise in patients with cardiorespiratory disease. *American Review of Respiratory Diseases, 133,* 21–25.

Lee, A. P., Ice, R., Blessey, R., & Sanmarco, M. E. (1979). Long-term effects of physical training on coronary patients with impaired ventricular function. *Circulation, 60,* 1519–1526.

Lentz, M. (1981). Selected aspects of deconditioning secondary to immobilization. *Nursing Clinics of North America, 16,* 729–737.

Leon, S. A. (1989). Patients with diabetes mellitus. In B. A. Franklin, S. Gordon, & G. C. Timmers (Eds.), *Exercise in modern medicine* (pp. 118–145). Baltimore: Williams & Wilkins.

Lertzman, M. M., & Cherniack, R. M. (1976). Rehabilitation of patients with chronic obstructive lung disease. *American Review of Respiratory Disease, 114,* 1145–1165.

Levine, S. A., & Lown, B. (1952). "Armchair" treatment of acute coronary thrombosis. *Journal of the American Medical Association, 148,* 1365–1369.

Mahler, D. A., Cunningham, D. P. E., & Curfman, G. D. (1986). Aging and exercise performance. *Clinics in Geriatric Medicine, 2,* 433–452.

Make, B. J. (1986). Pulmonary rehabilitation: Myth or reality? *Clinics in Chest Medicine, 7,* 519–540.

May, G. A., & Nagle, F. J. (1984). Changes in rate-pressure product with physical training of individuals with coronary artery disease. *Physical Therapy, 64,* 1361–1366.

McArdle, W. B., Katch, F. I., & Katch V. V. (1986). Training for anaerobic and aerobic power. In *Exercise physiology* (pp. 347–370). Philadelphia: Lea & Febiger.

Mcelvaney, G. N., Blackie, S. P., Morrison, N. J., Fairbarn, M. S., Wilcox, P. G., & Pardy, R. L. (1989). Cardiac output at rest and in exercise in elderly subjects. *Medicine and Science in Sports and Exercise, 21,* 293–298.

McGavin, C. R., Gupta, S. P., Lloyd, E. L., & McHardy, G. J. R. (1977). Physical rehabilitation for the chronic bronchitic: Results of a controlled trial of exercises in the home. *Thorax, 32,* 307–311.

McGavin, C. R., Gupta, S. P., & McHardy, G. J. R. (1976). Twelve-minute walking test for assessing disability in chronic bronchitis. *British Medical Journal, 1,* 822–823.

McHenry, P. L., Phillips, J. F., & Kroebel, S. B. (1972). Correlation of computer-quantitated treadmill exercise electrocardiography with arteriographic localization of coronary artery disease. *American Journal of Cardiology, 30,* 747–752.

Mertens, D. J., Shephard, R. J., & Kavanagh, T. (1978). Long-term exercise therapy for chronic obstructive lung disease. *Respiration, 35,* 96–107.

Miller, P. B., Johnson, R. L., & Lamb, L. E. (1964). Effects of four weeks of absolute bed rest on circulatory functions in man. *Aerospace Medicine, 35,* 1194–1197.

Miyashita, M., Mutoh, Y., Yoshioka, N., & Sadamoto, T. (1985). PWC 75% HRmax: A measure of aerobic work capacity. *Sports Medicine, 2,* 159–164.

Moritani, T., & de Vries, H. A. (1981). Neural factors versus hypertrophy in the time course of muscle strength gain in young and old men. *Journal of Gerontology, 36,* 294–297.

Mungall, I. P. F., & Hainsworth, R. (1980). An objective assessment of the value of exercise training to patients with chronic obstructive airways disease. *Quarterly Journal of Medicine, 49,* 77–85.

Myles, W. S., & Maclean, D. (1986). A comparison of response and production protocols for assessing perceived exertion. *European Journal of Applied Physiology, 55,* 585–587.

Naso, F., Carner, E., Blankfort-Doyle, W., & Coughey, K. (1990). Endurance training in the elderly nursing home patient. *Archives of Physical Medicine and Rehabilitation, 71,* 241–243.

Nelson, J. R., Prakash, C., & Deedwania, M. D. (1989). New exercise parameter for the identification of severe coronary artery disease. *Chest, 95,* 895–898.

Nicholas, J. J., Gilbert, R., Gabe, R., & Auchincloss, J. H. (1970). Evaluation of an exercise therapy program for patients with chronic obstructive pulmonary disease. *American Review of Respiratory Disease, 102,* 1–9.

Niederman, M. S., Clemente, P. H., Fein, A. M., Feinsilver, S. H., Robinson, D. A., Ilowite, J. S., & Bernstein, M. G. (1991). Benefits of a multidisciplinary pulmonary rehabilitation program: Improvements are independent of lung function. *Chest, 99,* 798–804.

O'Hara, W. J., Lasachuk, K. E., Matheson, P. C., Renahan, M. C., Schlotter, D. G., & Lilker, E. S. (1984). Weight training and back packing in chronic obstructive pulmonary disease. *Respiratory Care, 29,* 1202–1210.

O'Hara, W. J., Lasachuk, K. E., Matheson, P. C., Renahan, M. C., Schlotter, D. G., & Lilker, E. S. (1987). Weight training benefits in chronic obstructive pulmonary disease: A controlled crossover study. *Respiratory Care, 32,* 660–668.

Orlander, J., Kiessling, K. H., & Ekblom, B. (1980). Time course of adaptation to low intensity training in sedentary men: Dissociation of central and local effects. *Acta Physiologica Scandinavia, 108,* 85–90.

Paez, P. N., Phillipson, E. A., Masangkay, M., & Sproule, B. J. (1967). The physiologic basis of training patients with emphysema. *American Review of Respiratory Disease, 95,* 944–953.

Pardy, R. L., Hussain, S. N. A., & Macklem, P. T. (1984). The ventilatory pump in exercise. *Clinics in Chest Medicine, 5,* 35–49.

Pardy, R. L., Rivington, R. N., Despas, P. J., & Macklem, P. T. (1981). Inspiratory muscle training compared with physiotherapy in patients with chronic airflow limitation. *American Review of Respiratory Diseases, 123,* 421–425.

Peacock, E. E. (1963). Comparison of collagenous tissue surrounding normal and immobilized joints. *Surgical Forum, 24,* 440–441.

Petty, T. L. (1975). Pulmonary rehabilitation. *Basics of Respiratory Diseases, 4,* 1–6.

Pickering, T. G. (1987). Exercise and hypertension. In P. Hanson (Ed.), *Exercise and the heart* (pp. 311–318). Philadelphia: W. B. Saunders.

Pierce, A. K., Taylor, H. F., Archer, R. K., & Miller, W. F. (1964). Responses to exercise training in patients with emphysema. *Archives of Internal Medicine, 113,* 28–36.

Plowman, S. A., Drinkwater, B. L., & Horvath, S. M. (1979). Age and aerobic power in women: A longitudinal study. *Journal of Gerontology, 34,* 512–520.

Pollack, M. L., & Pels, A. E. (1984). Exercise prescription for the cardiac patient: An update Symposium on cardiac rehabilitation. *Clinics in Sports Medicine, 3,* 425–442.

Porcari, J., McCarron, R., Kline, G., Freedson, P. S., Ward, A., Ross, J. A., & Rippe, J. M. (1987). Is fast walking an adequate aerobic training stimulus for 30- to 69-year-old men and women? *The Physician and Sportsmedicine, 15,* 119–129.

Ray, J. F., Yost, L., Moallem, S., Sanoudos, G. M., Villamena, P., & Paredes, R. M. (1974). Immobility, hypoxemia, and pulmonary arteriovenous shunting. *Archives of Surgery, 109,* 537–541.

Rice, C. L., Cunningham, D. A., Paterson, D. H., & Rechnitzer, P. A .(1989). Strength in an elderly population. *Archives of Physical Medicine and Rehabilitation, 70,* 391–397.

Ries, A. L., Ellis, B., & Hawkins, R. W. (1988). Upper extremity exercise training in chronic obstructive pulmonary disease. *Chest, 93,* 688–692.

Risser, N. L. (1980). Preoperative and postoperative care to prevent pulmonary complications. *Heart and Lung, 9,* 57–67.

Robinson, S., Dill, D. B., Ross, J. C., Robinson, R. D., Wagner, J. A., & Tzankoff, S. P. (1973). Training and physiologic aging in man. *Federation Proceedings, 32,* 1628–1634.

Rodeheffer, R. J., Gerstenblith, G., & Becker, L. C. (1984). Exercise cardiac output is maintained with advancing age in healthy human subjects. Cardiac dilation and increased stroke volume compensate for a diminished heart rate. *Circulation, 69,* 203–206.

Ross, J., & Dean, E. (1989). Integrating physiological principles into the comprehensive management of cardiopulmonary dysfunction. *Physical Therapy, 69,* 255–259.

Rousseau, M. F., Brasseur, L. A., & Detry, J. R. (1973). Hemodynamic determinants of maximal oxygen intake in patients with healed myocardial infarction: Influence of physical training. *Circulation, 48,* 943–949.

Rubenstein, L. Z., Robbins, A. S., & Josephson, K. R. (1991). Falls in the nursing-home setting: Causes and preventive approaches. In P. R. Katz, R. L. Kane, & M. D. Mezey, (Eds.), *Advances in long-term care* (pp. 28–42). New York, Springer.

Rubin, M. (1988). The physiology of bed rest. *American Journal of Nursing, 88,* 50–56.

Ryback, R. S., Lewis, O. F., & Lessard, C. S. (1971). Psychobiological effects of prolonged bed rest (weightlessness) in young healthy volunteers (Study II). *Aerospace Medicine, 42,* 529–535.

Saltin, B., Blomqvist, G., Mitchell, J. H., Johnson, R. L., Wildenthal, K., & Chapman, C. B. (1968). Response to exercise after bed rest and after training. *Circulation, 38*(Suppl. 7), 1–78.

Saltin, B., Lindgarde, F., Houston, M., Horlin, R., Nygaard, E., Gad, P. (1979). Physical training and glucose tolerance in middle-aged men with chemical diabetes. *Diabetes, 28*(Suppl.), 30–32.

Samsoe, M. (1984). Prescription of exercise for the atypical patient with diabetes, obesity, or pulmonary disease. In L. K. Hall, G. C. Meyer, & H. K. Hellerstein (Eds.), *Cardiac rehabilitation: Exercise testing and prescription* (pp. 175–189). New York: SP Medical and Scientific Books.

Sandler, H. (1986). Cardiovascular effects of inactivity. In H. Sandler & J. Vernikos (Eds.), *Inactivity physiological effects* (pp. 11–47). New York: Academic Press.

Sandler, H., Popp, R. L., & Harrison, D. C. (1988). The hemodynamic effects of repeated bed rest exposure. *Aerospace Medicine, 59,* 1047–1054.

Sandu, H. S. (1986). Psychosocial issues in chronic obstructive lung disease. *Clinics in Chest Medicine, 7,* 629–642.

Seals, D. R., Allen, W. K., Hurley, B. F., Dalsky, G. P., Ehsani, A. A., & Hagberg, J. M. (1984a). Elevated high-density lipoprotein cholesterol levels in older endurance athletes. *American Journal of Cardiology, 54,* 390–393.

Seals, D. R., Hagberg, J. M., Hurley, B. F., Ehsani, A. A., & Holloszy, J. O. (1984b). Endurance training in older men and women: 1. Cardiovascular responses to exercise. *Journal of Applied Physiology, 57,* 1024–1029.

Selecky, P. A. (1987). Sexuality and the COPD patient. In J. E. Hodgkin & T. L. Petty (Eds.), *Chronic obstructive pulmonary disease: Current concepts* (pp. 215–226). Philadelphia: W. B. Saunders.

Sharkey, B. J. (1988). Specificity of exercise. In *Resource Manual for guidelines for exercise testing and prescription* (pp. 55–61). Philadelphia: Lea & Febiger.

Sheffield, L. T., & Roitman, D. (1977). Stress testing methodology. In E. H. Sonnenblick & M. Lesch (Eds.), *Exercise and heart disease* (pp. 145–161). New York: Grune & Stratton.

Shephard, R. J. (1976). Exercise and chronic lung disease. *Exercise and Sports Science Review, 4,* 263–296.

Shephard, R. J. (1991). Safety of exercise testing—the role of the paramedical exercise specialist. *Clinical Journal of Sports Medicine, 1,* 8–11.

Shephard, R. J., Allen, C., Benade, A. J. S., Davies, C. T. M., di Prampero, P. E., Hedman, R., Merriman, J. E., Myhre, K., & Simmons, R. (1968). Standardization of submaximal exercise test. *Bulletin of the World Health Organization, 38,* 765–775.

Siconolfi, S. F., Cullinane, E. M., Carleton, R. A., & Thompson, P. D. (1982). Assessing VO_2max in epidemiologic studies: Modification of the Astrand-Ryhming test. *Medicine in Science and Sports and Exercise, 14,* 335–338.

Sidney, K. H., & Shephard, R. J. (1976). Attitudes towards health and physical activity in the elderly: Effects of a physical training program. *Medicine and Science in Sports, 8,* 246–252.

Sidney, K. H., & Shephard, R. J. (1977). Activity patterns of elderly men and women. *Journal of Gerontology, 32,* 25–32.

Sidney, K. H., & Shephard, R. J. (1978). Frequency and intensity of exercise training for elderly subjects. *Medicine and Science in Sports, 10,* 125–131.

Sidney, K. H., Shephard, R. J., & Harrison, J. E. (1977). Endurance training and body composition of the elderly. *American Journal of Clinical Nutrition, 30,* 326–333.

Sinaki, M. (1989). Exercise and osteoporosis. *Archives of Physical Medicine and Rehabilitation, 70,* 220–229.

Sinclair, D. J. M., & Ingram, C. G. (1980). Controlled trial of supervised exercise training in chronic bronchitis. *British Medical Journal, 280,* 519–521.

Skinner, J. S. (1987). Importance of aging for exercise testing and exercise prescription. In J. S. Skinner (Ed.), *Exercise testing and exercise prescription for special cases* (pp. 67–75). Philadelphia: Lea & Febiger.

Skinner, J. S., & Strandness, D. E. (1967). Exercise and intermittent claudication: 2. Effect of physical therapy. *Circulation, 36,* 23–27.

Smith, E. L. (1981). Age: The interaction between nature and nurture. In E. L. Smith & R. C. Serfass (Eds.), *Exercise and aging: The scientific basis.* Hillside, NJ: Enslow.

Smith, E. L., & Gilligan, C. (1983). Physical activity prescription for the older adult. *The Physician and Sportsmedicine, 11,* 91–101.

Smith, E. L., Reddan, W., & Smith P. E. (1981). Physical activity and calcium modalities for bone mineral increase in aged women. *Medicine and Science in Sports and Exercise, 13,* 60–64.

Sobolski, J. C., Kolesar, J. J., Kornitzer, M. D., de Backer, G. G., Mikes, Z., Dramaix, M. M., Degre, S. G., & Denolin, H. F. (1988). Physical fitness does not reflect physical activity patterns in middle-aged workers. *Medicine and Science in Sports and Exercise, 20,* 6–13.

Stamford, B. A. (1972). Physiological effects of training upon institutionalized geriatric men. *Journal of Gerontology, 27,* 451–455.

Stamford, B. A. (1988). Exercise and the elderly. *Exercise and Sports Science Review, 16,* 341–379.

Stein, R. A. (1977). The effect of exercise training on heart rate during coitus in the post-myocardial infarction patient. *Circulation, 55,* 738–740.

Strasser, T. (1987). Cardiovascular care of the elderly. Geneva: World Health Organization.

Suominen, H., Heikkinen, E., & Parkatti, T. (1977). Effect of eight weeks' physical training on muscle and connective tissue of m. vastus lateralis in 69-year-old men and women. *Journal of Gerontology, 32,* 33–37.

Superko, H. R., & Haskell, W. H. (1987). The role of exercise training in the therapy of hyperlipoproteinemia. In P. Hanson (Ed.), *Exercise and the heart* (pp. 285–310). Philadelphia: W. B. Saunders.

Svanberg, L. (1957). Influence of position on the lung volumes, ventilation and circulation in normals. *Scandinavian Journal of Clinical Laboratory Investigations, 25*(Suppl.), 7–175.

Swerts, P. M. J., Mostert, R., & Wouters, E. F. M. (1990). Comparison of corridor and treadmill walking in patients with severe chronic obstructive pulmonary disease. *Journal of Physical Therapy 70,* 439–442.

Taniguchi, K., Itoh, H., Yajima, T., Doi, M., Niwa, A., & Marumo, F. (1990). Predischarge early exercise therapy in patients with acute myocardial infarction on the basis of anaerobic threshold (AT). *Japanese Circulation Journal, 54,* 1419–1425.

Thomas, S. G., Cunningham, D. A., Rechnitzer, P. A., Donner, A. P., & Howard, J. H. (1985). Determinants of the training response in elderly men. *Medicine and Science in Sports and Exercise, 17,* 667–672.

Tydeman, D. E., Chandler, A. R., & Graveling, B. M. (1984). An investigation into the effects of exercise tolerance training on patients with chronic airways obstruction. *Physiotherapy, 70,* 261–264.

Vallbona, C., & Baker, S. B. (1984). Physical fitness prospects in in the elderly. *Archives of Physical Medicine and Rehabilitation, 65,* 194–200.

Vandervoort, A. A., Hayes, K. C., & Belanger, A. Y. (1986). Strength and endurance of skeletal muscle in the elderly. *Physiotherapy Canada, 38,* 167–173.

Varnauskas, E., Bergman, H., Houk, P., & Bjorntorp, P. (1966). Haemodynamic effects of physical training in coronary patients. *Lancet, 2,* 8–12.

Vyas, M. N., Banister, E. W., Morton, J. W., & Grzybowski, S. (1971). Response to exercise in patients with chronic airway obstruction: 1. Effects of exercise training. *American Review of Respiratory Disease, 103,* 390–399.

Wall, J. C., & Charteris, J. (1981). Kinematic study of long-term habituation to treadmill walking. *Ergonomics, 24,* 531–542.

Ward, A., Malloy, P., & Rippe, J. (1987). Exercise prescription guidelines for normal and cardiac populations. In P. Hanson (Ed.), *Exercise and the heart,* (pp. 197–210). Philadelphia: W. B. Saunders.

Wasserman, K., Hansen, J. E., Sue, D. Y., & Whipp, B. J. (1987). *Principles of exercise testing and interpretation* (pp. 27–46). Philadelphia: Lea & Febiger.

Wasserman, K. (1990). Measures of functional capacity in patients with heart failure. *Circulation, 81*(Suppl. II), II1–II4.

Wasserman, K., & Whipp, B. J. (1975). Exercise physiology in health and disease. *American Review of Respiratory Diseases, 112,* 219–249.

Weber, K. T., Janicki, J. S., McElroy, P. A., & Reddy, H. K. (1988). Concepts and applications of cardiopulmonary exercise testing. *Chest, 93,* 843–847.

Weber, K. T., Janicki, J. S., Shroff, S. G., & Likoff, M. J. (1983). The cardiopulmonary unit: The body's gas transport system. *Clinics in Chest Medicine, 4,* 101–110.

Wenger, N. K. (1982). Early ambulation: The physiologic basis revisted. *Advances in Cardiology, 31,* 138–141.

West, J. B. (1990). *Respiratory physiology: The essentials* (4th ed.). Baltimore, Williams & Wilkins.

Whitley, J. D., & Schoene, L. L. (1987). Comparison of heart rate responses: Water walking versus treadmill walking. *Physical Therapy, 67,* 1501–1504.

Williams, R. S. (1985). Exercise training of patients with ventricular dysfunction and heart failure. In N. K. Wenger (Ed.), *Exercise and the heart,* (2nd ed., pp. 219–231). Philadelphia: F. A. Davis.

Williams, R. S., Conn, E. H., & Wallance, A. G. (1981). Enhanced exercise performance following physical training in coronary patients stratified by left ventricular ejection fraction. *Circulation, 64*(Suppl. 4), 186.

Williams, R. S., McKinnis, R. A., Cobb, F. R., Higginbotham, M. B., Wallace, A. G., Coleman, R. E., & Califf, R. M. (1984). Effects of physical conditioning on left ventricular ejection fraction in patients with coronary artery disease. *Circulation, 70,* 69–75.

Wilson, J. R. (1987). Exercise and the failing heart. In P. Hanson (Ed.), *Exercise and the heart,* (pp. 171–182). Philadelphia: W. B. Saunders.

Wolff, R. K., Dolovitch, M. B., Obminski, G., & Newhouse, M. T. (1977). Effects of exercise and eucapnic hyperventilation on bronchial clearance in man. *Journal of Applied Physiology, 43,* 46–50.

Wolf-Klein, G. P., Silverstone, F. L., Basavaraju, N., Foley, C. J., Pascaru, A., & Ma, P. H. (1988). Prevention of falls in the elderly population. *Archives of Physical Medicine and Rehabilitation, 69,* 689–691.

Woolf, C. R., & Suero, J. T. (1969). Alterations in lung mechanics and gas exchange following training in chronic obstructive lung disease. *Diseases of the Chest, 55,* 37–44.

Yano, K., Reed, D. M., Curb, J. D., Hankin, J. H., & Albers, J. J. (1986). Biological and dietary correlates of plasma lipids and lipoproteins among elderly Japanese men in Hawaii. *Arteriosclerosis, 6,* 422–433.

Yeng, J. E., Seals, D. R., Hagberg, J. M., & Holloszy, J. O. (1985). Effect of endurance exercise training on ventilatory function in older individuals. *Journal of Applied Physiology, 58*, 791–794.

Zadai, C. C. (1985). Rehabilitation of the patient with chronic obstructive pulmonary disease. In S. Irwin & J. S. Tecklin (Eds.), *Cardiopulmonary physical therapy*, (pp. 367–381). St. Louis: C. V. Mosby.

Zeimetz, G. A., Moss, R. F., & Butts, N. (1979). Support versus non support treadmill walking. *Medicine and Science in Sports and Exercise, 11*, 112–117.

Zubeck, J. P., & MacNeill, M. (1966). Effects of immobilization: Behavioral and EEG changes. *Canadian Journal of Psychology, 20*, 316–336.

ZuWallack, R. L., Patel, K., Reardon, J. Z., Clark, B. A., & Normandin, E. A. (1991). Predictors of improvement in the 12-minute walking distance following a six-week outpatient pulmonary rehabilitation program. *Chest, 99*, 805–808.

2
The Etiology, Prevention, and Treatment of Pressure Sores

Barbara J. Braden
Mildred G. Kemp
Mark H. Overton
Janet Cuddigan
Brenda Bergman

The occurrence of a pressure sore in any setting is viewed as a failure of care with potentially serious consequences. Some estimates of mortality rates for persons who develop pressure sores are as high as 60% (Vasile & Chaitin, 1972) and the presence of a pressure sore has been reported to increase the risk of death fourfold in elderly patients (Michocki & Lamy, 1976). The cost of treating a single pressure sore has been variously estimated from $1,000 to $20,000, depending on the depth of the ulcer and the method of calculating cost (Altrescu, 1989; Frantz, 1989). As a nation, the medical costs associated with treating pressure sores have been estimated to exceed $2 billion per year (Krouskop, Noble, Garber, & Spencer, 1983).

Consistent data concerning incidence and prevalence of pressure sores in the United States has been difficult to find and evaluate in the past because differences in methodology, sample size, definitions, and settings contribute to limitations (Allman 1989). Two recent multisite studies overcame some of these limitations. In a survey of 148 hospitals, clinicians identified (by direct observation) an overall prevalence of 9.2% (N = 34,987), when maternity patients were excluded, and newborn and neonatal nurseries were included (Mehan, 1990). In a second study, the rate of prevalence obtained by record review for residents of 51 nursing homes was also stable at 9.2% over the two year study period (Brandeis, Morris, Nash, & Lipsitz, 1990). In both cases, stage I ulcers were included in the prevalence rates. Brandeis and colleagues also found that point prevalence was highest at admission (17.4%) and declined to 8.1% by 2 years following admission while incidence of pressure sore formation in the first year following admission was 13.2%.

RISK FACTORS

Pressure sore formation is a complex phenomena, involving multiple etiological factors that contribute in varying degrees to either increased intensity and duration of pressure or decreased tissue tolerance for pressure. Although numerous factors may contribute to the development of a pressure sore, by definition, this type of lesion does not occur without the insult of pressure. Husain (1953) noted histological changes in the muscles of rats when externally applied pressure as low as 100 mm Hg was exerted for a period of as short as 1 hour. Kosiak (1959), in a similar study using mongrel dogs, observed pathological changes in tissues subjected to pressure as low as 60 mm Hg for only 1 hour.

To overcome limitations in other animals models, some investigators have used normal and paraplegic swine to explore the intensity-duration curve (Daniel, Priest, & Wheatley 1981; Dinsdale, 1974). Their findings continued to support the parabolic nature of the intensity-duration curve, but Daniel et al. were additionally able to demonstrate that muscle was much more susceptible to the destructive effects of pressure than normothermic skin, explaining instances of deep tissue damage that are obvious beneath the skin before actual skin breakdown. In this study, destruction was observed in muscle at 500 mm Hg of pressure applied over 4 hours; skin damage did not occur until the pressure increased to 800 mm Hg over 8 hours. In further investigations, skin over muscle was found to tolerate greater pressure than skin over bone before developing unacceptably low skin oxygen tension (Sangeorzan, Harrington, Wyss, Czernecki, & Matsen 1989; Seiler & Stahelin, 1979).

In clinical populations, persons with diminished mobility, activity, or sensory perception are more likely to be exposed to intense and prolonged pressure than those persons who can independently move in bed, ambulate and respond purposefully to pressure-related pain, and are, therefore, more likely to develop pressure sores (Allman, Laprade, Noel, et al., 1986; Barbenel, Jordan, Nicol, & Clark 1977; Ek & Boman, 1982; Manley, 1978; Moolten, 1972). In a survey of 10,571 hospital and home-bound patients in Scotland, Barbenel et al. found the highest prevalence of significant pressure sores (grade 2 or higher) in the chairfast and totally helpless group. A similar survey in Sweden found the highest prevalence of pressure sores among those immobilized or having neurological problems that interfered with activity or sensory perception (Ek & Boman, 1982). Manley (1978), in a third survey conducted in South Africa, found a strong inverse relationship between the distribution of degrees of mobility in the total survey population and in those who developed pressure sores.

In contrast, Patterson and Fischer (1986), after continually monitoring the sitting pressure patterns of five quadriplegic subjects, reported no pressure sore formation despite widely varying and sometimes multihour periods of exposure to sitting pressures exceeding the usual acceptable intensity level. Merbitz, King, Bleiberg, and Grip (1985), in a similar study of spinal cord–injured subjects also found wide variability in sitting pressure patterns between subjects. This type of variability has prompted scientists to consider other factors that may interact with pressure to increase or decrease the tolerance of tissue for pressure.

Those factors that diminish tissue tolerance for pressure can be divided into two categories, intrinsic and extrinsic, according to the site at which they produce their effect. Extrinsic factors are those physical factors that weaken the outer layers of the skin, thus diminishing the skin's tolerance for pressure. Intrinsic factors are primarily physiological factors that influence the supporting structures of the skin in such a way that tissue injury occurs at lower external pressures.

The extrinsic physical factors that affect tissue tolerance for pressure are friction, shear, and exposure to moisture. Dinsdale (1974) conducted experiments designed to investigate the amount of pressure required to produce a pressure sore when skin had been pretreated with light friction. In one experiment using normal swine Dinsdale found that, in the absence of friction, a pressure of 290 mm Hg was required to produce ulceration, whereas a pressure of only 45 mm Hg would produce ulceration in skin also subjected to friction. Friction is commonly experienced by patients who cannot lift or be lifted sufficiently during a position change to avoid dragging the skin over the rough surface of bed linens. Casts and other orthopedic devices are frequent sources of friction. Friction may also be a problem with agitated or spastic patients who are also bedfast or chairfast.

Shear forces are another factor in diminishing tissue tolerance for pressure. Shear forces occur when an external pressure load is applied at the same time that substantial movement of superficial layers of the skin is effected, leading to deformation and destruction of the vascular bed. Though several authors (Newell, Thornburgh, & Fleming, 1970); (Reichel, 1958) mention shear forces as a major cause of pressure sores, few controlled investigations have been done because of instrumentation problems. Recent developments in technology and mathematical modeling have, however, allowed investigators to explore shear as a factor in pressure sore formation (Bennett, Kavner, Lee, Trainor, & Lewis 1984). Bennett et al. examined shearing and pulsatile blood flow in normal, geriatric, and paraplegic sujects. Findings included the propensity of geriatric and paraplegic subjects to develop substantially greater shearing forces (accompanied by decrements in pulsatile blood flow) than normal subjects.

Exposure of the skin to moisture is frequently mentioned as a risk factor. Moisture appears to have been a factor in pressure sore formation among the 147 patients with existing pressure sores studied by Andersen and Kvorning (1982). The sources of moisture most frequently mentioned are urine and feces, though perspiration and drainage from wounds or moist packs may also be significant sources. Flam (1987) also contends that as much as 200 g of insensible moisture vapor is transmitted through the skin of the supine patients, sufficient to cause overhydration of the stratum corneum in nonexposed areas. Allman et al. (1986) found that fecal incontinence was a strong predictor of pressure sore formation but that urinary catherization was more strongly associated with pressure sore formation than urinary incontinence.

Certain intrinsic factors can change the architecture of the skin or the oxygen-delivery capabilities of the blood and vascular bed to such an extent that external mechanical load will cause ischemia at lower levels of applied pressure. Examples of these factors are undernutrition, aging, low arteriolar pressure, and elevations in body temperature.

The nutritional deficiences most frequently related to pressure sores are protein-calorie, iron (Bergstrom & Braden, 1990; Moolten, 1972; Vasile & Chaitin, 1972), ascorbic acid (Hunter & Rajan, 1971), and trace mineral deficiencies, particularly zinc and copper (Prasad, 1982). All of these deficiences can be related to a decrease in the quality and integrity of the components of soft tissue, particularly collagen.

Protein nutriture as reflected by serum albumin and red blood cell hemoglobin concentrations has been related to the presence of pressure sores (Allman et al., 1986; Artique & Hyman, 1976; Moolten, 1972; Ryan, 1979; Vasile & Chaitin, 1972). Moolten (1972) studied 50 patients with pressure sores using data available from patient records. Eight of the 31 patients with available hemoglobin levels were profoundly anemic, demonstrating a mean hemoglobin concentration of 10 g/dl. Twenty-four of the 50 subjects had moderate or worse protein depletion as evidenced by low serum albumin levels. Similarly, Allman et al. (1986) surveyed 634 adult hospitalized patients, identifying 30 with existing pressure sores and 78 who were at risk for pressure sores. Serum albumin levels were significantly lower among patients with pressure sores than those at risk.

There is some concern that loss of serum proteins through wound exudate contributes to the low serum albumin levels seen among patients with existing pressure sores. Bergstrom and Braden (1990), in a prospective study designed to overcome this concern, followed 200 nursing home residents older than age 65 who were at risk (Braden score ≤ 17) for pressure sores for 12 weeks following admission to determine factors related to the development and healing of pressure sores. They found that, of the 143 (73.5%) subjects who developed stage I or deeper pressure sores, 86 (58.5%) subsequently healed. Those subjects who developed pressure sores had a significantly lower intake of calories and protein than those who did not develop pressure sores or those whose sores healed. Likewise, serum albumin was significantly lower ($p < .001$) among those who developed pressure sores (M

= 3.0 g%) than among those who did not (M = 3.2 g%). Although total protein and iron were also lower for those who developed pressure sores, these differences were not clinically significant.

In a different vein, Trumbore and associates (1990) examined 40 patients on low-fat, low-cholesterol, tube-fed diets and found a significant correlation between hypocholesterolemia and pressure sores. In fact, low cholesterol proved to be a better predictor of pressure sores than albumin. There is theoretical and clinical evidence that deficiencies in essential fatty acids affect skin integrity. Linoleic acid is an essential component of the water-proof barrier within the stratum corneum, and deficiencies produce a scaly hyper-keratosis (Roe, 1986). Further investigation may be warranted regarding the role of essential fatty acid and cholesterol deficiencies in pressure sore development.

Ascorbic acid deficiency can impair wound healing in animals and humans (Irwin and Hutchins, 1976; Ringsdorf & Cheraskin, 1982), probably as a result of its role in the formation and maintenance of collagen. Vitamin C supplementation (1,000 mg/day) has been shown to increase the blood concentration of vitamin C and to increase the rate of healing of pressure sores to an extent not found in controls (Taylor, Rimmer, Day, Butcher, & Dymock, 1974). It has been hypothesized that vitamin C may have a role in the prevention of pressure sores (Ringsdorf & Cheraskin, 1982; Taylor et al., 1974), but this hypothesis has not been tested.

Certain trace minerals, such as zinc and copper, have been related to the quality of collagen formed in the body, and deficiencies in these (Prasad, 1983). Bergstrom and Braden (1990) found that dietary intake of zinc was significantly lower among elderly nursing home residents who developed pressure sores that did not heal (M = 37% recommended daily allowance [RDA]) than among those who did not develop sores (M = 51% RDA) or those whose sores healed (52% RDA). Serum zinc levels were also lower, but this difference was not significant. In addition, zinc supplementation has been shown to increase wound healing in elderly persons with statis ulcers of the leg (Haeger, Lannez, & Magnusson, 1974; Hallbook & Lanner, 1972; Prasad, 1983).

Certain changes occurred in the skin and its supporting structures as a result of aging (Kenney, 1982). Elastin fibers become more rigid, and normal mechanical stress causes the fibers to fray and fragment. The mechanical properties of collagen fibers also change so that distensibility and elasticity are impaired. These changes allow for a greater degree of transfer of mechanical load from externally applied pressure to the underlying vasculature, leading to ischemia (Krouskop, 1983). The effect on blood flow is supported by Bennett et al. (1984) who compared normal males to male paraplegic and geriatric subjects with respect to shear and skin blood flow in the area of the ischial tuberosities while sitting on a hard instrumented seat. Paraplegic and geriatric subjects had median blood flow rates that were roughly three times smaller than those found in the normal subjects. That aging increases susceptibility to pressure sore formation is also supported in several clinical survey studies (Anderson & Kvorning, 1982; Ek & Boman, 1982; Manley, 1978) and, even within an elderly population (R = 66 to 95, M = 80, SD = 7), those developing pressure sores were found to be significantly older than those who did not (Bergstrom & Braden, 1990).

A low arteriolar pressure diminishes tissue tolerance for pressure by creating a situation in which less pressure is required to effect vascular closure (Seiler & Stahelin, 1979). Larsen, Holstein, and Lassen (1979), in studying the relationship between ischemia and external pressure, found that subjects who were hypertensive could withstand higher external pressures before vascular occlusion occurred than those subjects who were normotensive. In one retrospective study, more than 20% of the subjects with pressure sores had a systolic blood pressure below 100 mm Hg (Moolten, 1972), whereas Gosnell, (1973), using a prospective design, found that a diastolic blood pressure below 60 mm Hg seemed to predispose elderly subjects to pressure sore development.

Another recent development is exploration of the association of psychosocial issues with pressure sore formation. Pressure sore development, for example, has been related to factors that influenced the patients motivation and emotional energy to deal with their self-care needs (Anderson & Andberg, 1979). A relationship between stress and pressure sore formation has been hypothesized based on the potentially deleterious effect of cortisol, the primary glucocorticoid secreted with stress, on mechanical properties of the skin. Braden (1990) explored this link in a prospective study of 26 elderly, pressure sore–free, nursing home residents during the first 5 weeks following their admission. When other causes of excessive cortisol secretion were controlled, either statistically or through exclusion criteria, significantly higher levels of serum cortisol were found to be exhibited by those elderly nursing home residents who developed a pressure sore than by those who did not.

Evidence that smoking may contribute to pressure sore formation is beginning to accumulate. Certainly the effect of smoking on wound healing is supported in animal model studies (Mosley, Finseth, & Goody 1978). Some investigators reported that cigarette smoking was significantly correlated with pressure sores in a group of spinal cord–injured patients, and that the incidence and extent of existing sores were greater in those patients with higher pack-year histories (Lamid & Ghatit, 1983).

Several investigators have demonstrated an association between disease states and pressure sore formation. In a prospective study of 78 at-risk paitents conducted by Allman (1986), fractures emerged as a significant predictor of pressure sore formation. Berlowitz and Wilking (1989) identified diabetes and cerebrovascular accident (CVA) as significant factors in a pro-spective study of chronic care patients. In a retrospective study of 131 spinal cord–injury patients, Hassard (1975) found a significant association between heterotopic ossification and pressure sore development. With the possible exception of diabetes, these conditions lead to immobility and probably do not represent independent risk factors.

RISK ASSESSMENT

Prevention of pressure sores is dependent on the clinician's ability to estimate the degree to which the patient is at risk and to intervene appropriately. Screening tests facilitate prevention by formalizing estimates of risk and discriminating those who are at risk for developing pressure sores from among the many who are not, thus allowing for judicious allocation of resources. Rating scales are the most common screening tools used by nurses to identify patients at risk for pressure sore. Rating scales have the advantage of being low cost and noninvasive, but a critical evaluation of their reliability and predictive validity is necessary before implementation in a clinical set-ting. Some data concerning the three most commonly used rating scales are available, but further research regarding performance of these scales in various populations is needed (Jahnigan, 1989).

The commonly accepted measures of predictive validity for screening tests are sensitivity, specificity, predictive value of positive results (PVP), and predictive value of negative results (PVN) (Larson, 1986; Lilienfeld & Lilien-feld, 1980). Sensitivity and specificity are somewhat better gauges of predic-tive validity because these figures are less susceptible to the influence of prevalence rates among different patient populations (Wasson, Sox, Neff, & Goldman 1985). Sensitivity measures, among all subjects who developed a pressure sore (PS+), the proportion of those who were identified by the screening tool as being at risk. Specificity measures, among all subjects who did not develop a pressure sore (PS–), the proportion of those who were identified by the screening tool as being at low or no risk. Sensitivity and the PVN are both influenced by the number of false negatives, whereas the number of false positives influences specificity and the PVP.

The ideal screening test would be 100% sensitive and 100% specific, but this is rarely achieved—even by tests intended for diagnosis rather than screening. This ideal is still less likely to be achieved when the condition is preventable. These performance estimates are, nevertheless, essential to de-termining appropriate usage in clinical decision making. Several instruments designed to predict the risk of pressure sores have been reported in the literature (Bergstrom, Braden, Laguzza, & Holman, 1987; Gosnell, 1973; Norton, McLaren, & Exton-Smith, 1962). These instruments use summative rating scales based on contributing factors and specify critical scores for identifying patients at risk.

The Norton scale has been studied extensively (Goldstone & Goldstone, 1982; Goldstone & Roberts, 1980; Lincoln, Roberts, Maddox, Levine, & Patterson, 1986). This tool consists of five parameters: physical condition, mental state, activity, mobility, and incontinence, each rated from 1 to 4, with one or two word descriptors for each rating. Scores range from 5 to 20, with a score of 14 indicating the "onset of risk" and a score of 12 or below indicating a high risk for pressure sore formation.

In a study of 59 orthopedic patients older than age 60, Goldstone and Roberts (1979) found that 32 patients received scores below 14, and 12 of these patients developed pressure sores more serious than erythema. A sensitivity of 92%, a specificity of 57%, a PVP of 37.5%, and a PVN of 96% can be calculated from these data. These investigators trained a team of nurses to rate the patients but did not report interrater reliability.

Goldstone and Goldstone (1982) replicated this study using only one rater and reported that among 40 patients older than age 60 admitted to an orthopedic ward, 30 were judged to be at risk, and 16 of these at-risk patients developed pressure lesions. This resulted in a sensitivity of 89%, a specificity of 36%, a PVP of 53%, and a PVN of 80%. Goldstone and Goldstone did not define pressure lesions, but likely included skin erythema that may account for the improved prediction.

Lincoln et al. (1986) also conducted an evaluation of the Norton scale. In testing for interrater reliability, these investigators found a low percent agreement among registered nurse (RN) raters (39.7%) and disagreement among experts concerning face validity. In their study of 50 patients, the two patients judged to be at risk did not develop a pressure sore, whereas five patients judged at no risk did develop a pressure sore. This resulted in a sensitivity of 0%, a specificity of 94%, a PVP of 0%, and a PVN of 85%.

A second tool for assessing patient risk for pressure sore development was reported in 1973 by Gosnell. It consists of five parameters or subscales: mental status, continence, mobility, activity, and nutrition. Two- or three-sentence descriptive statements were provided for each rating on each subscale. Gosnell assessed several additional variables such as temperature, blood pressure, skin tone, and sensation, but these additional variables were not weighted. The range of possible scores was from 5 to 20 and a score < 16 was considered indicative of risk. In a later revision (Gosnell, 1989), the scoring has been reversed (high scores denote high risk) and testing to determine cutoff score is reported to be in progress.

Gosnell (1973) validated her instrument in a study of 30 patients older than age 65 admitted to extended care facilities. On admission, 21 patients received scroes of 16 or above, and 9 patients received scores below 16. At the conclusion of the study, 4 patients had experienced skin breakdown, 2 with admission scores of 16 or better and 2 with scores below 16. In this limited sample of elderly patients, then, the Gosnell scale demonstrated a sensitivity of 50%, specificity of 73%, a PVP of 22%, and a PVN of 90%. Subsequent testing demonstrated a percent agreement of 90 when used by RNs (Gosnell, 1988).

A third instrument, the Braden scale (Bergstrom, Braden, Laguzza, & Holman, 1987; Bergstrom, Demuth, & Braden, 1987; Braden & Bergstrom, 1989) has also been developed to predict the risk for pressure sore development. The Braden scale is composed of six subscales reflecting sensory perception, skin moisture, activity, mobility, nutritional intake, and friction and shear. All subscales are rated from 1 to 4, with the exception of the friction and shear subscale, which is rated from 1 to 3. Each rating is accompanied by a description of criteria for rating. Potential scores range from 4 to 23.

Two studies of reliability have been carried out in two extended care facilities (Bergstrom, Braden, Laguzza, & Holman, 1987). The purpose of the first study was to estimate interrater reliability between a graduate student research asistant and RNs trained in the use of the tool. The Pearson product moment correlation among 86 pairs of observation scores was $r = .99$ ($p < .001$), and the percent agreement was 88%. In no case was the total score assigned by the two raters more than 1 point different. The purpose of the second study was to determine the reliability of the scale when used by licensed practical nurses and nurse aides who were not trained in the use of the tool. Pearson product moment correlations among 53 pairs of scores ranged from $r = .83$ to $r = .87$ ($p < .001$), but percent agreement ranged from 11% to 19%.

Studies of predictive validity have been conducted using patient populations admitted to a general nursing unit, a critical care step-down unit and an adult intensive care unit, all in tertiary care settings. In the first two studies ($n = 99$, $n = 100$), the tool demonstrated 100% sensitivity and PNP in both groups, and 90% and 64% specificity, respectively, at a cutoff score of 16 (Bergstrom, Braden, Laguzza, & Holman, 1987). The PVP was only 50% and 19%, however. In the third study of 60 subjects admitted to an adult intensive care unit (Bergstrom, Demuth, & Braden, 1987), the scale demonstrated a sensitivity of 83%, a specificity of 64%, a PVP of 61%, and a PVN of 85% at a critical cutoff score of 16 or below.

The differences in predictive validity when using the tool in different settings probably occur as a result of variances in subject age, caregiver-patient ratios, and severity of illness. Although a score of 16 or below seems to be a more appropriate predictor for an adult-hospitalized population, a higher cutoff score may be necessary in nursing homes where age, severity of illness, and sparse staffing patterns may add to risk of pressure sore formation.

Whatever the setting, risk assessment should be repeated 24 to 48 hours following admission and repeated when the patients condition changes. It is wise to specify an interval for reassessment in the nursing protocols that reflects the rapidity with which patients condition changes in that setting (e.g., daily in intensive care units, weekly in extended care facilities, and monthly in most nursing homes). None of these tools require more than 30 seconds to complete when the nurse is familiar with the patient, and frequent assessment should not be burdensome.

PREVENTION

Methodological difficulties make clinical trials of multivariate prevention protocols difficult, and none has been reported. Preventive protocols must, therefore, be formulated from research related to individual etiological factors and from collective clinical wisdom. The first priority when a patient is determined to be at risk for pressure sore development is to reduce the intensity and duration of pressure to which the skin may be subjected. Issues related to managing interface pressure are discussed in another section of this chapter, but a supersoft surface in combination with a turning schedule that substitutes a 30-degree turn for the usual 90-degree turn for lateral positioning is the backbone of a preventive protocol (Seiler & Stahelin, 1985). In addition, the head of the bed should not be raised higher than 30 degrees to avoid exposure to excessive pressure and shear in the sacral area.

Other preventive interventions should be tailored to the individual risk factors exhibited by the patient. Aggressive nutritional repletion and support should be undertaken, and vitamin supplementation may be warranted. When moisture is a problem, measures should be taken to control the source and protect the skin. The use of barrier creams, and fecal or urinary incontinence devices may be indicated, though a urinary catheter should be used only when absolutely necessary. The skin should be kept clean and dry, and feces should be kept away from the skin as much as possible. When diarrhea is also a problem, control should be aggressively pursued. Diarrhea should never be considered an inevitable consequence of tube feedings, and appropriate adjustments in volume, osmolality, or fiber content of the tube feedings should be undertaken.

MANAGEMENT

When health care providers take on the challenge of managing pressure sores, they must address two distinct issues. First, they must carefully assess each patient and identify factors that have contributed to the pressure sore and institute care that will minimize or alleviate these factors. Second, they must assess each pressure sore and develop a wound care protocol that addresses the characteristics and needs of the pressure sore. Although standardized procedures for managing pressure sores help maintain consistency of care, going a step further and individualizing this procedure to patient and pressure sore will increase the likelihood of a positive outcome. Tailoring care to both patient and pressure sore will also contain costs through judicious use of supplies and time.

Contributing Factors

While it is universally accepted that pressure at the skin or support surface interface is a prime factor in the etiology of pressure sores, what is not clear is the most effective way of managing this pressure. For example, does pressure need to be relieved completely before a pressure sore will heal, or does interface pressure only need to be decreased to promote healing? If decreasing interface pressure is a viable alternative, how far must it be decreased? Does the extent to which interface pressure must be reduced before healing occurs depend on the stage and size of the pressure sore, the length of time the pressure is sustained, or the general condition of the patient? These are only a few of the questions that health care providers confront when they develop a plan of care. Although there are many who would advise on these questions, there is a paucity of scientifically sound research to support the advice.

The value of 32 mm Hg is widely promoted as the gold standard for evaluating the clinical efficacy of pressure-reducing and -relieving devices. There are several factors, however, that should be considered when using this value to make clinical decisions. First, 32 mm Hg was the value recorded for arteriolar capillary pressure in human finger nailbeds (Landis, 1930). Second, the link between 32 mm Hg and the etiology of pressure sores is based on an assumption that when external pressures exceeded this value, complete tissue ischemia and ultimate necrosis would result (Kosiak, 1959).

Subsequent studies of the relationship between cutaneous perfusion and necrosis challenge this assumption (Bennett et al., 1979; Daniel et al., 1981; Holstein, Nielsen, & Barras, 1979; Seiler & Staehelin, 1979). Third, pressures measured at the interface of muscle and bone—the site where deep pressure sores originate—may be five times greater than pressures between the skin and support surface (Le et al., 1984). Finally interface pressure can vary with the age and general condition of the subjects (Clark & Rowland, 1989) and the recording device and protocol (Cochran, 1985; Krouskop & Garber, 1989; Reger et al., 1988).

In addition to the problems associated with trying to establish a specific therapeutic level for interface pressure, to date, there is only one randomized, controlled clinical trail that has examined the therapeutic effects of different pressure-reducing devices (Allman et al., 1987). Sixty-five adult patients with pressures sores hospitalized in an acute care setting were randomly assigned to an air-fluidized bed or an alternating air-mattress covered with a foam pad. The average length of treatment was 13 days. Although the pressure sores of patients nursed on an air-fluidized bed were more likely to improve than the pressure sores of patients nursed on an alternating air mattress, there was no significant difference between the two groups in the number of pressure sores that healed or the number of pressure sores that showed a 50% decrease in total surface area. Furthermore, there was no significant difference between the two groups in the number of patients who developed new skin breakdown while on the pressure-reducing devices. Other investigators have also reported new skin breakdown in patients treated on pressure-reducing devices (Jackson et al., 1988; Parish & Witkowski, 1980).

The role of pressure-reducing devices in long-term care settings is also poorly studied. A retrospective review of the medical records of 95 nursing home patients with severe pressure sores treated on an air-fluidized bed found that much time was required to even achieve a 50% decrease in pressure sore size (Bennett, Bellantoni, & Ouslander, 1989). During the first 30 days of treatment, only two small ulcers (< 2 cm^2) healed, and no ulcer achieved at least a 50% reduction in size. Overall, only 11 ulcers healed, and 42 of 95 decreased at least 50% in size. The median treatment period was 79 days. Because there was no control group, we can conclude nothing about the role the pressure-reducing device played in healing these pressure sores. Although they provide limited information about the role of pressure-reducing devices in managing pressure sores, these studies reiterate what others have noted (Dewis, Caplan, & Pache, 1968): Pressure sores heal slowly. Given the high costs associated with some pressure-reducing devices, prolonged healing rates can become a major financial constraint.

Although there is some evidence that patients with multiple, large pressure sores heal faster when nursed on "high-tech" beds, more research is needed before these devices become standard treatment for all patients. Controlled, randomized clinical trials to ascertain the extent to which pressure-reducing devices promote healing and to identify characteristics of both patients and devices that independently or together effect healing are indicated. Meanwhile, many patients with superficial pressure sores may be managed initially with less expensive foam and static air-mattress overlays (Allman, 1989) coupled with frequent changes in position, positioning techniques that reduce interface pressure over bony prominences (Garber, Campion, & Krouskop, 1982; Seiler & Stehelin, 1985), and positioning aides to lift pressure sores off support surfaces (Stewart & Wharton, 1976). Using the frequency of turning as a criteria for determining the density of foam overlays (Krouskop & Garber, 1987) and routinely monitoring devices for evidence of "bottoming out" will also enhance the effectiveness of foam and air-mattress overlays.

Regardless of the device used, caregivers must institute a scheduled, systematic program of skin assessment. Caregivers must also be taught how to recognize signs of wound healing as well as early signs warning that previously healthy skin is in danger of breaking down. Areas of erythema that do not resolve when pressure is relieved should be noted and the plan for managing pressure adjusted.

While instituting measures to decrease interface pressure is necessary to facilitate the healing of pressure sores, it is not sufficient. In those cases in which friction and shear, inadequate nutrition, moisture, and acute or chronic medical conditions have contributed to the etiology of the pressure sore, these factors must also be addressed.

WOUND CARE
Dressings

Although there is little research to help clinicians determine the best method of managing pressure, research on the topical management of pressure sores is growing steadily. In particular, the use of occlusive dressings has elicited increasing interest and research. Occlusive dressings are made of materials that keep tissues hydrated. In both animal and human models, when compared with wounds dressed with wet to dry gauze or exposed to air, wounds dressed with occlusive dressings reepithelialized significantly faster and demonstrated significantly greater rates of collagen synthesis (Alvarez, Mertz, & Eaglstein, 1983; Geronemus & Robins, 1982; Hinman & Maibach, 1963; Leipziger et al., 1985; Rovee et al., 1972; Winter, 1962; Winter & Scales, 1963). This phenomenon of enhanced epithelial migration is similar to that seen under intact blisters (Krawczyki, 1971). Although the enhanced rate of healing seen under occlusive dressings may be linked to the moist environment they provide, there is also evidence that by promoting the growth of fibroblasts, factors within the fluid contained over the wound may also facilitate healing (Alper, Tibbetts, & Sarazen, 1985).

A variety of occlusive dressings including polyurethane films, hydrocolloids, hydrogels, and foams are available, and several authors (Alvarez, 1988; Eaglstein, 1985; Eaglstein, Mertz, & Falanga, 1987) have written comprehensive articles discussing their characteristics and use. As the interest in moist wound healing grows, manufacturers are modifying the current generation of occlusive dressings. Unlike the present polyurethane films, "second-generation" film dressings can absorb and contain wound fluid without leaking (Carr, Lalagos, & Upman, 1989)—a feature that could protect healthy skin on the edge of pressure sores from macerating. Responding to studies tentatively linking debris found in intracellular vesicles and macrophages with residue from dressing materials (Reuterving et al., 1989), manufacturers have begun promoting non–gel-forming hydrocolloid dressings that are less likely to leave residue in the wound bed. Clinical studies of these second-generation dressings are limited (Watts & Shipes, 1988), and it is unclear where they will fit in the arena of occlusive dressings.

Although many support using occlusive dressings to treat noninfected, superficial pressure sores, occlusive dressings are not without their problems. Several investigators (Alvarez et al., 1983; Leipziger et al., 1985; Zitelli, 1984) have noted stripping of newly formed epidermis with both polyurethane film and hydrocolloid dressings, although this reinjury has been more common with the polyurethane films. A concern that was voiced with the early research on occlusive dressings (Hinman & Maibach, 1963) and continues to be addressed today (Alvarez, 1988) is infection. In addition to facilitating reepithelialization and collagen synthesis, the moisture under an occlusive dressing provides an environment that supports growth of resident and pathogenic bacteria (Friedman & Su, 1984; Gilchrist & Ree, 1989; Katz, McGinley, & Leyden, 1986; Mertz & Eaglstein, 1984; Varghese et al., 1986).

Despite the fact that bacteria are found under these dressings, investigators who have treated chronic wounds with occlusive dressings (Alm et al., 1989; Friedman & Su, 1984; Gilchrist & Reed, 1989; Gorse & Messner, 1987; Mulder, Albert, & Grimwood, 1985; Sebern, 1986; Yarkony et al., 1984) report few episodes of wound infection. Of the 195 chronic wounds these investigators treated, only 4 became infected (Alper et al., 1983; Oleske et al., 1986). In one case, the patient was receiving an average of 168 mg of hydrocortisone daily (Oleske et al., 1986). In the case of the three other chronic wounds, cellulitis developed and resolved with antibiotic therapy (Alper et al., 1983). Finally, in this series of studies, several investigators noted healing occurred in the presence of known colonization (Alper et al., 1983; Friedman & Su, 1984; Gilchrist & Reed, 1989).

Several factors may help understand the low incidence of infection reported with occlusive dressings. First, viable neutrophils and significantly increased lysozyme levels have been found in the wound fluid under occlusive dressings (Buchan et al., 1980–1981; Varghese et al., 1986). This suggests that the same environment that supports healing and the growth of bacteria also supports the body's natural defenses against bacterial invasion. Second, although the wounds may be colonized, there is evidence that it is its not the presence of bacteria, but the intensity of exposure and pathogenicity of the bacteria that delays or inhibits healing. In a study examining the clinical efficacy of gentamicin in treating pressure sores, only those pressure sores with bacterial counts that fell below 1,000,000/ml healed (Bendy et al., 1965). Similar relationships between quantitative bacterial counts from tissue biopsies and spontaneous healing of chronic wounds and successful skin grafts have been reported (Robson et al., 1968). In this work, the critical value was 100,000 per gram. Finally, the low incidence of infection in wounds dressed with occlusive dressings may also be attributed to the careful screening of patients—a lesson that should be carried over into clinical practice. Investigators who have used these dressings to treat chronic wounds usually limit the wounds they select to those in which there are no clinical signs or symptoms of infection, or in which infection has been treated successfully.

An issue related to but separate from supporting the growth of bacteria that have already colonized a pressure sore is that of protecting wounds from invading bacteria. There is evidence that occlusive dressings may be an effective barrier against bacteria (Mertz, Marshall, & Eaglstein, 1985)—a property to consider when selecting a dressing for patients who are incontinent.

Debridement

Pressure sores containing necrotic tissue will not heal and need to be debrided. The technique that is selected will depend on the type and amount of necrotic tissue present and the resources that are available. Surgical debridement is a quick method of excising eschar and loose, obviously nonviable fibrinous tissue. Serial surgical debridement is often required to clean a pressure sore. Transient bacteremia has been reported during surgical debridement of pressure sores (Glenchur, Patel, & Pathmarajah, 1981), prompting several authors to suggest antibiotic coverage during debridement especially in patients with large and deep pressure sores or compromised resistance to infection (Glenchur et al., 1981) or patients with valvular heart disease (Allman, 1989) or artificial joints.

Between episodes of surgical debridement, pressure sores are often packed with wet coarse gauze that is allowed to dry before removing. Although this technique entraps necrotic debris and wound exudate, there are several drawbacks. In addition to causing pain, removing gauze that has adhered to the pressure sore nonselectively debrides granulation and epithelial tissue as well as necrotic debris. Allowing gauze dressing to dry out also subjects regenerating tissue to further injury from desiccation.

Topical enzyme preparations can also be used to debride necrotic tissue. Because some of these preparations are inactivated by other wound care products, are pH dependent, or can produce side effects (Boxer et al., 1969; Cohen, 1985; Lee & Ambrus, 1975; Varma, Bugatch, & Germon, 1973), clinicians must read product information and directions carefully. Topical enzymes need to be applied at least daily and work slowly.

Hydrophillic dressings like dextranomer and those made from alginates are used to absorb exudate, necrotic debris, and bacteria away from the surface of pressure sores. In the process, the dressing material next to the pressure sores forms a gel that keeps the wound moist (Engdahl, 1980; Freeman, Carwell, & McCraw, 1981; Jeter & Tintle, 1990; Thomas, 1985). Hydrophillic dressings are designed for wounds with moderate to heavy exudate. If there is not enough moisture in the wound, these dressing materials can be difficult to remove. In the case of the calcium alginate fiber dressing, histological examination revealed intact fibers with subsequent foreign body reaction 14 days postwounding (Barnett & Varley, 1987). Cases of dextranomer dressings material plugging sinus tracts in wounds and eliciting serious infections have also been reported (Freeman, Carwell, & McCraw, 1981).

Irrigating a pressure sore is yet another method of removing necrotic tissue and debris. Irrigation pressures of 8 pounds per square inch (psi) or higher (high-pressure irrigation) can remove small particulate matter and bacteria from wounds (Rodeheaver et al., 1975). A ½-inch, 19-gauge needle attached to a 35-ml syringe can deliver fluid to the surface of a pressure sore at 8 psi (Wheeler et al., 1976). Because of the potential for inhibiting tissue defenses, however, it is recommended that high-pressure irrigation be limited to heavily contaminated wounds (Wheeler et al., 1976). Furthermore, because of its nonselective action, irrigation may wash out granulation tissue (Goode & Allman, 1989).

Whirlpool treatments have long been an adjunct to surgical and enzymatic debridement (Doughty, 1988; Longe, 1986). Although the additional costs of mobilizing and transporting patients and disinfecting equipment coupled with concern about dehydrating normal skin (Braden & Bryant, 1990) may speak against long-term use of Hubbard tanks, they may still be indicated in patients with multiple, extensive, necrotic pressure sores. In these instances, this type of therapy may decrease the time required for debridement, cleansing, and dressing changes. Because of similarities between irrigation and whirlpool, the possibility of the later washing out granulation tissue also supports limiting its use to necrotic wounds.

Infection

When a pressure sore is assessed and infection is identified as a real or potential problem, topical antiseptics may be ordered. Using tissue cultures and animal models, investigators (Breenan & Leaper, 1985; Brennan, Foster, & Leaper, 1986; Kozol, Gillies, & Elgebaly, 1988; Niedner & Schopf, 1986; Van Den Broek, Buys, & Furth, 1982) have studied the effects of a variety of topical antiseptics on the microenvironment of wounds. Although the extent to which some of these agents adversely affect microcirculation, fibroblasts, granulocytes, monocytes, and endothelial cells depends on the concentration, overall, the results suggest a fine balance between bacteriocidal and cytotoxic activities that should be considered when antispectics are used (Brennan & Leaper, 1985). Investigators (Lineaweaver et al., 1984) studied the effects of serial dilutions of 1% povidone-iodine, 0.25% acetic acid, 3% hydrogen peroxide, and 0.5% sodium hypochlorite on the viability of cultured human fibroblasts and *Staphylococcus aureus* as well as the rate at which wounds reepithelialized. At concentrations of 0.001% and 0.005%, 1% povidone-iodine and 0.5% sodium hypochlorite, respectively, were noncytoxic while retaining their bacteriocidal activity. At all dilutions studied, the fibroblast toxicity of 3% hydrogen peroxide and 0.25% acetic acid exceeded bacterial toxicity. Reepithelialization was delayed in wounds irrigated with 1% povidone-iodine, 0.25% acetic acid, and 0.5% sodium hypochlorite.

The extent to which results of studies conducted in vitro or with animal models can be reproduced in studies of pressure sores is uncertain. Quantitative bacterial counts have been used to evaluate treatment response in chronic pressure sores treated at random with silver sulfadiazine cream, povidone-iodine (Betadine) solution, or normal saline (Kucan et al., 1981). Although over time, the number of pressure sores with bacterial counts $< 10^5$ was greater for sores treated with silver sulfadiazine cream, only the difference in bacterial counts between pressure sores treated with silver sulfadiazine cream and povidone-iodine was significant.

In addition to considering the local effects of topical antispetics, clinicians must also be alert to potential systemic effects. Case studies that link iodide toxicity (Aronoff et al., 1980; D'Auria, Lipson, & Garfield, 1990; Dela Cruz et al., 1987) and deafness (Johnson, 1988; Kelly, Nilo, & Berggren, 1969) to applying povidone-iodine and neomycin, respectively, to pressure sores suggest clinicians think carefully when prescribing topical antiseptics. Although some authors (Brennan et al., 1986; Parish & Witkowski 1989) suggest using certain topical antispetics early and briefly to debride and reduce bacterial counts in grossly necrotic or infected pressure sores, the practice of using topical antiseptics in clean, granulating pressure sores is becoming more difficult to support (Kozol, Gillies, & Elgebaly, 1988; Lineaweaver et al., 1985; Rodeheaver et al., 1982).

The use of topical antibiotics in the treatment of pressure sores has been widely discouraged for several reasons—the most prominent being the lack of proven efficacy (Bendy, 1964; Morgan, 1975; Noble, 1971). Topical antibiotics have not been shown to reduce the quantitative bacterial counts in pressure sores or to penetrate into the tissues. Indeed, there is evidence (Morgan, 1975) that topical antibiotics may promote the growth of resistant organisms. Furthermore, topical gentamicin, neosporin, and bacitracin may lead to allergic skin reactions (Linneaweaver et al., 1985; Longe 1986). Metronidazole typifies the status of topical antibiotics. Although the Food and Drug Administration has approved metronidazole topical therapy (Pierleoni, 1984), data from randomized, double-blind, clinical trials are not available. Studies of this nature are needed to establish firmly the role of topical antibiotics in the management of pressure sores.

Systemic antibiotics are reserved for treating the infectious complications of pressure sores. The most common clinical uses are associated with the most serious complications—sepsis and osteomyelitis. Cellulitis, abscesses, and foul-smelling, draining pressure sores that deteriorate despite good local therapy also indicate the need for systemic antibiotics. This last category of pressure sores also warrants a careful search for osteomyelitis (Lewis et al., 1988; Shea, 1975; Sugarman et al., 1983).

In addition to when to use systemic antibiotics, there is the question of what antibiotic to use. Cefazolin, cephalothin, and penicillin do not penetrate into pressure sores and are not clinically effective in combination with aminoglycosides (Chow, 1977). Clindamycin and aminoglycosides, however, do penetrate necrotic tissue (Berger et al., 1978, 1981). Although some clinicians recommend various newer antibiotics, such as third-generation cephalosporins, semisynthetic penicillins, monobactams, and quinolones (Jones, 1990; Longe, 1986; Yoshikawa, 1989), none of these antibiotics has been studied systematically in pressure sores or necrotic tissues.

The polymicrobial nature of pressure sores makes choosing antibiotics difficult. Poorly healing sores are, more likely to have bacteria from the Proteus, Pseudomonas, and Bacteroides families present (Daltrey, 1981). This suggests systemic aminoglycosides as the drug of choice in these wounds. In other poorly healing pressure sores where staphylococcus or enterococcus have been cultured, clinicians frequently recommend vancomycin.

The time course for systemic antibiotic therapy varies with the complication being treated. If there is only local soft-tissue infection, 7 to 10 days is commonly recommended. If muscle and deep fascia are infected or sepsis is found, 14 to 21 days is the usual regimen, with an investigation into possible systemic or cardiac complications. Joint infections and osteomyelitis require 6 weeks of systemic antibiotics and usually a surgical procedure on the affected bone or joint (Agris & Spira, 1979; Sugerman et al., 1983).

Investigators continue seeking ways to facilitate healing of pressure sores. A steadily growing number of topical agents including growth factors (Barbul et al., 1988; Knighton et al., 1990) and drugs that increase local circulation to the wound (Janssen et al., 1989) as well as various types of electrical stimulation (Biedebach, 1989) have been studied. Although we cannot be certain whether these treatments and others that follow will become part of routine care of pressure sores, we can be certain that practitioners will have many more options from which to develop a plan of care. As their options increase, so does the challenge to practitioners. We must examine the scientific merit of research, question the clinical significance findings, consider the feasibility of delivering and monitoring care, and calculate cost-benefit ratios. Informed choices are the cornerstone of clinically and cost-effective treatment.

REFERENCES

Agris, J., & M. Spira. (1979). Pressure ulcers: Prevention and treatment. *CIBA Clinical Symposia, 31,* 2–32.

Allman, R. M. (1989a). Epidemiology of pressure sores in different populations. *Decubitus, 2,* 30–33.

Allman, R. M. (1989b). Pressure ulcers among the elderly. *New England Journal of Medicine, 320,* 850–853.

Allman, R. M., Laprade, C. A., Noel, L., et al. 1986. Pressure sores among hospitalized patients. *Annals of Internal Medicine, 105,* 337–342.

Allman, R. M., Walker, J. M., Hart, M. K., Laprade, C. A., Noel, L., & Smith, C. R. (1987). Air-fluidized beds or conventional therapy for pressure sores. *Annals of Internal Medicine, 107,* 641–648.

Alm, A., Hornmark, A., Fall, P., et al. (1989). Care of pressure sores: A controlled study of the use of a hydrocolloid dressing compared with wet saline gauze compresses. *ACTA Dermato-Venereologica (Stockh), 149* (Suppl.), 3–10.

Alper, J. C., Welch, E. A., Ginsberg, M., Bogaars, T., & Maguire, P. (1983). Moist wound healing under a vapor permeable membrane. *Journal of the American Academy of Dermatology, 8,* 347–353.

Alper, J. C., Tibbetts, L. L., and Sarazen, A. A. (1985). The in vitro response of fibroblasts to the fluid that accumulates under a vapor-permeable membrane. *Journal of Investigative Dermatology, 84,* 513–515.

Altrescu, V. (1989). The financial costs of inpatient pressure ulcers to an acute care facility. *Decubitus, 2,* 14–23.

Alvarez, O. (1988). Moist environment for healing: Matching the dressing to the wound. *Ostomy/Wound Management, 21,* 64–83.

Alvarez, P. M., Mertz, O. M., & Eaglstein, W. H. (1983). The effect of occlusive dressings on collagen synthesis and re-epithelialization in superficial wounds. *Journal of Surgical Research, 35,* 142–148.

Andersen, K. E., & Kvorning, S. A. (1982). Aspects of the decubitus ulcer. *International Journal of Dermatology, 21,* 265–270.

Anderson, T. P., & Andberg, M. M. (1979). Psychosocial factors associated with pressure sores. *Archives of Physical Medicine and Rehabilitation, 60,* 341–346.

Aronoff, G. R., Friedman, S. J., Doedens, D. J., & Lavelle, K. J. (1980). Increased serum iodide concentration from iodine absorption through wounds treated topically with povidone-iodine. *American Journal of the Medical Sciences, 279,* 173–176.

Artique, R. S., & Hyman, W. A. (1979). The effect of myoglobin on the oxygen concentration in skeletal muscle subjected to ischemia. *Annals of Biomedical Engineering, 4,* 128–137.

Barbenel, J. C., Jordan, M. M., & Nicol, S. M. (1977). Incidence of pressure-sores in the greater Glasgow health board area. *Lancet, 2,* 548–550.

Barbul, A., Pines, E., Caldwell, M., & Hunt, T. K. (Eds.). (1988). *Growth factors and other aspects of wound healing: Biological and clinical implications.* New York: Liss.

Barnett, S. E., & Varley, S. J. (1987). The effects of calciumalginate on wound healing. *Annals of the Royal College of Surgeons of England, 69,* 153–155.

Bendy R. H., Jr., Nuccio, P. A., Wolfe, E., et al. (1965). Relationship of quantitative wound bacterial counts to healing of decubiti: Effect of topical gentamicin. *Antimicrobial Agents Chemotherapy, 4,* 147–155.

Bennett, L., Kavner, D., Lee, B. Y., Trainor, F. S., & Lewis, J. M. (1984). Skin stress and blood flow in sitting paraplegic patients. *Archives of Physical Medicine and Rehabilitation, 65,* 186–190.

Bennett, L., Kavner, D., Eng, D., Lee, B. K., & Trainer, F. A. (1979). Shear vs. pressure as causative factors in skin blood flow occlusion. *Archives of Physical Medicine and Rehabilitation, 60,* 309–314.

Bennett, R. G., Bellantoni, M. F., & Ouslander, J. G. (1989). Air-fluidized bed treatment of nursing home patients with pressure sores. *Journal of the American Geriatrics Society 37,* 235–242.

Berger, S. A., Barza, M., Haher, J., et al. (1978). Penetration of clindamycin into decubitus ulcers. *Antimicrobial Agents and Chemotherapy, 14,* 498–499.

Berger, S. A., Barza, M., Haher, J., et al. (1981). Penetration of antibiotics in decubitus ulcers. *Journal of Antimicrobial Chemotherapy, 7,* 193–195.

Bergstrom, N., & Braden, B. J. (1990). Nutritional status during the development and resolution of pressure sores. *Key aspects of recovery: Improving mobility, rest, and nutrition.* New York: Springer.

Bergstrom, N., Braden, B., Laguzza, A., & Holman, A. (1987). The Braden Scale for predicting pressure sore risk. *Nursing research, 36,* 205–210.

Bergstrom, N., Demuth, P. J., & Braden, B. (1987). A clinical trial of the Braden scale for predicting pressure sore risk. *Nursing Clinics of North America, 22,* 417–418.

Berlowitz, D. R., & Wilking, S. V. (1989). Risk factors for pressure sores: A comparison of cross-sectional and cohort-derived data. *Journal of the American Geriatrics Society, 37,* 1043–1050.

Biedebach, M. C. (1989). Accelerated healing of skin ulcers by electrical stimulation and the intracellular physiological mechanisms involved. *International Journal of Acupuncture & Electrotherapeutic Res., 14,* 43–60.

Boxer, A. M., Getterman, N., Bernstein, H., & Mandl, I. (1969). Debridement of dermal ulcers and decubiti with collagenase. *Geriatrics, 24,* 75–86.

Braden, B. J. (1990). Emotional stress and pressure sore formation among the elderly recently relocated to a nursing home. *Key aspects of recovery: Improving mobility, rest, and nutrition.* New York: Springer.

Braden, B. J., & Bergstrom, N. (1987). A conceptual schema for the study of etiological factors in pressure sore formation. *Rehabilitation Nursing, 12,* 8–16.

Braden, B. J., & Bryant, R. (1990). Innovations to prevent and treat pressure ulcers. *Geriatric Nursing, 11,* 182–186.

Brandeis, G. H., Morris, J. N., Nash, D. J., & Lipsitz, L.A. (1990). The epidemiology and natural history of pressure ulcers in elderly nursing home residents. *Journal of the American Medical Association, 264,* 2905–2909.

Brennan, S. S., & Leaper, D. J. (1985). The effect of antiseptics on the healing wound: A study using the rabbit ear chamber. *British Journal of Surgery, 72,* 780–782.

Brennan, S. S., Foster, M. E., & Leaper, D. J. (1986). Antiseptic toxicity in wounds healing by secondary intention. *Journal of Hospital Infection, 8,* 263–267.

Buchan, I. A., Andrews, J. K., Lang, S. M., Boorman, J. G., Kemble, J. V. H., & Lamberty, G. H. (1980–1981). Clinical and laboratory investigation of the composition and properties of human skin wound exudate under semi-permeable dressings. *Burns, 7,* 326–334.

Burnakis, T. G. (1989). Topical metronidazole for decubitus ulcers. *Hospital Pharmacy, 24,* 961–962.

Carr, R. D., Lalagos, D. E., & Upman, P. J. (1989). Comparative study of occlusive wound dressings on full thickness wounds in domestic pigs. *Wounds, 1,* 53–61.

Chow, A. W., Galpin, J. E., & Guze, L. B. (1977). Clindamycin for treatment of sepsis caused by decubitus ulcers. *Journal of Infectious Diseases, 135* (Suppl.), S65–68.

Clark, M., & Rowland, L. B. (1989). Preventing pressure sores: Matching patient and mattress using interface pressure measurements. *Decubitus, 2,* 34–35, 38–39.

Cochran, G. V. B. (1985). Measurement of pressure and other environmental factors at the patient-cushion interface. In B. Y. Lee (Ed.), *Chronic ulcers of the skin,* (pp. 23–37). New York: McGraw-Hill.

Cohen, M. R. (1985). Topical treatment of pressure sores. *Hospital Pharmacy 20,* 451–457.

D'Auria, J., Lipson, S., & Garfield, J. M., (1990). Fatal iodine toxicity following surgical debridement of a hip wound: Case report. *Journal of Trauma, 30,* 353–355.

Daniel, R. K., Priest, D. L., & Wheatley, D. C. (1981). Etiologic factors in pressure sores: An experimental model. *Archives of Physical Medicine and Rehabilitation, 62,* 492–498.

Daniel, R. K., Priest, D. L., Wheatley, D. C., & Eng, B. (1981). Etiological factors in pressure sores: An experimental model. *Archives of Physical Medicine and Rehabilitation, 62,* 492–498.

Dela Cruz, F., Brown, D. H., Leikin, J. B., Franklin, C., & Hryhorczuk, D. O. (1987). Iodine absorption after topical administration. *Western Journal of Medicine, 146,* 43–45.

Dewis, L. S., Caplan, H. I., & Pache, H. L. (1968). Treatment of decubitus ulcers by use of a water mattress. *Archives of Physical Medicine Rehabilitation 49,* 290–293.

Dinsdale, S. M. (1974). Decubitus ulcers: Role of pressure and friction in causation. *Archives of Physical Medicine and Rehabilitation, 55,* 147–152.

Doughty, D. (1988). Management of pressure sores. *J. Enterostom. Ther., 15,* 40–44.

Eaglstein, W. H., Mertz, P. M., & Falanga, V. (1987). Occlusive dressings. *American Family Physician, 35,* 211–216.

Eaglstein, W. H. (1985). Experiences with biosynthetic dressings. *Journal of the American Academy of Dermatology, 12,* 434–440.

Ek, A. C., & Boman, G. (1982). A descriptive study of pressure sores: The prevalence of pressure sores and the characteristics of patients. *Journal of Advanced Nursing, 7,* 51–57.

Engdahl, E. (1980). Clinical evaluation of Debrisan on pressure sores. *Current Therapeutic Research, 28,* 377–380.

Flam, E. (1987). Optimum skin aeration in pressure sore management [Abstract]. *Proceedings, Annual Conference of England in Medicine and Biology, 29,* 84.

Frantz, R. (1989). Pressure ulcer costs in long term care. *Decubitus, 2,* 56–57.

Freeman, B. G., Carwell, G. R., & McCraw, J. B. (1981). The quantitative study of the use of dextranomer in the management of infected wounds. *Surgery, Gynecology and Obstetrics, 153,* 81–86.

Friedman, S. J., & Su, W. P. D. (1984). Management of leg ulcers with hydrocolloid occlusive dressing. *Archives of Dermatology, 120,* 1329–1336.

Geronemus, R. G., & Robins, P. (1982). The effect of two new dressings on epidermal wound healing. *Journal of Dermatologic Surgery and Oncology, 8,* 850–852.

Gilchrist, B., & Reed, C. (1989). The bacteriology of chronic venous ulcers treated with occlusive hydrocolloid dressings. *British Journal of Dermatology, 121,* 337–344.

Glenchur, H., Patel, B. S., & Pathmarajah, C. (1981). Transient bacteremia associated with debridement of decubitus ulcers. *Military Medicine, 146,* 432–433.

Goldstone, L. A., & Goldstone, J. (1982). The Norton score: An early warning of pressure sores? *Journal of Advanced Nursing, 1,* 419–426.

Goldstone, L. A., & Roberts, B. V. (1980). A preliminary discriminant function analysis of elderly orthopaedic patients who will or will not contract a pressure sore. *International Journal of Nursing Studies, 17,* 17–23.

Gomolin, I. H., & Brandt, J. L. 1983. Topical metronidazole therapy for pressure sores of geriatric patients. *Journal of the American Geriatric Society, 31,* 710–712.

Goode, P. S., & Allman, R. M. (1989). The prevention and management of pressure ulcers. *Medical Clinics of North America, 73,* 1511–1524.

Gorse, G. J., & Messner, R. L. (1987). Improved pressure sore healing with hydrocolloid dressings. *Archives of Dermatology, 123,* 766–771.

Gosnell, D. J. (1973). An assessment tool to identify pressure sores. *Nursing Research, 22,* 55–59.

Gosnell, D. J. 1988. Assessing client risk for pressure sores. In C. F. Waltz & O. L. Strickland (Eds.), *Measuring client outcomes.* New York: Springer.

Gosnell, D. J. 1989. Pressure sore risk assessment: A critique. *Decubitus, 2,* 32–38.

Haeger, K., Lanner, E., & Magnusson, P. (1974). Oral zinc sulphate in the treatment of venous ulcers. *Vasa, 1,* 62.

Hallbook, T., & Lanner, E. (1972). Serum zinc and healing of venous leg ulcers. *Lancet, 2,* 780–782.

Hassard, G. H. (1975). Heterotopic bone formation about the hip and unilateral decubitus ulcer in spinal cord injury. *Archives of Physical and Medical Rehabilitation 56,* 355–358.

Hinman, C. D., & Maibach, H. (1963). Effect of air exposure and occlusion on experimental human skin wounds. *Nature, 200,* 377–378.

Holstein, P., Nielsen, P. E., & Barras, J. P. (1979). Blood flow cessation at external pressure in the skin of normal human limbs. *Microvascular Research, 17,* 71–79.

Hunter, T., & Rajan, K. T. (1972). The role of ascorbic acid in the pathogenesis and treatment of pressure sores. *Paraplegia, 8,* 211–216.

Husain, T. (1953). An experimental study of some pressure effects on tissues, with reference to the bed-sore problem. *Journal of Pathology and Bacteriology, 66,* 347–358.

Irwin, M. I., & Hutchins, B. K. (1976). A conspectus of research on vitamin C requirements in man. *Journal of Nutrition, 106,* 823–879.

Jackson, B. S., Chagares, R., Nee, N., and Freeman, K. (1988). The effects of a therapeutic bed on pressure ulcers: An experimental study. *J. Enterostom. Ther., 15,* 220–226.

Janssen, P. A. J., Janssen, H., Cauwenbergh, G., et al. (1989). Use of topical ketanserin in the treatment of skin ulcers: A double-blind study. *Journal of the American Academy of Dermatology, 21,* 85–90.

Jeter, K. F., & Tintle, T. E. (1990). Early experience with a calcium alginate dressing. *Osmoty/Wound Mangagement, 28,* 75–77, 79–81.

Johnson, C. A. (1988). Hearing loss following the application of topical neomycin. *Journal of Burn Care Rehabilitation, 9,* 162–164.

Jones, S. R. (1990). Infections in frail and vulnerable elderly patients. *American Journal of Medicine, 88* (Suppl. 3c), 3c305–3c335.

Katz, S., McGinley, K., & Leyden, J. J. (1986). Semipermeable occlusive dressings: Effects on growth of pathogenic bacteria and re-epithelialization of superficial wounds. *Archives of Dermatology, 122,* 58–62.

Kelly, D. R., Nilo, E. R., & Berggren, R. B. (1969). Deafness after topical neomycin wound irrigation. *New England Journal of Medicine, 280,* 1338–1339.

Kenney, R. A. (1982). *Physiology of aging: A synopsis.* Chigago: Year Book Medical.

Knighton, D. R., Ciresi, K., Fiegel, V. D., Schumerth, S., Butler, E., & Cerra, F.

(1990). Stimulation of repair in chronic, nonhealing, cutaneous ulcers using platelet-derived wound healing formula. *Surgery, Gynecology and Obstetrics, 170,* 56–60.

Kosiak, M. (1959). Etiology and pathology of ischemic ulcers. *Archives of Physical Medicine and Rehabilitation, 40,* 62–68.

Kozol, R. A., Gillies, C., & Elgebaly, S. A. (1988). Effects of sodium hypochlorite (Dakin's solution) on cells of the wound module. *Archives of Surgery, 123,* 420–423.

Krawczyki, W. S. (1971). A pattern of epidermal cell migration during wound healing. *Journal of Cellular Biology, 49,* 247–263.

Krouskop, T. A. (1983). A synthesis of the factors that contribute to pressure sore formation. *Medical Hypotheses, 11,* 255–267.

Krouskop, T. A. & Garber, S. L. (1987). The role of technology in the prevention of pressure sores. *Ostomy/Wound Management, 16,* 44–45, 48–49, 52–54.

Krouskop, T. A., & Garber, S. L. (1989). Interface pressure confusion. *Decubitus, 2,* 8.

Krouskop, T. A., Noble, P. C., Garber, S. L., Spencer, W. A. 1983. The effectiveness of preventive management in reducing the occurrence of pressure sores. *Journal of Rehabilitation, 20,* 74–83.

Kucan, J. O., Robson, M. C., Heggers, J. P., & Ko, F. (1981). Comparison of silver sulfadiazine, povidone-iodine and physiological saline in the treatment of chronic pressure ulcers. *Journal of the American Geriatric Society, 29,* 232–235.

Lamid, S., & El Ghatit, A. Z. (1983). Smoking, spasticity and pressure sores in spinal cord injured patients. *American Journal of Physical Medicine, 62,* 300–306.

Landis, E. (1930). Studies of capillary blood pressure in human skin. *Heart, 15,* 209–228.

Larsen, B., Holstein, P., & Lassen, N. A. (1979). On the pathogenesis of bedsores. *Scandinavian Journal of Plastic and Reconstructive Surgery, 13,* 347–350.

Larson, E. (1986). Evaluating validity of screening tests. *Nursing Research, 35,* 186–188.

Le, K. M., Madsen, B. L., Barth, P. W., Ksander, G. A., Angell, J. B. & Vistnes, L. M. (1984). An in-depth look at pressure sores using monolithic silicon pressure sensors. *Plastic and Reconstructive Surgery, 74,* 745–754.

Lee, L. K., & Ambrus, J. L. (1975). Collagenase therapy for decubitus ulcers. *Geriatrics, 30,* 91–93, 97–98.

Leipziger, L. S., Glushko, V., DiBernardo, B., et al. (1985). Dermal wound repair: Rold of collagen matrix implants and synthetic polymer dressings. *Journal of the American Academy of Dermatology, 12,* 409–419.

Lewis, V. L., Bailey, M. H., Pulawski, G., et al. (1988). The diagnosis of osteomyelitis in patients with pressure sores. *Plastic and Reconstructive Surgery, 81,* 229–232.

Lilienfeld, A. M., & Lilienfeld, D. E. (1980). *Foundations of epidemiology* (2nd ed.). New York: Oxford University Press.

Lincoln, R., Roberts, R., Maddox, A., Levine, S., Patterson, C. (1986). Use of the Norton pressure sore risk assessment scoring system with elderly patients in acute care. *J. Enterostomal Ther., 13,* 17–23.

Lineaweaver, W., Howard, R, Soucy, D., et al. (1985). Topical antimicrobial toxicity. *Archives of Surgery, 120,* 267–270.

Longe, R. L. (1986). Current concepts in clinical therapeutics: Pressure sores. *Clinical Pharmacy, 5,* 669–681.

Manley, M. T. (1978). Incidence, contributory factors, and costs of pressure sores. *South African Medical Journal, 53,* 217–222.

Mehan, M. (1990). Multisite pressure ulcer prevalence survey. *Decubitus, 3,* 14–17.

Merbitz, C. T., King, R. B., Bleiberg, J., Grip, J. C. (1985). Wheelchair push-ups:

Measuring pressure relief frequency. *Archives of Physical and Medical Rehabilitation, 66,* 433–438.

Mertz, P. M., & Eaglstein, W. H. (1984). The effect of a semiocclusive dressing on the microbial population in superficial wounds. *Archives of Surgery, 119,* 287–289.

Mertz, P. M., Marshall, D. A., & Eaglstein, W. H. (1985). Occlusive wound dressings to prevent bacterial invasion and wound infection. *Journal of the American Academy of Dermatology, 12,* 662–668.

Michocki, R. J., & Lamy, P. P. (1976). The problem of pressure sores in a nursing home population: Statistical data. *Journal of the American Geriatric Society, 24,* 323–328.

Moolten, S. E. (1972). Bedsores in the chronically ill patient. *Archives of Physical and Mental Rehabilitation, 53,* 430–438.

Morgan, J. E. (1975). Topical therapy of decubitus ulcers. *Surgery, Gynecology and Obstetrics, 141,* 945–947.

Mosley, L. H., Finseth, F., & Goody, M. (1978). Nicotine and its effects on wound healing. *Plastic and Reconstructive Surgery,*

Mulder, G. D., Albert, S. F., & Grimwood, R. E. (1985). Clinical evaluation of a new occlusive hydrocolloid dressing. *Cutis, 35,* 396–397, 400.

Newell, P. H., Thornburgh, J. D., & Fleming, W. C. (1970). The management of pressure and other external factors in the prevention of ischemic ulcers. *Journal of Basic English, 92,* 590–596.

Niedner, R., & Schopf, E. (1986). Inhibition of wound healing by antiseptics. *Br. J. Dermatol., 155* (Supplement 31), 41–44.

Noble, W. C., & Savin, J. A. (1971). Gram negative infections of the skin. *British Journal of Dermatology, 85,* 286–289.

Norton, D., McLaren, R., & Exton-Smith, A. N. (1962). *An investigation of geriatric nursing problems in hospitals.* London: National Corporation for the Care of Old People.

Oleske, D. M., Smith, X. P., White, P., Pottage, J., & Donovan, M. I. (1986). A randomized clinical trial of two dressing methods for the treatment of low-grade pressure ulcers. *J. Enterostom. Ther., 13,* 90–98.

Parish, L. C., & Witkowski, J. A. (1980). Clinitron therapy and the decubitus ulcer: Preliminary dermatologic studies. *International Journal of Dermatology, 19,* 517–518.

Parish, L. C., & Witkowski, J. A. (1989). The infected decubitus ulcer. *International Journal of Dermatology, 28,* 643–647.

Patterson, R. P., & Fisher, S. V. (1986). Sitting pressure-time patterns in patients with quadriplegia. *Archives of Physical and Mental Rehabilitation, 67,* 812–814.

Pierleoni, E. E. (1984). Topical metronidazole for infected decubitus ulcers. *Journal of the American Geriatric Society, 32,* 775.

Prasad, A. S. (1982). *Clinical, biochemical, and nutritional aspects of trace elements.* New York: Liss.

Reger, S. I., McGovern, T. F., Chung, K., & Stewart, T. P. (1988). Correlation of transducer systems for monitoring tissue interface pressures. *Journal of Clinical Eng., 13,* 365–370.

Reichel, S. M. (1958). Shearing force as a factor in decubitus ulcers in paraplegics. *Journal of the American Medical Association, 166,* 762–763.

Reuterving, C., Argen, M. S., Soderberg, T. A., Tengrup, I., & Hallmans, G. (1989). The effects of occlusive dressings on inflammation and granulation tissue formation in excised wounds in rats. *Scandinavian Journal of Plastic and Reconstructive Surgery, 23,* 89–96.

Ringsdorf, W. M., & Cheraskin, E. (1982). Vitamin C and human wound healing. *Oral Surgery, Oral Medicine, Oral Pathology, 53,* 231–236.
Robson, M. C., Lea, C. E., Dalton, J. B., & Heggers, J. P. (1968). Quantitative bacteriology and delayed wound closure. *Surgical Forum, 19,* 501–502.
Rodeheaver, G. T., Pettry, D., Thacker, J. G., Edgerton, M. T., Edlich, R. F. (1975). Wound cleansing by high pressure irrigation. *Surgery, Gynecology and Obstetrics, 141,* 357–362.
Rodeheaver, G., Bellamy, W., Kody, M., et al. (1982). Bactericidal activity and toxicity of iodine-containing solutions in wounds. *Archives of Surgery, 117,* 181–185.
Roe, D. A. (Ed.). (1986). *Nutrition and the skin.* New York: Liss.
Rovee, D. T., Kurowsky, C. A., Labun, J., & Downes, A. M. (1972). Effect of local wound environment on epidermal healing. In H. L. Maibach & D. T. Rovee (Ed.), *Epidermal wound healing* (pp. 159–181). Chicago: Year Book Medical.
Ryan, T. J. (1979). Blood supply and decubitus ulcers. *International Journal of Dermatology, 18,* 123–124.
Sangeorzan, B. J., Harrington, R. M., Wyss, C. R., Czernecki, J. M., & Matsen, F. A. (1989). Circulatory and mechanical response of skin to loading. *Journal of Orthopaedic Research, 7,* 425–431.
Sebern, M. D. (1986). Pressure ulcer management in home health care: Efficacy and cost effectiveness of moisture vapor permeable dressing. *Archives of Physical and Mental Rehabilitation, 67,* 726–729.
Seiler, W., & Staehelin, H. (1979). Skin oxygen tension as a function of imposed skin pressure: Implication for decubitus ulcer formation. *Journal of the American Geriatrics Society, 27,* 298–301.
Seiler, W., & Staehlein, H. B. (1985). Decubitus ulcers: Preventive techniques for the elderly patient. *Geriatrics, 40,* 53–58, 60.
Shea, J. D. (1975). Pressure sores: Classification and management. *Clinical Orthopaedics and Related Research, 112,* 89–100.
Stewart, P., & Wharton, G. W. (1976). Bridging: An effective and practical method of preventive skin care for the immobilized person. *Southern Medical Journal, 69,* 1469–1473, 1475.
Sugarman, B., Hawes, S., Musher, D. M., et al. (1983). Osteomyelitus beneath pressure sores. *Archives of Internal Medicine, 143,* 683–688.
Taylor, T. V., Rimmer, S., Day, B., Butcher, J., & Dymock, I. W. (1974). Ascorbic acid supplementation in the treatment of pressure sores. *Lancet, 2,* 544–546.
Thomas, S. (1985). Use of a calcium alginate dressing. *Pharmaceutical Journal, 235,* 188–190.
Trumbore, L. S., Miles, T. P., Henderson, C. T., Benya, R., Fisher, L. V., & Mobarhan, S. (1990). Hypocholesterolemia and pressure sore risk with chronic tube feeding. *Clinical Research, 38,* 706A.
Van Den Broek, P. J., Buys, L. F. M., & Furth, R. V. (1982). Interaction of povidone-iodine compounds, phagocytic cells, and microorganisms. *Antimicrobial Agents and Chemotherapy, 22,* 593–597.
Varghese, M. C., Balin, A. K., Carter, M., & Caldwell, D. (1986). Local environment of chronic wounds under synthetic dressings. *Archives of Dermatology, 122,* 52–57.
Varma, A. O., Bugatch, E., & German, F. M. (1973). Debridement of dermal ulcers with collagenase. *Surgery, Gynecology and Obstetrics, 136,* 281–282.
Vasile, J., & Chaitin, H. (1972). Prognostic factors in decubitus ulcers of the aged. *Geriatrics, 27,* 126–129.
Wasson, J. H., Sox, H. C., Neff, R. K. & Goldman, L. (1985). Clinical prediction

rules: Applications and methodological standards. *New England Journal of Medicine, 313,* 793–799.

Watts, C., & Shipes, E. (1988). A study to compare the overall performance of two hydrocolloid dressings on partial thickness wounds. *Ostomy/Wound Management, 21,* 28–31.

Wheeler, C. B., Rodeheaver, G. T., Thacker, J. G., Edgerton, M. T., & Edlich, R. F. (1976). Side-effects of high pressure irrigation. *Surgery, Gynecology and Obstetrics, 143,* 775–778.

Winter, G. D. (1962). Formation of the scab and the rate of epithelization of superficial wounds in the skin of the young domestic pig. *Nature, 193,* 293–294.

Winter, G. D., & Scales, J. T. (1963). Effect of air drying and dressings on the surface of a wound. *Nature, 197,* 91–92.

Yarknoy, G. M., Kramer, E., King, R., Lukane, C., & Carle, T. V. (1984). Pressure sore management: Efficacy of a moisture reactive occlusive dressing. *Archives of Physical and Mental Rehabilitation, 65,* 598–600.

Yoshikawa, T. T. (1989). Pneumonia, UTI, and decubiti in the nursing home: Optimal management. *Geriatrics, 44,* 32–40.

Zitelli, J. A. (1984). Delayed wound healing with adhesive wound dressing. *Journal of Dermatologic Surgery and Oncology 10,* 709–710.

3
Disturbed Behavior in the Long-Term Care Setting

William E. Reichman
Hilary Hanchuk
Linda Feins

A substantial proportion of long-term care residents suffer from clinically significant psychopathology and associated behavioral problems. To date, a variety of studies suggest that dementia, mood and anxiety disorders, psychosis, sleep disorders, and nonspecific disturbances such as restlessness or aggression are significant sources of disturbed behavior in long-term care facilities (Borson, Liptzin, Nininger, & Rabins, 1987). Psychiatric morbidity in the nursing home is frequently overlooked or mistreated and leads to increased functional disability and dependence. The purpose of this chapter is to review the phenomenology, assessment, and management of psychiatric and behavioral disturbances in the long-term care setting. Attention will be directed to nonpharmacologic treatment strategies, and guidelines will be suggested for determining the appropriate indications and monitoring of psychotropic drug use in this setting.

BACKGROUND

Psychiatric Morbidity in the Nursing Home

Rovner et al. (1991) recently reported the prevalence of depressive disorder in the nursing home setting to be 12.6%; an additional 18.1% of residents were found to suffer varying numbers of depressive symptoms. Most of these cases eluded detection by facility staff despite an association between the presence of major depression and increased mortality at 1 year follow-up. In a study of psychosis in the long-term care setting, Morriss, Rovner, Folstein, and German (1990) noted that 21% of newly admitted residents to nursing homes were delusional. Most of this sample was comprised of demented patients.

Although data remain incomplete, recent figures suggest that nearly 70% of those residing in long-term care settings meet diagnostic criteria for dementia (Rovner, German, Broadhead, et al., 1990). In a related study, Zimmer and colleagues (1984) noted that in a group of 42 skilled-nursing facilities, almost two thirds of residents had significant behavioral problems; nearly one quarter of all residents had such problems labeled as "serious." Although two thirds of these patients had diagnoses indicating organic brain syndrome, very few had specific psychiatric diagnoses applied. Observed "serious" behavioral problems were actually documented by the attending physician in only 9.7% of cases. Psychiatric consultation was requested for only 14.8% of these serious cases.

Although the prevalence of psychiatric and behavioral problems in the nursing home is, in part, a consequence of the growth and increased availability of long-term care to the aged population, other factors are undoubtedly implicated. During the past quarter-century, because of state and federal policies of deinstitutionalization, greater numbers of mentally ill patients, previously cared for in state hospitals, began to reside in the community. Many of these chronically mentally ill elderly, increasingly physically infirm, have been reinstitutionalized in nursing homes (Zimmer, Watson, & Treat, 1984). Recently, Steele, Rovner, Chase, and Folstein (1990) examined predictors of nursing home placement and concluded that after controlling for cognitive ability, higher scores on standardized psychiatric rating scales (greater psychopathology) correlated with higher rates of placement.

Psychotropic Drug Use in the Nursing Home

Residents of long-term care facilities often receive a variety of psychoactive drugs including sedative-hypnotics, neuroleptics, and antidepressants. The adequacy of documentation of the indications for such psychotropic drug use in the nursing home has come under growing public scrutiny.

Buck (1988) examined the administration of psychotropic medication in Medicaid-recipient nursing home residents during the course of 1 year. Of these residents, 20,037 (60%) received at least one such medication. In a longitudinal study of psychotropic prescriptions in a teaching nursing home, Lantz, Louis, Lowenstein, and Kennedy (1990) reported that 50% of residents were placed on at least one such medication within a 5-year period. Nearly 25% of these patients were continuously receiving psychotropics.

Beardsley, Larson, Burns, Thompson, and Kamerow (1989), using data collected from the 1984 National Nursing Home Survey Pretest, examined the prescribing of psychotic drugs for elderly patients in a random sample of 150 nursing homes. The prevalence of a mental disorder including dementia was 69%. Of those residents receiving a psychotropic medication, however, 21% did not have a documented psychiatric diagnosis or symptom compatible with such treatment.

In a recent study of nearly 9,000 randomly sampled elderly nursing home residents, Garrard and colleagues (1991) noted that 21% were administered neuroleptics. Only half of the indications for these drugs were found to be acceptable under the 1989 Omnibus Budget Reconciliation Act (OBRA); federal guidelines were developed to monitor psychotropic drug use in Medicare- and Medicaid-certified nursing homes (Health Care Financing Administration, 1989). These guidelines include mandatory documentation of a psychiatric diagnosis indicating neuroleptic use, restrictions on the use of these agents if only certain behaviors are identified, prohibition of their use on an "as-needed" basis, and mandatory gradual dosage reductions accompanied by nonpharmacological management techniques.

Finally, Sloane et al. (1991) found that "pharmacologic restraints," defined as a standing order of a major or minor tranquilizer or combined use of these with an antidepressant, were routinely used in 45.3% of dementia care unit residents and 43.4% of traditional nursing home unit residents. Predictors of pharmacological restraint use included physically abusive behavior, severe mental status impairment, and frequent family visitation. Advanced patient age, nonambulatory status, and large nursing home size seemed to protect against such use.

As a group, these studies demonstrate significant prescribing of psychoactive medication in the long-term care setting and much variability in the adequacy of documentation of appropriate indications for such treatment.

EVALUATION AND MANAGEMENT
OF BEHAVIORAL DISTURBANCES
General Principles of Evaluation

Identification of troublesome behaviors involves careful and systematic preliminary inquiry directed to the patient's family, floor nurse, aides, head nurse, recreational therapist, and social worker. The resident is extensively interviewed to the extent this is possible, and a thorough mental status examination is completed. A complete review of the resident's nursing home chart is also essential so that the clinical features of the behavior are clearly identified (see Table 3.1).

In every patient with acquired cognitive impairment, a specific dementia diagnosis is warranted. If a dementia evaluation, including bloodwork and neuroimaging has been completed in the past, an appropriate summary and diagnosis should be clearly documented in the patient's records. Once this information is garnered, it is necessary to establish whether the patient's

TABLE 3.1 Essential Steps in Evaluation of Disturbed Behavior

---

Identify the specific disturbed behavior.

Identify the first onset of the behavior.

Ascertain the temporal nature of the behavior including duration and diurnal variation.

Identify all behavioral triggers such as the activities of other residents, particular settings, response to hallucinations or delusions, or comprehension difficulties.

Search for any concomitant medical or neurological illnesses including pain that may be causing or exacerbating the behavior.

Assess the effects of the patient's psychotropic and nonpsychotropic medications on the behavior.

Identify those approaches to date that have shown some efficacy in the management of the particular behavior (pharmacological and nonpharmacological).

---

present behavior and mental status is, in fact, compatible with this diagnosis.

Clear documentation of previously administered mental status and cognitive assessments significantly ameliorate many of the difficulties often experienced in evaluating the course of dysfunctional behavior in the nursing home setting. As a result, we advocate the regular use of standardized assessment tools such as the Mini-Mental State Exam (MMSE) (Folstein, Folstein, & McHugh, 1975) for cognitive evaluation, and the Brief Psychiatric Rating Scale (BPRS) (Overall & Gorham, 1962), Overt Aggression Scale (OAS) (Yudofsky et al., 1986), Geriatric Depression Scale (GDS) (Yesavage et al., 1983) and Hamilton Depression Scale (HAM-D) (Hamilton, 1960) to evaluate pertinent psychopathology. These scales refine initial and follow-up assessment technique and provide quantitative measures to evaluate outcome of treatment.

Often, with easily identified environmental triggers, corresponding solutions to certain pathological behaviors may be quite easily effected. Simple events such as an undesirable room or dining mate and excessive concern regarding significant others are frequent precipitants of dysfunctional resident behavior that are often easily dealt with by nursing home staff. It is usually through a well-designed and organized team approach involving all appropriate staff that dysfunctional resident behavior is best prevented, identified, and treated.

Approaches to Understanding the Patient

Thorough and effective assessment of dysfunctional behavior in the long-term care setting frequently involves the psychiatric evaluation of individuals with sensory or cognitive impairment. Before implementing a course of treatment, one must attempt to appreciate the role of these deficits in the person's behavior. For example, it is essential to evaluate the contribution of visual or auditory impairment to the development and maintenance of paranoia or aggression. Likewise, deficits in language comprehension may lead the resident to misconstrue nonthreatening staff queries or directives, and, as a result, behave inappropriately.

Especially important in the evaluation and management of disturbed behavior in the nursing home is assessment of the resident's verbal and nonverbal communications from a biological, psychological, and social perspective. This multidimensional approach has been referred to as the biopsychosocial model. In keeping with this approach, it is worthwhile to develop an appreciation of the patient's premorbid personality and interpersonal style. This information can help nursing home staff feel more comfortable in relating to a specific individual. Communal living, such as that exemplified in nearly all long-term care facilities, can be especially problematic for residents with paranoid, schizoid, or avoidant (socially phobic) personality styles. Some nursing home residents experienced significant authority and responsibility at work during their earlier, vocationally productive years, whereas others needed or even resisted the structure provided by supervisors. These previously experienced patterns of interpersonal relations must be considered in attempting to understand a resident's ability or inability to accept the regimentation and structure of long-term care living.

Previously dominant family dynamics may also be recapitulated by the manner in which the resident relates to the nursing home staff and other residents. An understanding and acceptance of these psychological processes can only aid communication between residents and staff.

As patients with dementia often tend to dwell in the past, knowledge of the individual's childhood and psychological traumas may enhance understanding of their present concerns and psychological adjustment to the nursing home. Unfortunately, simple assessment of a resident's interests, likes, dislikes, characteristic sources of stress, and methods for dealing with anxiety are often lacking in initial evaluations. Finally, knowledge of any previous personal or familial psychiatric illnesses or treatment is mandatory in considering the roots of disturbed behavior.

Psychiatric Consultation in the Nursing Home

The central task for the consultant psychiatrist is to assess cognitive function and mental status, diagnose dementia or delirium if previously overlooked, and identify and offer treatment guidelines for various other psychiatric illnesses. These include enduring personality disorders, adjustment-related difficulties, and primary mood, anxiety, and psychotic disorders. In addition, the psychiatrist may effectively identify and resolve family or staff issues that may be complicating the resident's adjustment to nursing home living.

In the long-term care setting, consultation to a psychiatrist can originate from several sources. It may be initiated by the resident's family, the primary attending physician, the nursing staff, or social worker. Occasionally, it is the long-term care facility's administration that arranges psychiatric consultation.

Loebel et al. (1991) recently described their experience examining 197 patients at six nursing homes. They found seven clusters of reasons generating psychiatric consultation: (a) behavioral problems, (b) mood-related problems, (c) requests by involuntary treatment services, (d) psychotic features, (e) physical signs, and (f) impaired activities of daily living (ADLs). Interestingly, they concluded that requests for psychiatric referral were weak predictors of diagnosis. Once such consultation is requested, the psychiatrist should become a member of the nursing home resident's evaluation and treatment team. Unfortunately, several obstacles in the long-term care setting may limit the consulting psychiatrist's usefulness. In some instances, in their zeal to fulfill OBRA regulations regarding psychotropic drug use, nursing home staff may request psychiatric consultation without a clear indication. The staff member initiating the consultation on behalf of the patient may actually know little about the patient's relevant symptoms or history. Additionally, there may be little or no discussion in physician or nursing notes related to the presenting behavioral or psychiatric problem. In many cases, if the patient or his or her family has not been previously informed that such a consultation has been requested, there is enhanced room for clinical error, mistrust, and miscommunication.

Once these initial obstacles are overcome and a workable differential diagnosis is established by the consultant, such information needs to be coherently shared with attendant staff, and further evaluation and treatment is determined. This approach will often include education of the staff and family, and specific therapy recommendations for the patient including behavioral modification, psychotherapy, and pharmacological intervention. In reality, only rarely are all these necessary approaches explored as treatment becomes excessively psychopharmacological.

MANAGEMENT OF BEHAVIORAL DISTURBANCES IN THE NURSING HOME DEMENTIA

Acquired intellectual impairment poses several difficulties for afflicted patients and atendant nursing home staff. Attention must often be directed to accompanying alterations in the patient's personality and mood, the development of significant anxiety or psychosis, and emerging combativeness and agitation. In addition, behavioral problems associated with dementia may exacerbate impairment in ADL and lead to increased caretaker stress.

Impairment in ADL

Assessment of Impaired ADL

Accurate evaluation of levels of functioning can give the nursing home staff valuable information as to what the resident is able and not able to do. This helps to preserve as high a level of function as possible and maintains self-esteem. Expecting too much of a resident can lead to heightened anxiety and agitation (a catastrophic reaction). Conversely, staff expectations that are set too low contribute to learned helplessness and a decline in resident self-image. Necessary areas for assessment of ADL include bathing, dressing, grooming, use of the telephone, eating, and toileting. Such assessments should be updated every 6 months and integrated into a comprehensive care plan that is made available to all nursing home staff and consultants.

Management of Impaired ADL

There are certain general principles that may be helpful if followed in the care of patients with declines in ADL. Whenever feasible, the patient should be given a choice of available options. An example includes providing a choice of two potential garments when helping the patient to dress. Only if a patient is too impaired to make such a decision should the caretaker provide more structure and limit decision making (Burnside, 1981). Independence should be actively encouraged with residents attending to as much of their own care as possible. In fact, with sufficient prompting and coaching, many patients can be talked through the many necessary steps of dressing, bathing, and toileting. Positive reinforcement and thoughtfully timed compliments support a resident's strivings toward functional independence.

Management Guidelines for Specific ADL

Communication with Demented Patients

Difficulty communicating with an aphasic patient can be demanding and stressful for staff. Additionally, patients may become increasingly anxious and agitated if they are misunderstood. If followed, some general principles may foster enhanced communication with demented patients and ease their management (see Table 3.2).

Dietary Disturbance

A demented person's appetite may pathologically increase or decrease. Sometimes, demented patients develop paranoid beliefs around eating and think the food is poisoned. Other patients may eat excessively or attempt to swallow nonfood items that look like food. Rigid likes and dislikes for certain

TABLE 3.2 Communicating with Demented Patients

Do not automatically assume demented patients are unable to comprehend what is said in front of them.

Remember that demented patients are often aware and sensitive to the emotional tone of what is said.

Sentences should be brief and simple.

Use proper names in place of pronouns.

Staff should be easily seen and at eye level when speaking with aphasic patients.

Give patients time to listen and understand.

Background noise and distractions should be minimized.

Idiomatic phrases such as "why don't you jump in the shower" should be avoided.

If a communicated message is not understood, it should be restated or rephrased.

Provide verbal cues when patients are having word-finding pauses.

Provide visual cues when directing patients to an activity.

food items may also result. Occasionally, demented patients eat very quickly or gorge on food, eating everything in sight (Carroll, 1989).

General Management Techniques

Mealtimes should be well structured and predictable (Aronson, 1988). It is helpful to have a staff member at each table to serve as a role model as demented patients are often imitative. A staff member should attempt to get the patient's attention and pick up the utensil and commence eating as often the patient will follow (Carroll, 1989). Additionally, condiments should be kept out of reach of very demented patients because they are unable to judge reasonable quantities. For example, impaired patients may eat mustard out of a jar or put multiple spoons of sugar in their coffee. Meal-related behavioral disturbances can be successfully managed by adhering to some general principles (see Table 3.3).

Dressing Difficulties

Many demented patients will become especially combative during dressing. Successful management techniques include using garments that can be worn easily (pullover tops, velcro fasteners), laying out clothes in the order that they are to be put on, and eliminating buttons or difficult snaps. Apraxic patients and those with gait difficulties require additional reassurance and aid.

Bathing Difficulties

Baths and especially showers can be very frightening to a demented patient. Often such impaired patients cannot remember or execute the necessary

TABLE 3.3 Management Techniques for Reducing Disturbed Behavior at Meals

Disorientation
　Announce what meal is to be served next.
　Present one course, one food item, and one utensil at a time.
　Dishes should be a different color than the place mat.
　Focus the patient's attention on eating.
　Monitor the rate of eating and size of each bite.
　Try to avoid using restraints in the dining room—try holding the patient's hand.
　Do not argue with the patient in the midst of a catastrophic reaction—use distraction or remove the patient from the dining area.
Persistent craving for food
　Distract the patient with walks or low-calorie snacks.
　Monitor weight gain closely.
Inability to grasp eating utensils properly and repeated spilling of food or liquid
Use
　Finger foods
　Straws
　Snorkel cups
　High-rim plates
　Suction cups
　Weighted spoons
　Double-handed cups
　One-handed cutlery
　Scooper dishes
Difficulty initiating chewing of food
　Apply light pressure to lips and underside of chin to push up the tongue.
　Verbally remind patient to swallow and wait until swallowing before giving the next bite of food.
　If the patient "squirrels" or pockets food in the cheek, gently rub the cheek to initiate chewing or remove food manually.
　Use chopped, softer foods that can be mashed with the tongue. Use gravy or sauce to moisten.
　Avoid foods with tough skins, or those that are dry or sticky.
Choking on food, liquid, or saliva
　Sit patient in an upright position when eating and for 45 minutes following the meal.
　Keep the patient's head straight and not tilted backward.
　Staff should be aware of aspiration techniques and the Heimlich maneuver.

steps to accomplish these tasks. In general, the patient should be clearly told that it is bath time and led to the appropriate area. Each step should be described to the patient during the procedure in a calm and relaxed manner (Carroll, 1989). The patient can be given a washcloth even if staff is bathing him. If the patient becomes agitated, the procedure should be promptly stopped. If a set pattern, ritual, and time of day are established, the demented patient may better tolerate bathing. Often the promise of a reward such as a walk or a favorite food will enhance compliance.

Toileting Difficulties

Incontinence has a negative psychological impact on most demented in-dividuals. It contributes to a loss of self-esteem in patients whose self-image is already compromised by the inability to do many things and by diminished cognitive functioning. Incontinence contributes to dependence and leads to further social isolation in patients who are already excessively alone. Medical causes of incontinence such as urinary tract infection, prostatic enlargement, medication, and stroke should be evaluated first. Lack of a toileting schedule and inability to remember the location of the bathroom all contribute to incontinence. Successful approaches to aiding toileting and avoiding associ-ated agitation or confusion depend on establishing a regular schedule, giving frequent directions, and distracting the resident (Carroll, 1989) (see Table 3.4).

Alterations in Personality Accompanying Dementia

In dementia, there may be characteristic alterations in demeanor accompany-ing intellectual decline. Petry, Cummings, Hill, and Shapira (1988) com-pared personality traits in 30 patients with dementia of the Alzheimer type (DAT) with 30 nondemented retirees by questionnaires completed from spouse interviews. Changes in personality were found in 12 of 18 measures for patients with DAT and none for the control retirees. These results suggested that patients with DAT were more passive, coarse, and less spontaneous compared with their premorbid personalities. These alterations also appeared early in the dementia process.

Rubin and Kinscherf (1989) suggested that in mild dementia of the Alzheimer type, increasing passivity is seen in the earliest stages and intensi-fies slightly over time. Excessive self-centeredness was also noted in their mild dementia patients and found to increase in degree as intellectual impair-

TABLE 3.4 Management Techniques for Toileting the Demented Patient

---

Establish and maintain a 2–4-hour schedule.
Encourage bowel movements in the morning as peristalsis is greater then.
Look for clues that the patient needs to be toileted
    Restlessness
    Searching behaviors
    Fingering of zippers in men
    Rocking
    Pacing
Overcome resistence to toileting by using distraction. Instead of asking the patient if
    he needs the bathroom, state- "let's take a walk" and lead to the proper area.
Point out where the commode and paper is in the bathroom. Talk the patient through
    the process—"lower your pants, sit down."

---

ment progressed to moderate levels. Low levels of interest, concentration, and energy were also characteristic of this patient group.

Certain degenerative diseases such as Pick's disease and its variants and other frontal lobe disorders resulting from tumor, stroke, or trauma can produce striking personality changes. Afflicted patients may be exceptionally passive and apathetic or quite disinhibited, emotionally labile, and sexually inappropriate. In such patients, there may or may not be an associated mood disturbance.

MOOD DISORDERS IN THE NURSING HOME

Depression

Assessment of Depression

The assessment of depressive symptoms in the institutionalized elderly must consist of surveillance for adjustment-related difficulties and comorbid somatic conditions that may commonly predispose to depression such as stroke (Eastwood, Rifat, Nobbs, & Ruderman, 1989; Starkstein, Robinson, Berthier, & Price, 1988), Parkinson's disease (Sano et al., 1989; Starkstein, Preziosi, Bolduc, & Robinson, 1990), and hypothyroidism. Additionally, all medications must be reviewed to exclude the possibility of a toxic mood disturbance such as that caused by steroids, centrally acting antihypertensives, and β-adrenergic blockers.

Parmelee, Katz, and Lawton (1991) studied the association between pain and depression in a study of 598 nursing home and congregate apartment residents. Intensity and number of complaints of pain were positively correlated with depression severity. In the nursing home setting, they concluded that in the presence of a somatic illness, chronic pain is exacerbated when there is a coexistent depressive disorder.

The loss of functional independence and self-esteem, and the disconnection from family that is so often experienced by newly admitted residents to long-term care facilities clearly lowers the threshold for the development of depressive symptoms. Residents may express feelings of abandonment and loss of control over their lives. Many old friends and family have died, highlighting feelings of isolation and loneliness. In addition, the regimentation of institutionalized living and the tendency of some nursing home staff to depersonalize residents encourages feelings of hopelessness, helplessness, and worthlessness.

Depression in the elderly is a spectrum disorder in which there may be a variety of clusters of symptoms. A depressed patient may have dysthymic disorder (chronic feelings of dysphoria) or a major depressive episode (unipolar or bipolar). Additionally, if depressed feelings are clearly stressor-related and milder in severity than major depression, the patient is most accurately diagnosed with an adjustment disorder with depressed mood. When an identifiable medical condition or medication is etiologically related to the disturbed mood state, the patient is suffering from an organic mood syndrome. Occasionally, a given patient may have overlapping diagnoses with several factors contributing to the depressed state.

Depression and Dementia

The assessment of depression in the nursing home resident frequently involves attempts to distinguish depression from dementia. The relationship between dementia and depression is complex and not fully understood. Both syndromes may coexist and share a common etiology (Dementia of Alzheimer's Type—DAT, cerebrovascular disease, Parkinson's disease) or may arise from different causes in the same patient (e.g., a demented patient who is receiving a β-blocker). Finally, depression may cause dementia, a state termed depressive "pseudodementia." Patients with pseudodementia, or the "dementia syndrome of depression," have a readily identified major depressive episode and associated cognitive impairment that tends to resolve with antidepressant treatment. Before therapy, such patients are psychomotorically slowed, poorly attentive and motivated, and dilapidted in their cognitive performance. There is often a previous personal or family history of mood disturbance as well (Wells, 1979).

There is a consistently documented association between Senile Dementia of Alzheimer's Type (SDAT) and depressive symptoms. Although nonspecific clusters of depressive symptoms are frequently encountered in the disease, full-blown major depression, as defined in the revised third edition of the Diagnostic and Statistical Manual of Mental Disorders (DSM-IIIR) (American Psychiatric Association, 1987) appears to be much less common (Wragg & Jeste, 1989). Recently, Burns, Jacoby, and Levy (1990) reported that in 178 patients with DAT, 63% endorsed at least one depressive symptom. Trained observers reported 24% of the cohort to be depressed. Interestingly, interviewed family members rated 43% of these patients as significantly depressed. Mackenzie, Robiner, and Knopman (1989) discovered a similar trend toward lack of agreement between family and patient reports of depression. In their review, 14% of DAT patients self-reported depression compared with 50% of their family member's reports of the patient's mood state. It is our own observation that famiy members occasionally attribute the passivity and withdrawal that characterizes altered personality in DAT to depression, despite the absence of depressed mood or anhedonia. It has also been argued that overburdened family members of DAT patients occasionally assign their own depressed feelings to the patient.

An assessment of neurovegetative features such as sleep, appetite, and energy impairment is also an important part of this evaluation. Because complaints in these areas are so often endorsed by elderly subjects whether or not they actually feel depressed, Rapp and Vrana (1989) have advocated the substitution of nonsomatic symptoms in the evaluation of depression in this group. As a result, attention should be preferentially directed to the patient's feelings of diminished self-esteem, hopelessness, and the desire to die. Standardized depression assessment tools such as the HAM-D and GDS are often helpful adjuncts to the evaluation. Snowden (1990) recently found that the GDS had an 83% specificity and 93% sensitivity for major depression as defined in DSM-IIIR. Earlier, Lesher (19860 had demonstrated the validity of the GDS in nursing home residents.

Treatment of Depression

There are many recent reviews of recommended approaches to the treatment of geriatric depression (Fitten, Morley, Gross, Petry, & Cole, 1989). Depression in this population is often effectively treated with a combination of psychotherapy and somatic approaches such as pharmacotherapy or electroconvulsive therapy. There remains a paucity of literature, however, addressing the best treatment modalities for depression in the long-term care setting.

The psychotherapeutic approach to depression in the nursing home often involves supportive therapy directed at restoring the resident's sense of control over his life and empathizing with his concerns and losses. Specifically, the patient is helped to identify activities and interests that are still fulfilling (e.g., socializing, reading, family visits) and that reinforce a sense of autonomy and self-worth. These interventions often include cognitive and psychoeducational techniques directed to the patient, his family, and nursing home staff. Other therapeutic interventions involve increased resident participation in day programming and social activities.

Antidepressant Treatment   Generally, antidepressant medication is indicated in the treatment of depression when depressed mood or anhedonia are unremitting, and accompany neurovegetative features and suicidality. The choice of an appropriate antidepressant is guided by the clinical features of the depression and any previous history of response to a particular agent or susceptibility to side effects. In patients whose depressions include prominent anxiety, agitation, or diminished sleep, standard clinical practice is to prescribe more sedating antidepressants such as doxepin or trazodone. In patients with depressions manifested by prominent anergia, psychomotor slowing, and excessive sleep, more activating agents such as fluoxetine, desipramine, and buproprion are indicated. Nortriptyline is a well-tolerated drug that may demonstrate activating or sedating properties in the elderly.

An advantge of this agent is that serum levels can be monitored to assess the likelihood of response. Because elderly patients are exceptionally sensitive to anticholinergic side effects (dry mouth, urinary retention, constipation, confusion, cardiac conduction, and rate changes) and orthostasis, the tertiary amines, imipramine and amitriptyline, should be used with additional precaution.

Many clinicians use monoamine oxidase inhibitors (MAOIS) such as phenelzine, tranylcypromine, and, more recently, selegeline in geriatric depression. These agents are generally well tolerated by the elderly despite a significant risk of orthostasis. Treated patients must conform to a tyramine-restricted diet to avoid the potentially lethal "hypertensive crisis" associated with these agents (see Table 3.5).

Reynolds, Kupfer, Hoch, et al. (1986) point to a more favorable outcome with treatment for depression in the elderly in the setting of greater initial depressive symptomatology, higher cognitive function, and early morning awakening. Joyce and Paykel (1989) have recently argued that, in fact, across all age groups, there are no consistent predictors of response to antidepressant therapy. However, when major depression is complicated by psychotic features, treatment responsiveness is improved when a neuroleptic is combined with a chosen antidepressant.

Reifler et al. (1989) reported their experience with antidepressant treatment in 28 patients with DAT and depression, and 33 patients with DAT

TABLE 3.5 Use of Antidepressant Medications

Antidepressant	Starting Daily Dose (mg)	Monitor
Tricyclics Nortriptyline Desipramine Doxepin	10–25	Confusion, sedation, electrocardiographic changes, orthostasis, anticholinergic side effects, serum levels
Trazodone	50	Orthostasis, confusion, priapism in men
Fluoxetine	5–20	Insomnia, anxiety, restlessness, hyponatremia, anorexia, confusion
Buproprion	75	Insomnia, anxiety, confusion, seizures
Monoamine oxidase inhibitors Phenelzine Tranylcypromine Selegiline	5–15	Tyramine-restricted diet and medications, orthostasis, sedation, anxiety, impotence, confusion

without depression. Subjects were randomized into an 8-week double-blind trial of imipramine or placebo. HAM-D scale scores were recorded at baseline, and at 2, 4, 6, and 8 weeks. In both the antidepressant and placebo groups there was significant improvement in depressive symptoms noted. Interestingly, the difference between the imipramine- and placebo-treated groups did not reach statistical significance.

Greenwald et al. (1989) studied the response to antidepressant treatment in patients with major depression and major depression with dementia. Seventy-three percent of those patients with major depression alone responded to antidepressant therapy compared with 70% of the group with both depression and dementia. In this latter cohort, although test performance improved after treatment, cognitive deficits still remained.

Treatment of Refractorily Depression

Certain principles should be consistently applied in managing the treatment of refractorily depressed patient in the nursing home. Guscott and Grof (1991) have suggested that treatment failure is most often due to inadequate evaluation and therapy, and less often a consequence of patient variables. Factors that may contribute to treatment refractoriness include inadequate dosing, inappropriately short trial length, and coexistent somatic disorders.

Once these variables have been considered, antidepressant augmentation with lithium carbonate (Finch & Katona, 1989; Van Marwijk et al., 1990) or thyroid hormone (Bauer, Whybrow, & Winokur, 1990) may be tried. The use of lithium in the elderly must be done judiciously given the altered renal function in this age group. Additionally, commonly administered nonsteroidal antiinflammatory drugs such as ibuprofen can elevate serum lithium levels (Miller, 1989).

Some authors have advocated the use of stimulants in the medically ill, depressed elderly (Frierson, Wey, & Tabler, 1991). Agents such as methylphenidate (10–30 mg/day) are often used without significant side effects. Such drugs are given in the morning to avoid insomnia and demonstrate efficacy within 1 to 3 hours of administration. The combination of a heterocyclic antidepressant and stimulant may be successfully used in the treatment of refractorily depressed patient.

Electroconvulsive Therapy (ECT)   Although not typically an on-site treatment option in the long-term care setting, many seriously depressed patients who are unresponsive to antidepressant medication or intolerant of side effects should be referred for ECT. Numerous, well-designed, recent reports have demonstrated the efficacy of this technique in the treatment of geriatric depression (American Psychiatric Association, 1990; Benbow, 1989; Cattan et al., 1990; Hickie, Parsonage, & Parker, 1990; Pearlman, 1991; Zimmer & Price 1991). The most common side effects of ECT remain transient confusion and memory impairment (Benbow, 1989). ECT has also proved to be a viable and efficacious treatment for those patients with depression and dementia. Liang, Lam, and Ancill (1988) noted significant improvement in mood after ECT therapy with little additional cognitive impairment.

Mania

Background

Mania in the elderly can be the consequence of toxic effects of medication (steroids, antiparkinsonian agents, stimulants) or cerebral pathology (stroke, tumor) (Rundell & Wise, 1989). Stone (1989) in a review of 92 cases of mania in the elderly, found 26% to have no prior history of affective illness, 30% with a previous depression, and 15% with greater than three previous depressions. Those with a positive family history had an earlier onset of illness. Organic impairment was found in 24% of the cases studied.

Treatment of Mania

The treatment of mania involves supportive psychotherapy and limit setting, and the use of medication. Lithium carbonate remains the mainstay of acute and prophylactic treatment of mania. When acute mania is severe or includes psychotic features, the addition of a neuroleptic is indicated.

Abrupt discontinuation of lithium can result in rapid recurrence of mania (Mander & Loudon, 1988). Gelenberg and coworkers (1989) compared standard and low serum levels of lithium for maintenance treatment of bipolar disorder. Higher lithium doses were associated with more side effects but much lower recurrence of the underlying affective disorder. Because of the elderly's increased sensitivity to lithium's adverse side effects (polyuria, polydipsia, tremor, ataxia, and confusion) we recommend the use of lower doses and serum levels with close monitoring of clinical response. Although not extensively studied in the elderly, alternative agents include the anticonvulsants carbamazepine, valproic acid, and clonazepam.

Restlessness and Anxiety

Restlessness and anxiety in the long-term care setting may be nonspecific behavioral features of dementia or a mood disorder, or may represent reactions to a particular stressor. Medications, pain, and systemic illnesses such as cardiac arrhythmia, hyperthyroidism, and pulmonary insufficiency can produce nervousness and restlessness.

The management of these symptoms involves consistent reassurance of the patient, distraction, and identification and active treatment of the underlying cause. In cognitively intact patients, adjunctive relaxation techniques such as progressive muscle relaxation may afford some relief.

The pharmacological approach to anxiety and restlessness most often involves the use of benzodiazepines or the nonbenzodiazepine alternative, buspirone. Patients who experience panic attacks in which anxiety seems to have an episodic, abrupt onset with prominent physiological concomitants (rapid respirations and pulse, lightheadedness, gastrointestinal symptoms, and paresthesias) may selectively benefit from the use of alprazolam or any of the heterocyclic antidepressants.

The decision to use medication should be based on the underlying cause and duration and severity of symptoms. If benzodiazepines are selected, agents such as lorazepam (0.5–3 mg/day) or oxazepam (10–30 mg/day) are preferred given their advantageous volumes of distribution, metabolism, and half-lives. The continued use of these drugs in the elderly is limited by their tendency to cause confusion, dysarthria, ataxia, and lethargy. Patients may become dependent with long term use and experience withdrawal symptoms on discontinuation.

Wandering

Wandering is a common behavioral disturbance in dementia that can result from the patient becoming lost, disoriented, or excessively restless. At times, the patient may be searching for an undefinable person or place. Often, wandering behavior is a means of handling tension or stress (Hiatt, Merlino, & Ronch, 1987). If the patient has structured rest periods, is not losing weight, does not have a medical or psychiatrically treatable condition, and the behavior is confined to the long-term care facility, wandering behavior need not necessarily be discouraged. In general, there are no effective medications that selectively reduce wandering. As a result, management when indicated is essentially nonpharmacological (Carroll, 1989) (see Table 3.6).

Catastrophic Reactions

Catastrophic reactions are exaggerated emotional reactions to environmental events. Often, events such as dressing or undressing, bathing, language comprehension difficulties, confusion about the environment, or difficulty with manual dexterity precipitate such reactions. Occasionally, it is merely a break in the usual routine, awareness of incontinence, or an upsetting television program that elicits an emotional outburst. Fatigue or concurrent medical illness such as a urinary tract infection can lower a patient's threshold for such behavior.

During a catastrophic reaction the patient may look angry, cry abruptly, or become aggressive. Sometimes, there are initial signs that may herald the

TABLE 3.6 Techniques to Reduce Wandering Behavior

Assess wanderer's physical needs.
 Hunger
 Pain
 Need to be toileted
Increase structure, supervision, long walks, and recreational activities.
Distract with alternative activities.
 Squeezing balls
 Twirling tops
 Shaking bean bags
Enforce rest periods for 30 minutes every 4 hours by using gerichairs. Nursing staff
 should check feet for swelling and blisters.

onset of such behavior. The patient may back away, or turn his head or body away and avoid eye contact. He may appear fidgety with increased respiration, flushing, or pallor of the skin, and narrow or closed eyes; the voice may become high pitched.

Management Techniques

It must first be remembered that the behavior is not willful and under the patient's control (Gwyther 1985). The patient should be taken to a quiet area and distracted and encouraged to walk. Lengthy explanations should be avoided by attending staff. Caretakers should use a soothing voice during a catastrophic reaction and offer calming actions after it is over such as stroking the arm, holding the hand, or rubbing the back (Ronch, Doan, & Schwab, 1985). Often, the patient will become relaxed if the staff appears calm and in control. It is frequently helpful to monitor the time of day the patient typically has catastrophic reactions to help determine potential causes (Carroll, 1989).

PSYCHOSIS IN THE NURSING HOME
Background

Psychosis in the elderly may represent the late stages of a psychiatric disorder such as chronic schizophrenia, delusional disorder, or mood disturbance. In the long-term care setting, hallucinations and delusions are common manifestations of dementia or delirium. Structural brain lesions (trauma, tumor, or stroke) or toxic effects of medication can also cause hallucinations and delusions. Hallucinations can be olfactory or tactile, but are most often auditory or visual. In the elderly, sensory impairment may be the primary cause of such symptoms.

Delusions in the aged population are often persecutory in nature. In the context of dementia, such beliefs are generally not well elaborated and consist mostly of simple delusions of theft, infidelity, or abandonment. In less cognitively impaired patients, delusions can be quite systematized and elaborate with no obvious cause (delusional disorder). Pearlson et al. (1989) conducted a retrospective chart review to determine whether there were clinical diffrences betwen early- and late-onset schizophrenia. They compared the records of 54 schizophrenic subjects with late onset of illness (after age 45) with 54 young and 22 elderly subjects with early onset (before age 45). The late-onset schizophrenics were more likely to have had visual, tactile, and olfactory hallucinations. Additionally, they suffered predominantly persecutory delusions. They were also noted to have experienced less thought disorder (loosening of associations) and less affective flattening. Interestingly, the late-onset group also has more visual and auditory impairment than the early-onset patient groups. Of these patients 48.1% responded to neuroleptic treatment with complete remission of symptoms.

Treatment of Psychosis

The management of psychotic symptoms in the long-term care setting depends on accurate identification of the underlying causes and appropriate treatment. Such symptoms often cause significant distress for the patient mandating a supportive and empathic stance by attendant caregivers. Although it is inappropriate to agree with patient experiences or feelings that are clearly not reality based, it is also countertherapeutic to confront aggressively the patient's false beliefs or experiences. The treatment team should assume a neutral stance and reassure the patient that attention should be directed to the stress and anxiety such symptoms are causing the patient. If psychotic symptoms are sustained or cause subjective distress to the patient or to the milieu, then antipsychotic medications (neuroleptics) are indicated.

Use of Neuroleptics in the Long-Term Care Setting

Elderly patients are especially sensitive to the myriad side effects of neuroleptic medications. These side effects fall into two categories: acute and chronic. The relatively acute side effects of neuroleptics include extrapyramidal reactions such as akathisia, rigidity, tremor, ataxia, and bradykinesia (parkinsonism). This is particularly true of the higher potency agents such as haloperidol, fluphenazine, and thiothixene. Patients may also become increasingly confused with relatively low doses of these agents. In a recent study of the effects of haloperidol in the treatment of agitation and psychosis in dementia, Devanand, Sackeim, Brown, and Mayeux (1989) demonstrated that although effective, the use of haloperidol above 4 mg/day was associated with severe extrapyramidal reactions and cognitive decline.

With the lower potency drugs such as thioridazine or chlorpromazine, anticholinergic side effects and orthostasis may limit usefulness. The choice of an appropriate agent is guided by the patient's previous response to neuroleptics and sensitivity to side effects.

The longer term use of neuroleptics in the elderly is associated with an increased risk for the development of tardive dyskinesia and less common variants such as tardive dystonia and tardive akathisia. As a result, patients should be treated with the lowest possible effective doses of these medications and monitored for the emergence of side effects (see Table 3.7).

Treatment of Neuroleptic-Induced Side Effects

For the treatment of neuroleptic-induced acute extrapyramidal reactions, we recommend either an initial dosage reduction if clinically possible or the addition of an antiparkinsonian agent such as amantadine 100 mg twice to three times per day. Anticholinergic agents are generally avoided for this purpose as their side effects are particularly troublesome in the elderly. Neuroleptic-induced restlessness or akathisia may not adequately respond to conventional antiparkinsonian therapy. Relatively low doses of a short-acting benzodiazepine such as lorazepam 0.5 to 1 mg twice per day may afford relief. Propranolol may also be used to treat akathisia if the preceding interventions are unsuccessful. If these approaches are inadequate, the patient may need to be switched to a lower potency neuroleptic.

A universally accepted medication treatment for tardive dyskinesia is lacking. The initial approach should be to lower the patient's neuroleptic dose. In

TABLE 3.7 Use of Neuroleptic Agents

Agents	Starting Daily Dose (mg)	Side-Effects	
		Parkinsonian	Anticholinergic
High-potency			
Haloperidol	0.5–1	High	Low
Fluphenazine	1	High	Low
Middle Potency			
Trifluoperazine	1	Moderate	Moderate
Thiothixene	1	Moderate	Moderate
Low potency			
Thioridazine	10	Low	High
Chlorpromazine	10	Low	High

some cases, a transient worsening of the disorder may then be noted (withdrawal dyskinesia).

AGITATION, AGGRESSION, AND VIOLENCE
Background

Agitated behavior takes several forms and may thus require a variety of responses and interventions. Although clinical case histories and vignettes offer guidelines for treatment of disturbed behavior in nursing homes, these are primarily pharmacologically based and lack integration with nonpharmacological techniques. Examples of agitated verbal behavior include yelling or screaming, excessive repetition of a statement or request, or perseverative incomprehensible utterances. Agitation often includes self-directed behaviors such as hair pulling, scratching, or head banging. Agitated patients may direct violent behavior toward others by throwing things, striking out, grabbing, pushing, or groping. At times, agitated behavior may take the form of intense pacing and hand wringing.

Assessment and Management of Agitation

The agitated patient is most often communicating distress of one form or another to those around him. The observed behavior may be a reaction to pain, may represent drug-induced restlessness and discomfort (akathisia), or may be the consequence of a perceived threat or paranoid delusion. Occasionally, patients become agitated in resonse to hallucinations. Successful management of agitation is contingent on adequate consideration of all of these factors with treatment directed to the identified cause. Treatment initially consists of gentle reassurance and distraction away from any stressor. With combative patients, nursing home staff must ensure their own safety and remove any potentially dangerous objects. In some patients, these nonpharmacological techniques are often adequate. When such approaches fail to manage agitation successfully, however, restraint of the patient must be accomplished physically or pharmacologically.

Use of Mechanical Restraints

The use of physical restraints in the long-term care setting includes chairs with locking lap trays (geriatric chairs), Posey vests, and ankle and wrist cuffs. Mechanical restraint use in nursing homes has been increasing and may occur in 25% to 85% of residents (Evans & Strumpf, 1989; Folmar & Wilson, 1989; Sloane et al., 1991). Sloane et al. 1991), in a case-control study of 31 specialized dementia units and 32 traditional nursing home units, found that in the former setting, 18.1% of demented residents were restrained mechanically. In the latter setting, of those dementia patients who were out of bed, 51.6% were noted to be in restraints. Independent predictors of physical restraint use were found to include residence in a nonspecialized nursing home unit, nonambulatory status, mental status impairment, hip fracture, transfer dependency, and inadequate nursing staff-to-patient ratio.

Tinetti, Wen-Liang, Marottoli, and Ginter (1991) examined the patterns and risk factors for mechanical restraint use in residents of 12 skilled nursing facilities. Restraints were noted to be in use in 59% of residents at the beginning of the study. At 1-year follow-up, 31% of remaining residents were observed to be mechanically restrained. Although no particular features of the skilled nursing facilities studied predicted restraint use, resident characteristics associated with such use included older age, confusion, dependence in dressing, greater participation in social activities, and lack of antidepressant use. The most frequently cited reasons for using mechanical restraints were unsteadiness, agitated behavior, and wandering.

Despite frequent use, what remains unclear is whether physical restraints actually improve disturbed behavior or serve to reduce injury. It appears that physical restraints are acceptably used to prevent injury and falls, but may actually worsen agitation (Sloane et al., 1991; Werner, Cohen-Mansfield, Braun, & Marx, 1989).

Pharmacological Approaches to Agitation and Combativeness

The pharmacological approach to agitated and aggressive behavior has involved a wide variety of psychotropic medications. Neuroleptics, benzodiazepines, and, more recently, anticonvulsants, β-adrenergic blockers, lithium carbonate, and serotonergic agents have been used with mixed results. There remains, however, a paucity of double-blind placebo-controlled studies investigating the efficacy of such agents in dementia patients in the long-term care setting (Helms, 1985; Risse & Barnes, 1986).

The use of neuroleptics and benzodiazepines for disturbed behavior has been previously addressed. Neuroleptics are the most studied and effective medications for controlling severe acute aggressive behavior in dementia and chronic aggression associated with psychosis (Maletta, 1990; Yudofsky, Silver, & Schneider, 1987). Particularly in the context of acute aggression, high-potency neuroleptics such as haloperidol or thiothixene, or benzodiazepines such as lorazepam are the drugs of choice (Yudofsky et al., 1987). Coccaro, Kramer, Zemishlany, et al., (1990), in a double-blind 8-week trial, compared the effects of haloperidol, oxazepam, and diphenhydramine in the short-term management of behavioral disturbances. The study was conducted in 59 elderly dementia patients residing in the long-term care setting. Although modest efficacy was found with all the agents studied, oxazepam was found to be the least effective.

A literature has emerged that supports the use of alternative agents in the control of chronic, nonpsychotic agitated behavior and aggression. Although some patients may adequately respond to neuroleptics, for many others, the sustained use of these agents is often limited by side effects (extrapyramidal and cognitive) or lack of efficacy.

Alternative Agents for Control of Chronic Agitation

Anticonvulsants   Carbamazepine is the anticonvulsant agent that has been most extensively used to control agitation. Efficacy has been demonstrated in irritability, aggressivity, and impulsivity in patients with abnormal and normal electroencephalograms (Risse & Barnes, 1986). Patterson (1987), in an open pilot study of this drug, demonstrated improvement in assaultive behavior in eight brain-injured patients refractory to treatment with other agents. Earlier, Klein et al. (1984) reported the beneficial use of combined carbamazepine and haloperidol over haloperidol alone or placebo in agitated, psychotic patients. Mattes, Rosenberg, and Mays (1984), in an open trial and 8-week follow-up, demonstrated the efficacy of carbamazepine in 21 aggressive patients with a variety of diagnoses including dementia. In an additional study, he reported improvement in assaultive behavior in most of 34 aggressive patients treated with carbamazepine for 4 to 8 weeks (Mattes, 1984). As yet, there are no controlled, systematic studies of the use of this drug in agitated, elderly nursing home populations.

In the elderly, the use of carbamazepine carries some risks. These include ataxia, dysarthria, and increased confusion. Treated patients also need to be monitored for signs of bone marrow suppression including aplastic anemia (Maletta, 1990).

We generally recommend initiating dosing of carbamazepine at 100 mg twice per day. Serum levels should be monitored weekly while the dose is adjusted for the first month of treatment and monthly thereafter. Before starting treatment, a complete blood count (CBC) and liver function tests should be reviewed. The CBC should be monitored every 1 to 2 weeks for the first few months and monthly thereafter.

Sodium valproate, like carbamazepine, has demonstrated some efficacy in treating cyclic mood disorders and aggressivity. Kahn, Stevenson, and Douglas (1988) reported beneficial effects of sodium valproate in three patients with agitated behavior owing to organic brain disease. It use in agitated and aggressive elderly patients has not been systematically studied.

Diphenylhydantoin and primidone have generally demonstrated lack of efficacy in the treatment of aggressive or combative behavior (Yudofsky et al., 1987).

Serotonergic Agents   A variety of serotonergic agents have been used to treat behavioral disturbances in brain-injured and demented patients. Most studied in this regard is trazodone. Greenwald, Marin, and Silverman (1986) reported the successful use of a trazodone-tryptophan combination to treat repetitive screaming, and head and table banging in an 82-year-old moderately demented woman. Simpson and Foster (1986) reported the use of trazodone in four elderly nondepressed agitated patients who failed therapy with neuroleptics. The behavior of all four patients was noted to improve substantially with treatment. Pinner and Rich (1988) reported that three of seven demented patients treated for aggression with trazodone experienced complete cessation of such behavior. They speculated that the lack of response noted in another three of the seven patients may have been due to inadequate dosing. Additional scattered case reports and our own clinical experience confirm that a subset of demented, agitated patients may respond well to trazodone. We recommend initiating treatment at 50 mg per day and increasing the dose by this amount every 3 to 5 days until clinical response or the emergence of side effects (sedation, hypotension).

Other serotonergic drugs such as the anxiolytics buspirone and clonazepam may also have efficacy in treating combative or agitated patients. Ratey, Sovner, Parks, and Rogentine (1991) recently reported buspirone's effectiveness in six mild-moderately retarded adults with aggressive or self-injurious behavior. The drug was found to be well tolerated while its beneficial effects on aggressivity were not directly related to treatment of anxiety. Earlier, Tiller (1988) reported efficacy for buspirone in the treatment of disinhibited behavior in a demented elderly patient. In an additional case study, Levine (1988) reported beneficial effects of buspirone for agitation in a head-injured patient. Colenda (1988) reported the successful use of buspirone to control rocking, vocal grunts, oppositional behavior, and restlessness in a 74-year-old demented woman. The dose employed was 15 mg 3 times a day. Improvement was noted during a 2-month period.

Clonazepam reportedly has efficacy for behavioral problems associated with multiinfarct dementia (Smeraski, 1988). Sobin, Schneider, and McDermott (1989) reported the successful use of fluoxetine, a potent serotonin uptake inhibitor, in the treatment of combativeness and verbal agitation in a 48-year-old man with a traumatic brain injury.

β-Adrenergic Blockers Since Elliot (1977) first reported the effective use of proparnolol to treat assaultive behavior following acute brain injury in seven patients, there has been growing interest in this pharmacological role for β-adrenergic blockers. β-Blockers have been used successfully to control agitated behavior in a variety of conditions including chronic schizophrenia, Alzheimer's disease, stroke, and traumatic brain injury (Risse & Barnes, 1986; Yudofsky et al., 1987). Petrie and Ban (1981) reported the successful treatment of behavioral problems such as irritability, wandering, and assaultiveness with propranolol in three patients with Alzheimer's disease. Most studies reporting efficacy with propranolol focus on middle-aged and younger patients suffering from anoxia, traumatic brain injury, and stroke. Dosages employed range considerably (40–1,400 mg/day). Wide-scale study of the efficacy and safety of this agent in demented elderly patients has yet to be reported. At present, it is best to consider propranolol as an alternative agent for the treatment of behavioral disturbances in the nursing home given the risk of significant side effects in elderly patients. These include bradycardia, hypotension, diminished cardiac output, and worsening of chronic obstructive pulmonary disease. In addition, propranolol may cause increased confusion and depression in susceptible patients. The drug may also increase serum levels of concurrently administered neuroleptics and anticonvulsants. Its use is contraindicated in insulin-dependent diabetes mellitus, hyperthyroidism, and severe renal insufficiency (Risse & Barnes, 1986).

Dosing of propranolol for agitated, aggressive behavior in elderly demented patients has not been standardized. If this agent is to be used, dosing can be judiciously commenced at 10 mg twice a day. The dose can be adjusted upward every 3 to 5 days by 10-mg increments until clinical response or the emergence of side effects. Yudofsky et al. (1987) have published more specific dose recommendations for the use of propranolol in this setting. It appears that clinical efficacy may not become evident at the highest tolerated dose for 6 to 8 weeks.

SLEEP DISORDERS IN NURSING HOME
Background

Disturbed sleep among nursing home residents is often a great source of stress for the afflicted patient and attending staff. A variety of psychiatric conditions including depression, dementia, and delerium have disrupted sleep as a common symptom. The identification of underlying causes of impaired sleep and subsequent treatment can pose a formidable clinical challenge.

Estimates suggest that nearly 5 million elderly persons in this country suffer from a severe sleep disorder. Approximately 35% to 40% of prescribed sedative-hypnotics are for this age group (Moran, 1988). The precise prevalence of clinically significant sleep disorders in the nursing home setting is unknown. An early report of prescribing trends in nursing homes and other institutional settings revealed that as many as 90% of residents received a hypnotic on a regular basis (Reynolds, 1991; U.S. Public Health Service, 1976). James (1985) more recently reported that 35% of nursing home residents were receiving such medication.

In determining whether a patient is suffering from a sleep disorder requiring treatment, it is essential to gain familiarity with the expected changes in sleep that accompany normal aging. With advancing age, there may be a decrease in the overall quality and quantity of sleep. Although sleep latency (the time it takes to fall asleep) does not appreciably change with age, the number of nocturnal awakenings and their duration does (Moran, 1988). It also appears that the requirement for total daily sleep remains the same throughout the life cycle, whereas nocturnal sleep efficiency (percentage of time in bed actually spent asleep) declines (Moran, 1988).

With advanced age, other factors undoubtedly contribute to disturbed sleep such as concomitant medical illnesses involving nocturia, orthopnea, pain, and limited mobility. Other conditions such as sleep apnea, nocturnal myoclonus, and restless legs syndrome can contribute to sleep difficulties. Elderly patients in long-term care settings may particularly suffer from psychiatric conditions such as dementia, depression, or anxiety resulting in sleep problems. Boredom, loneliness, and adjustment-related stresses may also be contributory. Finally, administered medications, noise from other residents or staff, or inadequate lighting that encourages napping during the day can all result in insomnia in the nursing home setting (Reynolds, 1991).

Assessment and Management of Sleep Disturbances

In the nursing home, sleep problems that are transient (2–3 weeks duration) may be determined by particular environmental factors or psychological adjustment-related difficulties. The relatively sudden onset of disruption of the sleep-wake cycle in an elderly resident may herald the onset of delirium. All medical and psychiatric contributions to disrupted sleep should be initially considered, and if the disturbance continues without obvious cause, more aggressive evaluation such as referral to a sleep center is warranted. In most cases, an identifiable etiology, whether medical or psychiatric, is generally found. As treatment of the underlying condition is commenced, specific therapy for disrupted sleep may consist of nonpharmacological and pharmacolocigal interventions.

In many patients, simple improvement in sleep hygiene may be therapeutic. Residents should be discouraged from daytime napping, nocturnal eating or reading in bed, and the use of stimulant medications and caffeinated beverages in the afternoon and evening. A regular, individualized sleep time should be established and maintained. Unfortunately, excessive regimentation of sleep scheduling to serve the institution's staffing needs poses a formidable barrier to such interventions.

For those patients in whom an underlying cause for disturbed sleep is found, temporary use of hypnotic medication may be warranted with certain precautions. Benzodiazepines such as temazepam 15 mg and lorazepam 0.5 to 2 mg are often better tolerated than longer acting agents, minimizing the risk of daytime somnolence, confusion, dysarthria, or ataxia. These agents should be administered 1 hour before desired sleep onset. Although there is a relative lack of studies examining the chronic use of such agents in institutionalized elderly, consensus has emerged that numerous side effects do, in fact, limit utility. Patients with respiratory illnesses, including apnea, may experience significant worsening of associated symptoms with the use of benzodiazepines. In insomnia associated with Alzheimer's disease, the use of a benzodiazepine hypnotic may be especially problematic as a relationship between dementia severity and the occurrence of sleep apnea has been noted in women (Reynolds et al., 1985). With continued use of benzodiazepines for sleep, patients experience dependency, tolerance, increased somnolence during the day, impairment in ADLs, and insomnia and other withdrawal symptoms on drug discontinuation (Reynolds, 1991). After chronic therapy with benzodiazepines, discontinuation should involve gradual tapering over several days (Moran, 1988). In those elderly patients with dementia or chronic sleep difficulties unresponsive to nonpharmacological approaches, sedating antidepressants such as trazodone 50 to 200 mg or doxepin 20 to 100 mg may be effective, nonhabituating alternatives. In dementia with nocturnal agitation or psychosis, low doses of thioridazine (25–100 mg) is helpful to control disturbed sleep.

Chloral hydrate 500 to 1000 mg has some efficacy in treating insomnia in this population. One of the drug's principal metabolites, however, may potentiate the activity of other medications such as warfarin or phenytoin via displacement effects on protein binding. The resultant increased risk of toxicity of these drugs may limit the concurrent use of chloral hydrate in the elderly (Moran, 1988).

Antihistamines such as diphenhydramine or hydroxyzine are occasionally prescribed in the long-term care setting as hypnotics. These agents are not as efficacious as benzodiazepine hypnotics and may be apt to produce delirium in susceptible patients Gillin & Byerley, 1990; (Moran, 1988).

REFERENCES

American Psychiatric Association. (1987). *Diagnostic and statistical manual of mental disorders* (3rd ed., rev.). Washington, DC: American Psychiatric Association.

American Psychiatric Association Task Force on Electroconvulsive Therapy. (1990). *Recommendations for treatment, training, and privileging.* Washington, DC: American Psychiatric Association.

Aronson, M. K. (1988). *Understanding Alzheimer's disease.* New York: Scribner's.

Bauer, M. S., Whybrow, P. C., & Winokur, A. (1990). Rapid cycling bipolar affective disorder: 1. Association with grade I hypothyroidism. *Archives of General Psychiatry, 47,* 427–432.

Beardsley, R. S., Larson, D. B., Burns, B. J., Thompson, J. W., & Kamerow, D. B. (1989). Prescribing of psychotropics in elderly nursing home patients. *Journal of the American Geriatrics Society, 37,* 327–30.

Benbow, S. M. (1989). The role of electroconvulsive therapy in the treatment of depressive illness in old age. *British Journal of Psychiatry, 155*, 147–152.

Borson, S., Liptzin, B., Nininger, J., & Rabins, P. (1987). Psychiatry and the nursing home. *American Journal of Psychiatry, 144*, 1412–1418.

Buck, J. A. (1988). Psychotic drug practice in nursing homes. *Journal of the American Geriatrics Society, 36*, 409–418.

Burns, A., Jacoby, R., & Levy, R. (1990). Psychiatric phenomena in Alzheimer's disease: 3. Disorders of mood. *British Journal of Psychiatry, 157*, 81–86, 92–94.

Burnside, I. M. (1981). *Nursing and the aged.* New York: McGraw-Hill.

Carroll, D. L. (1989). *When your loved one has Alzheimer's.* New York: Harper & Row.

Cattan, R. A., Barry, P. P., Mead, G., Reefe, W. E., Gay, A., & Silverman, M. (1990). Electroconvulsive therapy in octogenarians. *Journal of the American Geriatric Society, 38*, 753–758.

Coccaro, E. F., Kramer, E., Zemishlany, Z., et al. (1990). Pharmacologic treatment of noncognitive behavioral disturbances in elderly demented patients. *American Journal of Psychiatry, 147*, 1640–1645.

Colenda, C. C. (1988). Buspirone in treatment of agitated demented patient [Letter to the editor]. *Lancet,* 1169.

Devanand, D. P., Sackeim, H. A., Brown, R. P., & Mayeux, R. (1989). A pilot study of haloperidol treatment of psychosis and behavioral disturbance in Alzheimer's disease. *Archives of Neurology, 46*, 854–857.

Eastwood, M. R., Rifat, S. L., Nobbs, H., & Ruderman, J. (1989). Mood disorder following cerebrovascular accident. *British Journal of Psychiatry, 154*, 195–200.

Elliott, F. A. (1977) Propranolol for the control of belligerent behavior following acute brain damage. *Annals of Neurology, 1*, 489–491.

Evans, L. K., & Strumpf, N. E. (1989). Tying down the elderly: A review of the literature on physical restraint. *Journal of the American Geriatrics Society, 37*, 65–74.

Finch, E., & Katona, C. (1989). Lithium augmentation in the treatment of refractory depression in old age. *International Journal of Geriatric Psychiatry, 4*, 41–46.

Fitten, L. J., Morley, J. E., Gross, P. L., Petry, S. D., & Cole, K. D. (1989). Depression [clinical conference]. *Journal American Geriatric Society, 37*, 459–472.

Folmar, S., & Wilson, H. (1989). Social behavior and physical restraints. *Gerontologist, 29*, 650–653.

Folstein, M. F., Folstein, S. E., & McHugh, P. R. (1975). "Mini-Mental State": A practical method for grading the cognitive state of patients for the clinician. *Journal of Psychiatric Research, 12*, 189–198.

Frierson, R. L., Wey, J. J., & Tabler, J. B. (1991). Psychostimulants for depression in the medically ill. *American Family Physician, 43*, 163–170.

Garrard, J., et al. (1991). Evaluation of neuroleptic drug use by nursing home elderly under proposed Medicare and Medicaid regulations. *Journal of the American Medical Association, 265*, 463–467.

Gelenberg, A. J. (1988). Lithium efficacy and adverse effects. *Journal of Clinical Psychiatry, 49*, 8–11.

Gillin, J. C., & Byerley, W. F. (1990). The diagnosis and management of insomnia. *New England Journal of Medicine, 322*, 239–248.

Greenwald, B. S., Kramer-Ginsberg, E., Marin, D. B., Laitman, L. B., Hermann, C. K., Mohs, R. C., & Davis, K. L. (1989). Dementia with coexistent major depression. *American Journal of Psychiatry, 146*, 1472–1478.

Greenwald, B. S., Marin, D. B., & Silverman, S. M. (1986). Serotonergic treatment of screaming and banging in dementia [Letter to the editor]. *Lancet, 2*, 1464–1465.

Guscott, R., & Grof, P. (1991). The clinical meaning of refractory depression: A review for the clinician. *American Journal of Psychiatry, 148,* 695–704.

Gwyther, L. P. (1985). *Care of Alzheimer's patients: A manual for nursing home staff.* Chicago: American Health Care Association and Alzheimer's Disease and Related Disorders Association.

Hamilton, M. (1960). A rating scale for depression. *Journal of Neurology, Neurosurgery and Psychiatry, 23,* 56–62.

Health Care Financing Administration. (1989). Medicare and Medicaid: Requirements for long term care facilities. Final rule with requests for comments. *Federal Register, 54,* 5316–5336.

Helms, P. M. (1985). Efficacy of antipsychotics in the treatment of the behavioral complications of dementia: A review of the literature. *Journal of the American Geriatrics Society, 33,* 206–209.

Hiatt, L. G., Merlino, M., & Ronch, J. (1987). *Innovations in the care of the mentally impaired elderly: Conference proceedings.* Albany: New York State Department of Health.

Hickie, I., Parsonage, B., & Parker, G. (1990). Prediction of response to electroconvulsive therapy: Preliminary validation of a sign-based typology of depression. *British Journal of Psychiatry, 157,* 65–71.

James, D. S. (1985). Survey of hypnotic drug use in nursing homes. *Journal of the American Geriatrics Society, 33,* 436–439.

Joyce, P. R., & Paykel, E. S. (1989). Predictors of drug response in depression. *Archives of General Psychiatry, 46,* 89–99.

Kahn, D., Stevenson, E., & Douglas, C. J. (1988). Effect of sodium valproate in three patients with organic brain syndromes. *American Journal of Psychiatry, 145,* 1010–1011.

Klein, E., et al. (1984). Carbamazepine and haloperidol versus placebo and haloperidol in excited psychosis. *Archives of General Psychiatry, 41,* 165–171.

Lantz, M. S., Louis, A., Lowenstein, G., & Kennedy, G. J. (1990). A longitudinal study of psychotropic prescriptions in a teaching nursing home. *American Journal of Psychiatry, 147,* 1637–1639.

Lesher, E. L. (1986). Validation of the Geriatric Depression Scale among nursing home residents. *Clinical Gerontologist, 4,* 21.

Levine, A. M. (1988). Buspirone and agitation in head injury. *Brain Injury, 2,* 165–167.

Liang, R. A., Lam, R. W., & Ancill, R. J. (1988). ECT in the treatment of mixed depression and dementia. *British Journal of Psychiatry, 152,* 281–284.

Loebel, J. P., Borson, S., Hyde, T., Donaldson, D., Van Tuinen, C., Rabbitt, T. M., & Boyko, E. J. (1991). Relationships between requests for psychiatric consultations and psychiatric diagnoses in long-term-care facilities. *American Journal of Psychiatry, 148,* 898–903.

Mackenzie, T. B., Robiner, W. N., & Knopman, D. S. (1989). Difference between patient and family assessments of depression in Alzheimer's Disease. *American Journal of Psychiatry, 146,* 1174–1178.

Maletta, G. J. (1990). Pharmacologic treatment and management of the aggressive demented patient. *Psychiatric Annals, 20,* 446–455.

Mander, A. J., & Loudon, J. B. (1988). Rapid recurrence of mania following abrupt discontinuation of lithium. *Lancet, 2*(8601), 15–17.

Mattes, J. A. (1984). Carbamazepine for uncontrolled rage outbursts. *Lancet, 11,* 1164–1165.

Mattes, J. A., Rosenberg, M. A., & Mays, D. (1984). Carbamazepine versus propranolol in patients with uncontrolled rage outbursts: A random assignment study. *Psychopharmacological Bulletin, 20,* 98–100.

Miller, L. G., Bowman, R. C., & Bakht, F. (1989). Sparing effect of sulindac on lithium levels. *Journal of Family Practice, 28,* 592–593.

Moran, M. G. (1988). Sleep disorders in the elderly. *American Journal of Psychiatry, 145,* 1369–1378.

Morriss, R. K., Rovner, B. W., Folstein, M. F., & German, P. S. (1990). Delusions in newly admitted residents of nursing homes. *American Journal of Psychiatry, 147,* 299–302.

Overall, J. E., & Gorham, D. R. (1962). The Brief Psychiatric Rating Scale. *Psychological Reports, 10,* 799–812.

Parmelee, P. A., Katz, I. R., & Lawton, M. P. (1991). The relation of pain to depression among institutionalized aged. *Journal of Gerontology, 46,* 15–21.

Patterson, J. F. (1987). Carbamazepine for assaultive patients with organic brain disease. *Psychosomatics, 28,* 579–581.

Pearlman, C. (1991). Electroconvulsive therapy: Current concepts. *General Hospital Psychiatry, 13,* 128–141.

Pearlson, G. D., Kreger, L., Rabins, P. V., Chase, G. A., Cohen, B., Wirth, J. B., Schlaepfer, T. B., & Tune, L. E. (1989). A chart review study of late-onset and early-onset schizophrenia. *American Journal of Psychiatry, 146,* 1568–1574.

Petrie, W. M., & Ban, T. A. (1981). Propranolol in organic agitation [Letter to the editor]. *Lancet, 1,* 324.

Petry, S., Cummings, J. L., Hill, M. A., & Shapira, J. (1988). Personality alterations in dementia of the Alzheimer type. *Archives of Neurology, 45,* 1187–1190.

Pinner, E., & Rich, C. L. (1988). Effects of trazodone on aggressive behavior in seven patients with organic mental disorders. *American Journal of Psychiatry, 145,* 1295–1296.

Rapp, S. R., & Vrana, S. (1989). Substituting nonsomatic for somatic symptoms in the diagnosis of depression in elderly male medical patients. *American Journal of Psychiatry, 146,* 1197–1200.

Ratey, J., Sovner, R., Parks, A., & Rogentine, K. (1991). Buspirone treatment of aggression and anxiety in mentally retarded patients: A multiple-baseline, placebo lead-in study. *Joural of Clinical Psychiatry, 52,* 159–162.

Reifler, B. V., Teri, L., Raskind, M., Veith, R., Barnes, R., White, E., & McLean, P. (1989). Double-Blind Trial of Imipramine in Alzheimer's Disease patients with and without depression. *American Journal of Psychiatry, 146, 1,* 45–59.

Reynolds, C. F. (1991). Sleep disorders. In J. Sadavoy, L. W. Lazarus, & L. F. Jarvik (Eds.), *Comprehensive review of geriatric psychiatry.* Washington, DC: American Association of Geriatric Psychiatry, American Psychiatric Press.

Reynolds, C. F., et al. (1985). Sleep apnea in Alzheimer's dementia: Correlation with mental deterioration. *Journal of Clinical Psychiatry, 46,* 257–261.

Reynolds, C. F., Kupfer, D. J., Hoch, C. C., et al. (1986). Two-Year Follow-Up of Elderly Patients With Mixed Depression and Depression. *Journal of the American Geriatrics Society, 34,* 793–799.

Risse, S. C., & Barnes, R. (1986). Pharmacologic treatment of agitation associated with dementia. *Journal of the American Geriatrics Society, 34,* 368–376.

Ronch, J., Doan, J., & Schwab, M. (1985, July–August). How to decrease wandering: A form of agenda behaviour. *Geriatric Nursing.*

Rovner, B. W., German, P. S., Brant, L. J., Clark, R., Burton, L., & Folstein, M. (1991). Depression and mortality in nursing homes. *Journal of the American Medical Association, 265,* 993–996.

Rovner, B. W., German, P. S., Broadhead, J., et al. (1990). The prevalence and management of dementia and other psychiatric disorders in nursing homes. *International Psychogeriatrics,* 147.

Rubin, E. H., & Kinscherf, D. A. (1989). Psychotherapy of very mild dementia of the Alzheimer type. *American Journal of Psychiatry, 146,* 1017–1021.

Rundell, J. R., & Wise, M. G. (1989). Causes of Organic Mood Disorder. *Journal of Neuropsychiatry and Clinical Neuroscience, 1,* 398–400.

Sano, M., Stern, Y., Williams, J. Cote, L., Rosenstein, R., & Mayeux, P. (1989). Coexisting dementia and depression in parkinson's disease. *Archives of Neurology, 46,* 1284–1286.

Simpson, D. M., & Foster, D. (1986). Improvement in organically disturbed behavior with trazodone treatment. *Journal of Clinical Psychiatry, 47,* 191–193.

Sloane, P. D., Mathew, L. J., Scarborough, M., Desai, J. R., Koch, G. G. & Tangen, C. (1991). Physical and pharmacologic restraint of nursing home patients with dementia: Impact of specialized units. *Journal of the American Medical Association, 265,* 1278–1282.

Smeraski, P. J. (1988). Clonazepam treatment of multi-infarct dementia. *Journal of Geriatric Psychiatry and Neurology, 1,* 47–48.

Snowdon, J. (1990). Validity of the Geriatric Depression Scale [Letter to the editor]. *Journal American Geriatric Society, 38,* 722–723.

Sobin, P., Schneider, L., & McDermott, H. (1989). Fluoxetine in the treatment of agitated dementia [Letter to the editor]. *American Journal of Psychiatry, 146,* 1636.

Starkstein, S. E., Preziosi, T. J., Bolduc, P. L., & Robinson, R. G. (1990). Depression in Parkinson's disease. *Journal of Nervous Mental Disorders, 178,* 27–31.

Starkstein, S. E., Robinson, R. G., Bertheir, M. L., & Price, T. R. (1988). Depressive disorders following posterior circulation as compared with middle cerebral artery infarcts. *Brain, 111,* 375–387.

Steele, C., Rovner, B., Chase, G. A., & Folstein M. (1990). Psychiatric symptoms and nursing home placement of patients with Alzheimer's disease. *American Journal of Psychiatry, 147,* 1049–1051.

Stone, K. (1989). Mania in the elderly. *British Journal of Psychiatry, 155,* 220–224.

Tiller, J. G. (1988). Short-term buspirone treatment in disinhibition with dementia. *Lancet, 1,* 1169.

Tinetti, M. E., Wen-Liang, L., Marottoli, R. A., & Ginter, S. F. (1991). Mechanical restraint use among residents of skilled nursing facilities: Prevalence, patterns, and predictors. *Journal of the American Medical Association, 265,* 468–471.

U.S. Public health Service (1976). Physician's drug prescribing patterns in skilled nursing facilities. Department of Health, Education and Welfare, Bethesda, Maryland.

Van Marwijk, H. W., Bekker, F. M., Nolen, W. A., Jansen, P. A., Van Nieuwkerk, J. F., & Hop, W. C. (1990). Lithium augmentation in geriatric depression. *Journal of Affective Disorders, 20,* 217–223.

Wells, C. F. (1979). Pseudodementia. *American Journal of Psychiatry, 136,* 895–900.

Werner, P., Cohen-Mansfield, J., Braun, J, & Marx, M. S. (1989). Physical restraints and agitation in nursing home residents. *Journal of the American Geriatrics Society, 37,* 1122–1126.

Wragg, R., & Jeste, D. V. (1989). An overview of depression and psychosis in Alzheimer's disease. *American Journal of Psychiatry, 146,* 577–587.

Yesavage, J. A., et al. (1983). Development and validation of a geriatric depression screening scale: A preliminary report. *Journal of Psychiatric Research, 17,* 37–49.

Yudofsky, S. C., et al. (1986). The Overt Aggression Scale: An operationalized rating scale for verbal and physical aggression. *American Journal of Psychiatry, 143,* 35–39.

Yudofsky, S. C., Silver, J. M., & Schneider, S. E. (1987). Pharmacologic treatment of aggression. *Psychiatric Annals, 17*, 397–405.

Zimmer, B., & Price, T. R. (1991). "It ain't over till . . . : ECT, depression, competency, and ethical dilemmas [letter to the editor]. *Journal of the American Geriatric Society, 39*, 438–439.

Zimmer, J. G., Watson, N., & Treat, A. (1984). Behavioral problems among patients in skilled nursing facilities. *American Journal of Public Health, 74*, 1118–1121.

4

Nurse Staffing in Nursing Facilities: Implications for Achieving Quality of Care

Mathy Mezey
Mary Knapp

With the lifetime risk of entering a nursing facility now estimated to be above 40% (Kemper & Murtaugh, 1991) a stay in a nursing facility is no longer an unexpected event for the elderly in American society. Among persons aged 85 or older, one out of every three will spend some time in a nursing facility.

It goes without saying that, in most instances, community residence, including small board and care facilities, or a stay on a rehabilitation or geriatric unit in acute care hospitals are preferable to nursing home placement. Nevertheless, even if such options were to increase substantially, they would not substitute for the need for additional nursing home care in the near future.

Already, a moratorium on new beds, the general increase in the number and disability of people 80 and older, and the substitution of a nursing facility stay for time previously spent in an acute care hospital have resulted in increased numbers and a sicker case mix of residents in nursing facilities (Kahn et al., 1990). This increase in acuity has received substantial attention in the lay and professional press. The consequences of these changes on quality of care have, however, received less scrutiny (Mezey, in press).

In the absence of better outcome criteria, nurse staffing is frequently used as a proxy for quality of care in nursing facilities. Yet, despite increased resident acuity, RN staffing has remained virtually unchanged. The purpose of this chapter is to review recent changes in resident acuity and what little is known about quality of care in the face of rising acuity. The relationship of quality of care and RN staffing are explored along with factors impeding the increase of RN staffing in nursing facilities.

CHANGING FACE OF NURSING FACILITIES

In contrast to only a few years ago, only the sickest of people now gain admission to nursing facilities.* The elderly in nursing homes are increasingly sicker in comparison with community residents and older peole using home health services (Shaughnessy & Kramer, 1990). This change in the case mix of residents has come about as a result of the convergence of several factors.

Restrictions on Bed Capacity

In 1988 there were 19,700 Medicare and Medicaid certified nursing facilities with a bed capacity of 1,624,200 beds (National Center for Health Statistics, 1989). Encouraged by reimbursement from both Medicaid and Medicare, starting in 1965 there was a rapid growth in nursing facility beds, with bed capacity increasing 38% by 1973–74 (National Center for Health Statistics, 1989).

Since the early 1980s, bed supply has failed to keep pace with increases in the elderly population. Twenty-five percent of states have placed moratoriums on adding new nursing home beds (Harrington, 1990). As a result, beds are in short supply. Nursing facility beds declined 2.8 beds per 1,000 population 65 and older between 1977 and 1988. HCFA data confirm minimal increases in nursing facility beds per 1,000 Medicare enrollees from 53.4 in 1981 to 55.3 in 1987 (HCFA, 1988). In 1984 nursing facilities operated at approximately 92% of capacity, in contrast to an occupancy rate of 85.6% in 1972 (National Center for Health Statistics, 1989).

Aging of Residents in Nursing Facilities

The high rate of bed occupancy and declines in bed supply must be viewed in light of current and projected increases in the population 85 years of age and older, who are proportionally higher users of nursing facilities. Those persons over age 65 who are 85 and older increased from 40% in 1977 to 45.2% in 1985. Demand for admission to nursing facilities among the very old has continued to rise. The median age of residents is now 81 years, and residents age 85 and older comprise 45% of all residents. Persons age 85 and older accounted for 76% of the 17% overall increase in nursing facility use between 1977 and 1985. Seventy-five percent of elderly residents are female, many of whom are widowed or never married, and more than 30% of whom

---

*This chapter is limited to a discussion of people 65 years of age and older confined to nursing facilities as defined by the Health Care Financing Administration.

have no surviving child (National Center for Health Statistics, 1989). Given that between 1990 and 2010 the age 85+ cohort will grow 3 to 4 times as fast as the general population, the demand for nursing facility beds will continue to rise.

By virtue of their increasing age, residents in nursing facilities are sicker and more disabled than was the case 10 years ago. As the age at admission has increased, so too has the overall functional, physical, and mental disability of residents (see Table 4.1). Of 4,000 new admissions to nursing facilities in 1985, 51% were dependent in five ADLs (Spector et al., 1988).

In addition to a very high level of functional disability, residents in nursing facilities experience frequent exacerbations of their multiple chronic illnesses as well as new episodes of acute illnesses. Residents have multiple medical diagnosis; more than 60% have some evidence of mental incapacity in addition to severe functional and physical disabilities (National Center for Health Statistics, 1989; Zimmer et al., 1988).

Describing only aggregate data, however, creates a false illusion of homogeneity among residents in nursing facilities. In fact, facilities serve diverse populations of both short- and long-stay residents. Although the overwhelming majority of all residents are older and sicker, one of the major reasons for the increased acuity is the influx of people for whom a stay in a nursing facility substitutes for time previously spent in hospital. These "short-stay" posthospital residents, who enter for both recuperative services, for example, following a stroke or hip fracture, and for terminal care, remain in the nursing facility for less than 90 days.

Since the introduction of prospective payment in hospitals in 1984, hospital lengths of stay for Medicare beneficiaries have fallen sharply, while, at the

TABLE 4.1 Percentage of Nursing Home Residents 65 Years of Age and Older by Type of Dependency in Activities of Daily Living

Type of Dependency	Total (%)	
	1977	1985
Requires assistance in bathing	88.6	91.2
Requires assistance in dressing	77.7	77.7
Requires assistance in using toilet room	54.8	63.3
Requires assistance in transferring		62.7
Continence difficulty with bowel or bladder control	47.3	54.5
Requires assistance in eating	33.6	40.4

Source: From E. Hing. (1987, May 14). *Use of nursing homes by the elderly: Preliminary data from the National Nursing Home Survey.* Advance Data from Vital and Health Statistics, No. 135 (DHHS Publication No. [PHS] 87-1250). Hyattsville, MD: Public Health Service, National Center for Health Statistics.

same time, nursing facility discharges from acute care hospitals as a percentage of all admissions have more than doubled. (American Hospital Association, 1988; Hing, 1989; Morrisey, Sloan, & Valvona, 1988) Posthospital admission to nursing facilities has risen 61% since 1986. (Densen, 1991). More than 50 percent of admissions to skilled nursing facilities (SNFs) in 1984 were Medicare patients (Lewis, Leake, & Leal-Sotelo, 1987; Specter, 1989). As an example, the probability of a hip fracture patient's transfer to a nursing facility was 17% in 1983 and 25% in 1985 (Fitzgerald, 1988). Moreover, there is evidence that a substantial portion of patients remain in the facility longer than originally anticipated (Fitzgerald, 1988).

Short-stay Medicare users of nursing facility care are among the sickest residents (Kramer, Shaughnessey, & Pettigrew, 1985; Morrisey, Sloan, & Valvona, 1988; Specter, 1989). Neu (1988) found SNF Medicare users to be the sickest patients in each DRG category; SNF admission was found probably to substitute for some part of hospital stay (Neu & Harrison, 1988). Morrisey, Sloan, and Valvona (1988) report that, in addition to being 75 and older, comorbidity substantially increases the probability of transfer from hospital to a nursing home (Morrisey, Sloan, & Valvona, 1988). In a study of changes reported by 66% of nursing facilities in Portland, Oregon, during a 1-year period, Lyles (1986) reports an 80% increase in acuity of illness, 60% or more increase in requests for admission too sick for the facility, and an increase of more than 50% in the use of oxygen, respiratory suction, tube feedings, and intravenous fluids (Lyles, 1986). Thus, most people in nursing facilities are now truly patients with multiple and complex chronic and acute functional, physical, and mental health problems. Questions remain, however, as to the impact of sicker residents on RN staffing and on quality of care.

STAFFING IN NURSING FACILITIES

Direct and indirect services in nursing facilities are delivered by 1.2 million Full-Time Equivalent (FTE) employees, 700,000 of whom provide some form of nursing or personal care. Nursing aides and orderlies, by far the largest group of employees providing personal care, account for more than 40% of a nursing home's total FTEs (American Nurses Association, 1986; National Center for Health Statistics, 1989). Of the estimated 1.5 million RNs in the United States only approximately 7% are employed in nursing facilities (American Nurses Association, 1990; National Center for Health Statistics, 1989).

While a variety of factors influence the number of RNs who work in nursing facilities, federal and state regulations exert the greatest impact on a nursing facility's RN work force. As of October 1, 1990, to replace differentiated staffing between nursing facilities providing skilled as opposed to intermediate services, the federal government mandated specific minimum professional nurse staffing requirements for all levels of care in nursing homes (OBRA, 1987). The specific requirements regarding nursing services and the associated interpretive guidelines are shown in Table 4.2. The new law sets high expectations for the way nursing care needs are to be met, and mandates that licensed nursing services be "sufficient" to meet the nursing care needs of residents (Mohler & Lessard, 1991).

**TABLE 4.2 Summary of Requirements for Nursing Facilities
Related to Nursing Services**

Nursing responsibilities
  Each comprehensive resident assessment must be conducted or coordinated by a registered nurse who signs and certifies the completion of the assessment.

  A comprehensive care plan must be developed within 7 days after completion of the comprehensive assessment prepared by an interdisciplinary team that includes the attending physician, a registered nurse with responsibility for the resident, and other appropriate staff in disciplines as determined by the resident's needs, and, to the extent practicable, the participation of the resident, and the resident's family or legal representative; and periodically reviewed and revised by a team of qualified persons after each assessment.

  A facility must maintain a quality assessment and assurance committee consisting of the director of nursing services, a physician designated by the facility, and at least three other members of the facility's staff.

Staffing
  The facility must have sufficient nursing staff to provide nursing and related services to attain or maintain the highest practicable physical, mental, and psychological well-being of each resident, as determined by resident assessments and individual plans of care.

  Except when waived, the facility must designate a licensed nurse to serve as a charge nurse on each tour of duty.

  Except when waived, the facility must use the services of a registered nurse for at least 8 consecutive hours a day, 7 days a week.

  Except when waived, the facility must designate a registered nurse to serve as the director of nursing on a full-time basis.

  The director of nursing may serve as a charge nurse only when the facility has an average daily occupancy of 60 or fewer residents.

Advanced nursing practice
  At the option of the physician, required visits of Skilled Nursing Facilities (SNFs) after the initial visit may alternate between personal visits by the physician and visits by a physician assistant, nurse practitioner, or clinical nurse specialist.

Required training of nurse aides

A facility must not use any individual working in the facility as a nurse aide for more than 4 months, on a full-time, temporary, per diem, or other basis, unless that individual has completed a training and competency evaluation program, or a competency evaluation program approved by the state, and that individual is competent to provide nursing and nursing-related services.

A facility must provide, for individuals used as nurse aides as of January 1, 1990, a competency evaluation program approved by the state and preparation necessary for the individual to complete the program by October 1, 1990.

A facility must check with all state nurse aide registries it has reason to believe contain information on an individual before using that individual as a nursing aide.

The facility must provide regular performance review and regular in-service education to ensure that individuals used as nurse aides are competent to perform services as nurse aides. In-service education must include training for individuals providing nursing and nursing-related services to residents with cognitive impairments.

The facility must ensure that nurse aides are able to demonstrate competency in skills and techniques necessary to care for resident's needs, as identified through resident assessments and described in the plan of care.

Nevertheless, while nursing facilities are required to have licensed nurses on duty 24 hours a day, they are only required to have an RN on duty 8 consecutive hours a day, 7 days a week. In 1987, an effort to require at last one RN on duty at all times in every nursing facility was defeated by a tie vote in the House Committee on Energy and Commerce (Mohler & Lessard, 1991). In 1990, Congress granted substantial waiver rights to nursing facilities for all or part of their nurse staffing requirements.

Consequently, many nursing facilities operate without an RN in the facility 16 out of 24 hours of the day. More than half of the states have no state minimum full-time RN requirement; 42.7% have full-time but not 24-hour RN requirements (HCFA, 1988). In 1985 there were 6.3 RNs per 100 beds (National Center for Health Statistics, 1989) and 80% of RNs worked in SNF or combined SNF and Intermediate Care Facility (ICF) certified nursing homes. Nationally, Medicare-certified facilities staff at higher levels than those not Medicare certified; on average, they have 6.1 RNs per facility and 17.3 beds per RN (National Center for Health Statistics, 1989).

In contrast to hospitals, which report an average of one RN for every eight patients, nursing facilities are staffed with one RN for every 49 residents, and, in 1985, residents in nursing facilities received on average 12 minutes or less of RN time per 24 hours. Nearly 40% (7,402) of facilities report 6 minutes or less of RN time per resident per day, and 60% of these report no RN hours during the past week. Voluntary and government facilities, and larger homes report higher ratios of RNs per 100 beds (Jones, et al., 1987).

Many nursing facilities are out of compliance with even these minimal standards. In a study of more than 15,000 Medicare and Medicaid facilities, using 1988 data, a third did not meet the 1990 licensed nurse requirement. Thirty-four percent were out of compliance with RN staffing requirement, 8% needed more licensed vocational nurses (LVNs) and 88 percent of facilities needed additional nursing assistants to comply with the new minimum federal and state regulations. The cost of full compliance with minimum RN staff requirements is estimated at an additional $173,201,431 (Mohler & Lessard, 1991). These projected costs are the most commonly cited reasons for lack of compliance with and for the congressional waivers of nurse staffing requirements.

The impact of so few RNs is of special concern because RNs are the only readily available health care professional in nursing facilities. Primary care physicians spend, on average, less than 2 hours a month in nursing facilities (Robert Wood Johnson, 1982). Very few facilities have a physician available on the premises at all times. Only 6% report a physician available on premise during weekdays. The most common coverage is physician availability on premises but only at scheduled times.

As a consequence of their limited numbers and the relative absence of physicians, RNs in nursing facilities spend less than 10% of their time on direct care to residents. Rather, their time is spent coordinating and completing the mandated resident assessment, assigning and supervising nursing staff, observing and charting information about residents, and determining, evaluating, and modifying resident care plans (American Nurses Association, 1986; Johnson & Connelly, 1990). Direct care is limited to administration of complex therapies. Lack of ready access to physicians results in additional RN time spent contacting physicians by telephone to report changes in patient status and to obtain new orders, or to arrange for patients to be transported to emergency departments.

Despite their wide range of responsibilities, salaries of RNs in nursing facilities are significantly lower than RNs working in hospitals. In 1986 dollars, the average wage of RNs was $10.56 per hour. At the higher end of the salary scale, nursing facility RNs had less than half the proportion earning $500 per week or more than is true for RNs in hospitals and other settings (Jones et al., 1987). This holds true despite the fact the RNs in nursing facilities have many more years of work experience and have been in the facilities longer than comparable RNs employed in hospitals.

Differences in the work environment and possibly lower salaries influence the type of nurse who chooses to work in nursing facilities. In comparison with RNs in hospitals, RNs in nursing facilities are older, more frequently widowed, divorced, or separated, predominantly diploma prepared, and more likely to have graduated from their nursing program 15 or more years ago (Cotler & Kane, 1988). Less than 10% of hospital-employed RNs are 55 years of age and older in comparison with just over 25 percent of nursing facility RNs in that age group (American Nurses Association, 1986). Forty-one percent of RNs have worked in the facility 5 or more years. Nearly 90% of RNs in supervisory positions are employed full time. Overall, however, nearly 45% of RNs are employed part time, in contrast to about 33% of RNs working in hospitals. The average number of hours worked by full-time RNs in nursing homes is 39.2 hours. Retention of RNs during a 1-year period is similar to that in hospitals: 73% for nursing facilities, 82% for hospitals, and 73% for other settings (American Health Care Association, 1988; American Nurses Association, 1986; Jones et al., 1987).

QUALITY OF HEALTH CARE IN FACE OF RISING ACUITY

Irrespective of setting, measurement of quality of health care follows Donebedian's (1981) model of structural, process, and outcome criteria. Outcome criteria are recognized as the best standard by which to assess quality of care. Commonly used outcome criteria include mortality; morbidity, in nursing facilities measured in terms of functional deficits and common health conditions such as decubiti, infections, falls; inappropriate use of hospitals or emergency departments; and patient satisfaction or complaints. In studies which assess the quality of care rendered by nurse practitioners (NPs), the degree to which NP care approaches physician care is often used as the marker of quality (Freund, in press).

Responsibility for monitoring quality in nursing facilities has fallen primarily to federal and state licensing and credentialing bodies. Unfortunately, the public's perception to the contrary, state and federal agency surveys measure only compliance with minimal standards, and to date, existing studies of quality of care in nursing homes rely almost exclusively on structural and process criteria. New OBRA regulation surveys will attempt to examine outcomes of care, but in pre-OBRA surveys there is substantial evidence that indicators are not sufficiently sensitive to capture many important aspects of quality (Shaughnessey & Kramer, 1990); in fact, none of the current methods for surveying nursing facilities profess to measure quality of care comprehensively.

Thus, there is a paucity of data on the impact of greater resident acuity on quality of care in nursing facilities. Studies have documented increased morbidity of residents: increased use of technology such as catheters and intravenous infusions, and more transfers from nursing facilities to hospitals. Several studies have also documented increased mortality in nursing facilities

(Kramer, Shaughnessey, & Pettigrew, 1985; Sager, Easterling, & Leventhal, 1989). Given changes in case mix, however, it is difficult to determine if this greater morbidity and mortality is an anticipated consequence or an untoward outcome of a sicker case-mix of residents.

In the absence of outcome criteria, level and skill mix of a home's staffing has been used as a measure of quality of care in nursing facilities (Mezey & Scanlon, 1988). In its landmark report, the Institute of Medicine (IOM) concluded that insufficient nurse staffing is an important factor related to poor quality care in nursing facilities (Institute of Medicine, 1986). Although high level of staffing cannot guarantee quality care, such care cannot occur in an atmosphere of low staffing (Mohler & Lessard, 1991).

Although often limited by small sample size and questionable endpoints, nevertheless a substantial body of literature supports the conclusion that nursing hours overall, and the ratio of professional to nonprofessional nursing staff in particular, provide a good indication of quality of care in nursing facilities (Fottler, Smith, & James, 1981; Kaeser, 1981; Kurrerow, 1990; Linn, Gurel, & Linn, 1977; Mech, 1980; Mitty, 1989; Munroe, 1990; Rango, 1985; Ulmann, 1985; U.S. Senate, 1976). In a study of more than 300 long-term care facilities in California, for example, using number of health care deficiencies (a questionable marker for quality) facilities with a higher ratio of RN hours to LVN hours per resident per day were found to have a higher quality of care. Every 25% increase in the ratio of RN hours to LVN hours resulted in a 0.53 decrease in the number of health related deficiencies. Similarly, RN staff turnover was associated with poor quality (Munroe, 1990).

Introducing nurses with advanced clinical skills into nursing facilities has shown to be effective in improving quality of care including some important resident level outcomes as well as use of hospitals and emergency departments (Garrard, Kane, & Ratner, et al. 1990; Shaughnessy, Kramer, & Hittle, 1990; Small & Walsh, 1988). Moreover, in a study to identify a "gold standard" assessment for new admissions to nursing facilities, nurse practitioners and physicians identified similar items, (Mezey et al., in press) and performed equally well in actually carrying out assessments on new admissions (Lavizzo-Mourey, Mezey, & Taylor, 1991).

Such findings suggest that, in the absence of better indicators, the number of skilled nursing hours are an effective "proxy" measure of nursing facility quality of care (Cohen & Bubay, 1990; Tellis-Nayak, 1988). Thus, in the face of rising resident acuity, for quality of care to be maintained, the number of skilled nursing hours would be expected to rise. Yet, there is very little evidence that resident acuity has had any substantial effect on RN staffing.

As was the case in 1975, RNs make up less than 7% of a nursing facility's total FTE employees (National Center for Health Statistics, 1989). In a study of more than 2,500 nursing facilities in Pennsylvania before and after the introduction of prospective payment, Konda and Mezey (1991) found that although, as expected, resident acuity had increased, RN staffing had either remained the same or in some instances had decreased somewhat because of decreased employment of part-time RNs. Although total nursing hours had increased this was primarily due to increases in nonprofessional nursing staff (LVNs and nursing assistants) (Konda & Mezey, 1991).

There is a beginning appreciation of the fact that nursing facilities are being asked to provide a level of care that exceeds their capability given current RN and total nurse staffing, and thus residents are receiving inadequate care (Sager, Easterling, & Leventhal, 1989). Monroe (1990), for example, found that as the number of residents requiring complex nursing care exceeded the number of knowledgeable and skilled nursing personnel, quality of care declined.

Such conclusions are, however, preliminary. Although methodology for tracking outcomes exists, it is expensive and difficult to implement, and is not incorporated into commonly collected data bases on care in nursing facilities. Moreover, several additional factors further compound the complex relationship between acuity, staffing, and quality.

RELATIONSHIP BETWEEN ACUITY, STAFFING, AND QUALITY OF CARE

There are three possible explanations as to why, despite major increases in resident acuity, nursing facilities have failed to increase their professional nursing staff and have thus jeopardized the quality of care they deliver: (a) Current resident classification systems, because they reflect primarily functional rather than composite health status, underestimate the health deficits of residents, and thus provide no incentive for federal and state government to raise minimum RN staffing levels; (b) low Medicaid reimbursement prevents nursing facilities from offering competitive salaries necessary to attract, hire, and retain more professional staff; and (c) By paying for hospitalization and emergency department use for any health deviation beyond the most routine, Medicare discourages nursing facilities from providing enhanced professional services.

Patient Classification and RN Staffing

All methods of resident classification, including state Medicaid case-mix systems, attempt to equate resident characteristics to the amount of time necessary to provide care. In contrast to hospitals, which use DRGs and other measures of disease and diagnosis as the basis for determining severity of illness and staffing needs, current classification methodologies in nursing facilities rely heavily on functional status to describe the health of residents for allocation of nursing personnel and in some instances for allocating reimbursement. Functional status, as measured by ADLs, is widely accepted as a better measure on which to base staffing in long-term care than either disease or diagnosis (Institute of Medicine, 1986; Solomon, 1988; Specter et al. 1988).

With the increase in acuity of residents, there are reasons to question how well methodologies based primarily on functional status depict initial or changes in health status; how accurately ADLs correlate with use of other health care resources, such as hospitalizations; and how useful ADLs are in predicting RN as opposed to LVN and nurse assistant staffing in nursing facilities.

Level of ADLs evidence a high degree of consistency in nursing facilities nationally. In 1987, the average ADL Index nationally for Medicare- and Medicaid-certified nursing facilities was 3.4, with a range among individual states of from 3.1 to 3.9 (HCFA, 1988). Case mix, when expressed by ADLs, remains remarkably stable over time, especially for long-stay residents. Eighty-five percent of residents have no or only one-level change in ADL over a 6-month period. Change from dependent to independent occurs in less than 10% of residents, whereas change from independent to dependent occurs in fewer than 20% of residents (Specter, 1989).

The stability of the ADL measures is partially accounted for by the fact that those who change (for better or worse) tend to be short-stay residents who leave the facility. Lack of variation in long-stay residents, conversely, is most likely attributable to the large number of ADL deficits exhibited by these residents on admission to a nursing facility. A typical example pertains to feeding. At the time of the first assessment following nursing home admission, only 10% of residents are able to feed themselves independently; the remaining 90% need some form of staff supervision or assistance. At the end of 6 months, 75% of residents remaining in the facility have had no change in their feeding ability, and of those residents whose eating or feeding changed it did so by only one ADL level (Specter, et al., 1988). Thus the extreme disability of residents on admission may be such that no change in ADL can be reasonably expected to occur, or ADLs may not be sufficiently sensitive to capture the small changes that do occur over time.

A further concern is that case mix based on ADLs does not correlate consistently with other measures of acuity, such as clinical complexity or diagnoses, for residents in nursing facilities. Spector et al. (1988), for example, found that in one sample, residents classified as clinically complex became more dependent in feeding over 6 months, while in another they became less dependent. Congestive heart failure correlated positively with dependency in transferring in one sample and negatively in another (Specter et al., 1988). The relative stability of ADLs as a proxy for health status is also at odds with variations in the use of other health care resources. One in three residents in nursing home facilities uses an emergency department in any one year; one in four is hospitalized (Aiken et al., 1985). Ray et al. (1987), for example, in a study of elderly Medicaid residents in three states, found that, although ADL levels were similar across states, there were pronounced interstate differences in use of medical care, particularly in relation to hospital use (Ray, et al. 1987).

Although ADLs show little variability, RN employment in nursing facilities varies widely from state to state and does not appear to correlate with a facility's case mix, as determined by level of ADL. The average number of Medicare- and Medicaid-certified beds per RN in 1988 was 17.3, with a range of 7.7 in New Hampshire to 89.8 in Texas.

Thus case mix as currently constructed varies from other health indicators and bears little relationship to RN staffing in nursing facilities. Several explanations for this phenomenon have been proposed including regional variations in hospital use, variations in the relationship of RN to non-RN staffing, practice limitations imposed on RNs in some states, facility size, and RN availability. Unfortunately, studies that examine the relationship between case mix and nurse staffing fail to differentiate between differing levels and roles of nursing personnel in nursing homes. Although the overall functional status of residents within a facility may be adequate to predict total hours of direct nursing care, which is delivered almost exclusively by nurse assistants, functional status may not be an adequate measure on which to base RN hours. Rather, RN hours may better be based on a combination of ADL and other measures of acuity, such as diagnosis, and level of stability and predictability of physical and mental health status (Kearnak, 1989; Mitty, 1989).

The better case-mix systems currently in operation in nursing facilities do, in fact, recognize specific health care problems that require the intervention by different levels of nursing personnel; professional nurses (RNs); licensed practical nurses; or certified nursing assistants (Deane, 1989; Kearnak, 1989; Mitty, 1989). Often missing from even the most sophisticated resident classification systems is the level of professional needed to perform the observation and assessment of residents who are "at risk" for developing additional health problems and the time necessary to react to those problems professionally. For instance, a resident recovering from a hip fracture with a surgical repair may be identified as being functionally dependent but stable. Based on this assessment, the resident will probably receive most of his or her day-to-day care from a certified nursing assistant. In any case, RN will not directly assess the resident's health status on a daily basis. In the early stages of recovery, however, this resident is at risk for the development of a wound infection, pneumonia, and deep vein thrombosis. The chances of these problems developing may be low, especially if the resident is ambulating, eating, and drinking adequate liquids. Nonetheless, the "potential for developing complications" can be predicted, and it is only through periodic professional assessment that a complication can be detected early and given the attention necessary to prevent further deterioration (Kearnak, 1989).

Thus, professional nurse staffing might better be based on a combination of a resident's functional and health status, and potential risk for developing complications, than on functional status alone. In 1989, a panel of experts proposed criteria for predicting nursing needs based on a combination of factors reflective of residents' functional status and "complex needs" (Kearnak, 1989). Using these criteria, three levels of nursing facility residents were identified.

Functionally Dependent with Complex Needs

Residents classified as functionally dependent with complex needs include those relatively stable persons who have been discharged from hospitals but still are acutely ill and require technologies such as ventilators and special feedings. Others who would be classified in this category include the medically fragile, those who continue to be dependent on technologies, individuals who are beginning long-term rehabilitation, and the terminally ill. Individuals requiring extended care services, either in hospitals or nursing homes, are classified in this category.

Five percent of residents currently in nursing facilities are thought to be functionally dependent with complex needs. This number is expected to increase to 10% by the year 2000, 15% by 2010, and 17% by 2020.

Functionally Dependent but Stable

Residents who are classified as functionally dependent but stable are frequently the frail and chronically ill, those with multiple diagnoses, and individuals who are mentally impaired. Measures to promote safety, and prevent and control infection are needed to protect this vulnerable population.

Nursing management for these residents is directed at maintaining and improving current health status, preventing further deterioration, and promoting appropriate available elements of quality of life. Because of multiple dependencies, these residents require more care than those who are functionally assisted, but the care is similar and predictable.

Most (55%) of the current residents in nursing facilities can be classified as functionally dependent but stable. The percentage is expected to increase to 60% in 2000, 65% in 2010, and 73% in 2020.

Functionally Assisted

Residents who are classified as functionally assisted need minimal nursing care, but do need assistance in one or more ADLs. Nursing care for these residents seeks to achieve the highest level of independent function.

Many of the residents in this category are frail and chronically ill; some have behavioral management problems; all are medically stable. To observe for changes, to provide support, to perform interventions, and to provide behavioral management, 24-hour RN coverage is needed.

While at present 40% of the total nursing facility population could be classified as functionally assisted, the panel believed that, in the future, fewer residents requiring functionally assisted care will be in nursing facilities, and that the stay of such residents will be much shorter. They will either be discharged, or their condition will change, thus requiring a different level of care. Alternative methods for providing care, such as adult day care, home care, community health programs, and congregate living setting would allow many of these residents to be cared for in the community. The percentage of all residents that will fit the functionally assisted category is expected to decrease to 30% by the year 2000, 20% in 2010, and 10% in 2020.

In summary, although appropriate for determining nonprofessional staffing levels, there is reason to question the reliability of residents' functional status as the basis for predicting RN staffing needs in nursing facilities. Functional assessments may underestimate or miss other health problems. Staffing derived solely from an ADL-based case-mix methodology may underestimate the number of RNs needed to monitor residents with complex functional, physical, and mental health deficits, resulting in poor quality of care.

Medicaid Reimbursement and RN Staffing

Reimbursement is a second factor often determining the number of professional mix of nurses in nursing facilities. The primary source of reimbursement for most nursing facilities (close to 50% of total revenues) comes from the resident or the resident's family as self-pay. Medicaid reimbursement is the second most common source of payment, accounting for 41% of payments at admission. Medicare pays less than 5% of direct costs for care in nursing facilities. As we will explore further, however, although not reimbursing directly for either health care or hotel services within the home itself, Medicare has a profound influence on the delivery of health care for people in nursing facilities.

State medicaid reimbursement programs often group nursing facility costs into four distinct areas: administrative and routine costs; ancillary and other costs; nursing service costs; and property costs. Nursing service costs, which include all costs associated with direct care of residents such as nursing supplies and direct nursing care hours, are the largest and most importnt of the four groupings, often accounting for close to 40% of all costs.

There are two primary methods for reimbursing nursing services (see Table 4.3) (National Governors Conference, 1989). One method is a resident-based reimbursement system that uses resident assessments to establish

TABLE 4.3 State Medicaid Nursing Facility Payment*

Methods

Prospective payment

Alabama	Florida	Missouri	Rhode Island
Alaska	Georgia	Montana	South Carolina
Arizona	Illinois	Nevada	South Dakota
Arkansas	Indiana	New Jersey	Texas
California	Iowa	New Mexico	Utah
Connecticut	Kentucky	New York	Vermont
Delaware	Louisiana	North Carolina	Wisconsin
District of Columbia	Minnesota	Oklahoma	Wyoming

Retrospective payment

Massachusetts	Pennsylvania	Tennessee

Combination of payments

Colorado	Nebraska	Oregon	Virginia
Idaho	Ohio		

Retrospective (Skilled Nursing Facility) /prospective (Intermediate Care Facility)

Maine	New Hampshire

Case-Mix States

Arizona	Maine	Montana	Ohio
Delaware	Minnesota	Nevada	South Carolina
Illinois	Missouri	New York	Texas

*Based on states that responded to National Governor's Association Survey, 1989.

a ceiling on allowable costs per day for each facility, so that costs can be reimbursed retrospectively up to the ceiling. Some ceilings are set as low as the median, and some states have also placed limits on the number of staff hours per resident day deemed reimbursable (Cohen & Bubay, 1990). The second method is based on preestablished prospective payment rates for each resident or service type. This method pays the facility on the basis of resident specific profiles or case mix. Both of these resident-based approaches require the reporting of resident assessment data to state Medicaid agencies. The retrospective ceiling approach uses quarterly or semiannual special assessment reports, whereas the prospective, case-mix system uses an invoice to report resident status. Both approaches also require the state agency to verify the accuracy of the assessments to avoid the overstatement of resident needs.

Despite a similarity as to process, there are great variations in Medicaid reimbursements to nursing facilities. For example, in 1989, the state Medicaid per diem rates for skilled nursing facilities ranged from a high of $173.51 in the District of Columbia to a low $33.24 in Georgia. In almost all states, Medicaid reimbursement for care in nursing facilities is lower than either private pay and Medicare (National Governor's Conference, 1989).

Inadequate Medicaid reimbursement is the most frequently cited *financial* explanation for low staffing and low salaries of RNs in nursing facilities. Faced with increasing Medicaid nursing facility expenditures, which in 1988 comprised just under 30% of total Medicaid expenditures, many states have been forced to contain costs, primarily by cutting reimbursement or restricting bed supply. States estimate that all the provisions of nursing home reform (OBRA, 1987) will cost states an additional $461.3 million in 1991 (Harrington & Shea, 1991).

Overall, nursing facilities adjust their nurse staffing mix to accommodate the chronic disability levels of residents; homes with higher disability tend to have more RNs and LVNs. Conversely, constraining Medicaid reimbursement results in lower nurse staffing levels (Cohen & Bubay, 1990; Halohan & Cohen, 1987). Nursing facilities in flat-rate reimbursement states, for example, have fewer nurses per bed than similar homes in cost-based reimbursement states (Cohen & Bubay, 1990). In states where Medicaid cost reduction incentives are especially strong, there is some suggestion that staffing is reduced beyond the apparently appropriate level, given the case mix (Cohen & Bubay, 1990).

In addition to restricting the overall number of RNs, Medicaid rates are also blamed for low salaries paid to RNs in nursing facilities in comparison with RNs in hospitals. Average salaries and benefits offered nursing personnel in hospitals and other care settings are approximately one third greater than average salaries and benefits offered in nursing facilities (Mohler & Lessard, 1991). In 1986, almost 10% of RNs in nursing homes made less than $300 per week, and only 17% made $500 per week or more (Jones et al., 1987). Moreover, retention was substantially linked to salary. One-year retention was 65% for nurses earning under $300 per week in comparison with 83% for those earning $500 or more per week. Low salaries also impede the ability of nursing facilities to retain younger nurses. RNs under the age of 35 have a retention rate of 77% in hospitals as compared with 51% in nursing facilities (Jones, et al., 1987).

Mechanisms for increasing RN salaries in nursing facilities has received little discussion in the literature. It is important to remember that the nursing home industry is a multibillion dollar business, with one of the highest growth rates in expenditures among all health services (Harrington & Shea, 1991). Proprietary facilities account for 75% of all nursing facilities and 69% of beds. Chain homes, those that are members of a group of facilities operating under one general authority of general ownership, make up 41% of total homes and 49.3% of total beds (National Center for Health Statistics,

1989). Nursing service is the largest and most flexible cost center in which to decrease expenses and thus increase profits.

Industry spokespeople have sought to encourage a passthrough of government funding to nursing facilities as a prerequisite to increasing RN salaries. The effect of previous passthroughs on RN salaries is unclear, however. Among other problems, it is difficult to monitor whether additional money goes toward RN salaries or the hiring of more RNs. Ullman (1985) found that careful selection of nursing personnel may achieve quality objectives without necessarily increasing operational costs (Ulmann, 1985). Mullinex and Cornelius (1988) computed the dollar figure necessary to increase RN salaries in facilities employing four FTE RNs. For most nursing facilities (average bed size 100 to 200 beds), upgrading salaries to equivalent salaries for supervisory RNs in hospitals would cost approximately $1 per day per nursing home resident. Such an increase could be easily allocated from a facilities operating budget (Mullinex & Cornelius, 1988).

Medicare Disincentives to Improving RN Staffing

By virtue of being a federal program, Medicare's eligibility and benefit structure in principal is similar throughout the United States. In direct payments, Medicare pays for less than 5% of nursing home care, covering long-term care services only when a need for skilled care can be demonstrated. The Medicare skilled benefit is limited to 100 days of service per spell of illness following a hospital stay of at least 3 days. Medicare pays for all routine care during a qualified skilled nursing stay up to 20 days. After day 20, the resident must pay a daily copayment. In addition, Medicare pays for ambulatory and in-hospital care of residents whose stay in the nursing facility is paid for by Medicaid (McMillan et al., 1987).

Although direct payment for nursing home care is small, indirectly Medicare pays for a substantial portion of the health care of nursing home residents. Medicare reimbursement encourages both early discharge of hospital patients to nursing facilities and discharge of nursing facility residents back to the acute care setting for the slightest change in health status. Thus, health problems beyond the most routine continue to result in the resident's transfer from the nursing facility to a physician's office, emergency department, or hospital. Lewis (1989) found that, for a nursing home admission cohort, approximately a half of all transfers are between nursing facility and a general hospital. (Lewis et al., 1987). This continuous "ping-pong" of patients between the nursing facility and hospital contributes to the backup in emergency departments and restricts access of others to hospitals, to say nothing of the negative consequences on the quality of care delivered within the nursing facility.

Several studies have documented that close to one third of hospital admissions generated by skilled nursing facilities could be avoided with better nurse and physician coverage in the nursing home (Holmes et al., 1991; Shaughnessy, Kramer, 1999; Van Buren, 1981). Until recently, the lack of qualified personnel capable of providing this specialized care precluded recommending any substitution of nursing facility for hospital care. Recent demonstration projects and practice arrangements, however, have shown that geriatric nurse practitioners markedly increase the ability of nursing facilities to care for sick residents (Garrard, et al. 1990; Mezey, in press; Shaughnessy, Kramer, & Hittle, 1990; Small & Walsh, 1988). Caring for residents in the facility during an episode of illness has the potential to both improve access and quality of health care.

Before recommending such a shift, however, Medicare must be convinced that change would be cost saving, or at best cost neutral. Medicare pays virtually the full bill for office, emergency department visits, and hospital care for residents in nursing facilities. Because they are dually insured, Medicare even reimburses for physician and acute care services of residents whose nursing facility stay is covered by Medicaid. Convincing Medicare to pay for care that is shifted from the hospital to nursing facility requires data as to the current total cost to Medicare for care of residents in nursing facilities. Unfortunately such data are largely unavailable.

Actual calculation of the total charges to Medicare parts A and B for all health care encounters of nursing facility residents over a period has not yet been done. A 1981 HCFA study of nursing facility residents eligible for both Medicare and Medicaid in four states estimated that these residents each used $2,909 of hospital care and $1,183 of physician care. Using these figures as a guide, Medicare part A and B costs for all nursing facility residents would be in the billions of dollars (Mezey & Scanlon, 1988). A study of hospital readmissions in the Medicare population suggested that in 1984; Medicare spent close to $8 billion on Medicare participant readmission to hospitals (Anderson & Steinberg, 1984). Several studies have imputed Medicare costs savings of between $3,000 and $4,000 per resident resulting from preventable hospitalizations of nursing home resident (Holmes, et al., 1991; Van Buren, 1981; Zimmer, et al., 1988).

Because there are no easily accessible data sets that provide an accurate determination of the total health care services, charges, and costs to Medicare for people who reside in nursing facilities, obtaining such information requires a prospective study that tracks a nursing facility cohort of residents over a set period, and records all ambulatory and acute care services, charges, and payer source. Although expensive, such a study is vital to the development of a rational system of long-term care services.

CONCLUSION

Concern about quality of care in nursing facilities is not new. Stronger regulations and oversight have been effective in correcting many of the past abuses. But the face of nursing facilties has changed dramatically. The acuity of residents in many facilities now resembles that seen on medical units in community hospitals.

Most nursing facilities are attempting to deliver sound care to their residents. But, hampered by inadequate measures of resident acuity and low Medicaid reimbursement, nursing facilities have been unable to convince payers that high resident acuity and low RN staffing is approaching the point that exceeds their ability to provide safe care.

The nursing home industry has fought legislation that would impose higher RN staffing levels without assurances of higher Medicaid and Medicare reimbursement. In the face of current reimbursement, nursing facilities prefer to keep RN staffing low and to transfer residents who evidence the slightest change in health status to hospitals and emergency departments. Despite the added cost and the burden to residents, Medicare reimbursement encourages and reinforces this behavior. Medicare now pays a substantial portion of the health care bill for residents in nursing homes, but it pays for these services in the most expensive setting, the hospital.

We are not alone in calling for better ways to provide quality health care in nursing homes (Kane & Kane, 1991). Basic to considering any change is an accurate accounting of Medicare's portion of the health care bill for residents in nursing facilities, including costs accrued in the facility, the hospital, and ambulatory, part B, costs. Such data would provide the basis for discussions of where health care can best be delivered.

Preliminary data has shown that, with augmented professional nurse and physician services, a substantial number of nursing facility residents currently transferred to hospitals can be cared for equally well in the nursing facility, at a much lower cost. The next step is to determine how generalizable these findings are and the extent to which care in nursing facilities can safely substitute for care in hospitals.

REFERENCES

Aiken, L., Mezey, J., Lynaugh, J., & Buck, C. (1985). Teaching nursing homes: Prospects for improving long-term care. *Journal of the American Geriatric Association, 33,* 223–229.

American Health Care Association. (1988, July). *AHCA manpower survey: Preliminary report* (Unpublished data). Washington, DC: American Hospital Association.

American Nurses Association. (1986). *Gerontological nurses in clinical settings: Survey analysis* (GE-11 1M). Kansas City, MO: American Nurses Association.

American Nurses Association. (1990). *Facts about nursing.* Kansas City, MO: American Nurses Association Nursing Information Bureau.

Anderson, G., & Steinberg, E. (1984). Hospital readmissions in the medicare population. *New England Journal of Medicine, 311,* 1349–1353.

Cohen, J., & Bubay, L. (1990). The effects of medicaid reimbursement method and ownership on nursing home costs, case mix, and staffing. *Inquiry, 27,* 183–200.

Cotler, M., & Kane, R. (1988). Registered nurses and nursing home shortages: Job conditions and attitudes among RNs. *Journal of Long Term Care Administration, 16,* 13–18.

Deane, R. T. (1989). Is your reimbursement system fair? *American Health Care Association Journal,* 41–56.

Densen, P. (1991). *Tracing the elderly through the health care system: An update: Research activities* (Publication No. 141). Washington DC: U.S. Department of Health and Human Services, PHS, Agency for Health Care Policy and Research.

Donebedian, A. (1981). Advantages and limitations of explicit criteria for assessing the quality of health care. *Milbank Quarterly, 59,* 99–104.

Fitzgerald, J., Moore, P., & Dittus, R. (1988). The care of elderly patients with hip fracture: Changes since implementation of the prospective payment system. *New England Journal of Medicine, 319,* 1392–1397.

Fottler, M., Smith, H., & James, W. (1981). Profits and patient care quality in nursing homes: Are they compatible? *The Gerontologist, 21,* 31–38.

Freund, C. (in press). Research findings on the use of nurse practitioners. In M. Mezey & D. McGivern (Eds.), *Nurses, nurse practitioners: The evolution of primary care.* New York: Springer.

Garrard, J., Kane, R., Ratner, E., & Buchanan, J. (1991). The impact of nurse clinicians on the care of nursing home residents. In P. Katz, R. Kane, & M. Mezey (eds.), *Advances in long-term care* (Vol. 1). New York: Springer.

Halohan, J., & Cohen, J. (1987). Nursing home reimbursement: Implications for cost containment, access, and quality. *The Milbank Quarterly, 65,* 111–147.

Harrington, C., Swann, J., & Grant, L. (1988). State medicaid reimbursement for nursing homes, 1978–86, *Health Care Financing Review, 9,* 33–50.

Harrington, C., & Shea, S. (1991). Effects of nursing reimbursement rates on access to care for medicare beneficiaries, particularly those who are underserved. Paper prepared for the American Nurses Association.

Health Care Financing Administration. (1988). Unpublished data.

Hing, E. (1989). *Effects of the prospective payment system on nursing homes* Department of Health and Human Services Publication No. [PHS] 89–1759). Washington, DC: U.S. Government Printing Office.

Holmes, D., Bloom, H., Teresi, J., Monaco, C., & Rosen, S. (1991). An examination of nursing home transfers to hospitals: Final report. New York: The United Hospital Fund.

Institute of Medicine. (1986). *Improving the quality of care in nursing homes.* Washington, DC: National Academy Press.

Johnson, M. A., & Connelly, J. R. (1990). *Nursing and gerontology: Status report.* Washington DC: Association for Gerontology in Higher Education.

Jones, D., Bonito, A., Gower, J., & Williams R. (1987). *Analysis of the environment for recruitment and retention of registered nurses in nursing homes.* Washington, DC: U.S. Government Printing Office, USDHS, PHS, HRSA, Bureau of Health Professions, Division of Nursing.

Kaeser, L. (1981). The relationship between patient care expenditures and quality of care. Unpublished doctoral thesis, Cornell University, Ithaca.

Kahn, J., Keeler, E. B., Sherwood, S. M. et al. (1990). Common outcomes of care before and after implementation of the DRG based prospective payment system. *Journal of the American Medical Association, 264,* 1984–1988.

Kane, R. L., & Kane, R. A. (1991). A nursing home in your future? *New England Journal of Medicine, 324,* 627–629.

Kearnsk, J. M. (1989, June). *Report of the 1989 Panel of Experts meeting to* review and update the criteria for the criteria-based model. Washington, DC: U.S. Government Printing Office, U.S. Department of Health and Human Services, PHS, HRSA, Bureau of Health Manpower, Division of Nursing.

Kemper, P., & Murtaugh, C. M. (1991). Lifetime use of nursing home care. *New England Journal of Medicine, 324,* 595–600.

Konda, K., & Mezey, M. (1991). Registered nurse staffing in Pennsylvania nursing homes: Comparison before and after implementation of Medicare's prospective payment system. *The Gerontologist, 31,* 318–324.

Kramer, A., Shaughnessey, P., & Pettigrew, M. (1985). Cost-effectiveness implication based on a comparison of nursing home and home health case mix. *Health Services Research, 20,* 388–403.

Kurrerow, R. (1990, April). *Resident abuse in nursing homes: Understanding and preventing abuse* (pp. 17–19). Washington, DC: U.S. Government Printing Office.

Lavizzo-Mourey, R., Mezey, M., & Taylor, L. (1991). Completeness of resident's admission assessments in teaching nursing homes. *Journal of the American Geriatric Society, 39,* 433–439.

Lewis, A., Leake, B., Leal-Sotelo, M., & Clark, V. (1987). The initial effects of the prospective payment system on nursing home patients. *American Journal of Public Health, 77,* 819–822.

Linn, M., Gurel, L., & Linn, A. B. (1977). Patient outcome as a measure of quality of nursing home care. *American Journal of Public Health, 67,* 337–344.

Lyles, L. (1986). Impact of Medicare diagnosis-related groups (DRGs) on nursing homes in the Portland, Oregon, metropolitan areas. *Journal of the American Geriatric Society, 34,* 573–577.

McMillan, A., et al. (1987, Winter). Nursing home costs for those dually entitled to Medicare and Medicaid. *Health Care Financing Review, 9,* 1–14.

Mech, A., (1980). Evaluating the process of nursing care in long-term care facilities. *Quality Review Bulletin, 6,* 24–30.

Mezey, M., & Scanlon, W. (1988). *Registered nurses in nursing homes: Secretary's Commission on Nursing.* Washington, DC: Department of Health and Human Services.

Mezey, M., Lavizzo-Mourey, R., Brunswick, J., & Taylor, L. (in press). The assessment of nursing home patients. *Nurse Practitioner.*

Mezey, M. (in press). Care in nursing homes: Patients' needs: Nursings' response. In L. Aiken & C. Fagin (Eds.), *Nursing in the 90s.* Philadelphia: J. P. Lippincott.

Mitty E. (1989) Response to institutional care: Caregivers and quality. *Indices of quality in long-term care research and practice.* New York: National League for Nursing.

Mohler, M., & Lessard, W. (1991, March). Nursing staff in nursing homes: Additional staff needed and cost to meet requirement and intent of OBRA '87. Washington DC: Nation Committee to Preserve Social Security and Medicare.

Morrisey, M., Sloan, F., & Valvona, J. (1988). Medicare prospective payment and posthospital transfers to sub-acute care. *Medical Care, 26,* 685–698.

Mullinex, C., & Cornelius, B. (1988). In M. Mezey & W. Scanlon (Eds.).

Munroe, D. (1990). The influence of registered nurse staffing on quality of nursing home care. *Research in Nursing & Health, 13,* 263–270.

National Association of State Budget Officers. (1991). *Cost estimates of enacted federal medicaid expansions.*

National Center for Health Statistics. (1989). *The National Nursing Home Survey: 1985 summary for the United States* (DHHS). Publication No. [PHS] 89-1758). Washington, DC: U.S. Government Printing Office.

National Governors Conference. (1989). Washington, DC: National Governors Association.

Neu, C. R., & Harrison, S. (1988). Posthospital care before and after the medicare prospective payment system. Santa Monica, CA: The RAND/UCLA Center for Health Care Financing Policy Research.

Rango, N. (1985). The nursing home resident with dementia: Clinical care, ethics and policy implications. *Annals of Internal Medicine, 102,* 835–839.

Ray, W., Federspiel, C., Baugh, D., & Dodds, P. (1987). Interstate variation in elderly medicaid nursing home populations. *Medical Care, 25,* 738–752.

Robert Wood Johnson Foundation. (1982). *Medical practice in the United States: A special report* (pp. 34–35) Princeton NJ.

Sager, M. Easterling, D., & Leventhal, E. (1989). An evaluation of increased mortality rates in Wisconsin nursing homes. *Journal of the American Geriatric Society, 37,* 774–776.

Shaughnessy, P., Kramer, A., & Hittle, D. (1990, March). *The teaching nursing home experiment: Its effects and implications (Study Paper 6).* Denver: University of Colorado, Center for Health Services Research.

Shaughnessy, P., & Kramer, A. (1990). The increased needs of patients in nursing homes and patients receiving home health care. *New England Journal of Medicine, 322,* 21–27.

Small, N., & Walsh, M. (1988). *Teaching nursing homes: The nursing perspective.* Owings Mill, MD: National Health Publishing.

Solomon, P. (1988). Geriatric assessment: Methods for clinical decision making. *Journal of the American Medical Association, 259,* 24–50.

Spector, W. D., Kapp, M., Eichan, A., Tucker, R. Rosenstein, R., & Katz, S. (1988). *Case-mix outcomes and resource use in nursing homes.* Providence RI: Brown University, Center for Gerontology and health Care Ressearch.

Specter, W. D. (1989). Reforming nursing home quality regulation: Impact on cited deficiencies and nursing home outcomes. *Medical Care, 8,* 789–801.

Tellis-Nayak, V. (1988). *Nursing home exemplars of quality.* Springfield, IL: Charles C Thomas Publisher.

Ulmann, S. (1985). The impact of quality on cost in the provision of long-term care. *Inquiry, 22,* 293–302.

U.S. Senate, Special Committee on Aging, Subcommittee on Long-Term Care. (1976, March). Major points of supporting paper No. 4 (Issued April 24, 1975). Nurses in nursing homes: The heavy burden (the reliance on untrained and unlicensed personnel). *Nursing home care in the United States: Failure of policy* (pp. XVIII–XIX). Washington, D.C.: U.S. Government Printing Office.

Van Buren, C. B. (1981). The acute-hospitalization of residents of skilled nursing facilities in Monroe County, New York. Unpublished master's thesis, University of Rochester, Department of Preventive Medicine and Rehabilitation, Rochester.

Zimmer, J, Eggert, G., Treat, A., & Brodows, B. (1988). Nursing homes as acute care providers. *Journal of the American Geriatric Society, 36,* 124–129.

5

The Changing Role of the Nursing Home Medical Director

Steven A. Levenson

In the past several years, the job of medical direction in long-term care has become much more visible, but is only now starting to receive the recognition, prestige, and compensation that it rightfully deserves. This chapter will consider why it is so important, what it entails, and how a physician can fulfill the role both for personal satisfaction and to meet the facility's and the resident's needs.

THE CHANGING FACE OF NURSING HOMES

Nursing homes have changed dramatically during the past decade, reflecting both an aging, increasingly disabled population in addition to a new regulatory focus on resident rights, quality of life, and comprehensive assessment. The nursing home has, for all intents and purposes, become a primary site for managing advanced old age, and the health problems accompanying and associated with aging. There are currently more people (1.5 million) in nursing home beds than in acute care hospital beds in the United States (American Medical Association Council on Scientific Affairs, 1990). Most nursing home residents are older than age 65 (mean age, 83 years), predominantly female (approximately two thirds), physically disabled with respect to basic ADLs, and cognitively impaired (Ouslander, 1989).

One fourth of those reaching age 65 will spend some time in a nursing home before they die. Because of shorter lengths of hospital stay under prospective payment reimbursement, nursing homes are receiving sicker patients and providing more medical care than ever before. More nursing home residents are dying within 30 days of admission including more terminally ill patients transferred to nursing homes just before death. Many nursing homes are having trouble providing this more intensive medical care complicated by insufficient staff, and adequate medical and rehabilitation programs and support systems (American Medical Association Council on Scientific Affairs, 1990).

The nursing home population is very diverse. Facilities and attending physicians must manage a broad spectrum of age groups, illnesses, functional problems, and goals of care. Nursing home residents range from those who enter very ill with a life expectancy of less than 6 months to those with a mix of physical and cognitive impairments who will remain institutionalized for many years (Ouslander, 1989).

Thus, American nursing homes are undergoing a major reorientation of their functions and relationships. They are shifting from a predominantly social model providing personal care toward a health care model managing illnesses and dysfunctions. Simultaneously, the roles of caregivers within nursing homes are changing.

MEDICAL DIRECTOR'S ROLES AND FUNCTIONS

Nursing home care challenges physicians and other caregivers in many ways. Physicians and nursing home staff and administration are starting to appreciate the medical director's critical role in dealing with these challenges effectively.

The medical director's role has evolved substantially since its inception. The nursing home medical director concept is less than 2 decades old (Reichel, 1983). In 1973, the American Medical Association published a list of basic job responsibilities entitled *Guidelines for a Medical Director in a Long-Term Care Facility.* In 1974, the Department of Health, Education and Welfare regulations required every skilled nursing facility to retain a full- or part-time medical director, either directly by the facility, or through arrangements with local physician groups, medical societies, or hospital medical staffs. These regulations contained little more for the medical director than a detailed job description. There were few mandatory responsibilities, and little enforcement of physician performance.

In 1977, the American Medical Association issued a booklet of articles about the medical director (American Medical Association, 1977). A 1978 study (Ingman, Lawson, & Carboni, 1978) reviewed the early development of this medical director role, and presented the views of more than 1,000 administrators, nurses, and physicians about the responsibilities, authority, and impact of the nursing home medical director. Most respondents agreed that medical directors should be primarily responsible for creating written policies for physician care, enforcing medical staff compliance with institutional and statutory regulations, participating in nursing and other professional and staff conferences, and contributing to the quality assurance program. The respondents, however, were divided on the desirability of more "activist" roles, such as negotiation with fiscal third parties on controversial denials of payment, initiation of educational programs, supervising rehabilitation care, deciding on the need for admission and placement of patients, conducting floor rounds, and having broader responsibilities for the social well-being of residents beyond strictly medical care. Many physicians were reluctant to have medical directors become a chief of service or act in a consultant role.

During the ensuing decade, most nursing homes continued to resemble the description of a 1957 study (Solon & Roberts, 1957) of being "divorced from the mainstreams of medical care." There was little further discussion of medical direction until articles and books about the medical director began to appear in the middle to late 1980s (Fanale, 1989; Levenson, 1988; Pattee, 1983; Staats, 1988).

The real impetus to the further evolution of the medical director's role, and the legal foundation for that role, has come from the extensively revised federal nursing home regulations ("Conditions of Participation for Medicare and Medicaid"). These have become known as the "OBRA '87" regulations, because the law mandating their revision was part of the 1987 federal OBRA Act.

The October 1, 1990, implementation of these regulations was the result of a process that began in the early 1980s. It has included the 1986 Institute of Medicine study on nursing home care (Institute of Medicine, 1986), the OBRA '87 law, the actual regulations, surveyor's guidelines, public comments, advisory committee meetings, drug reviews, internal HCFA reviews, surveyor training, development of the MDS, nurse's aide training, and many ancillary rules. The first draft of these regulations did not appear until 1989, and they were not final until late 1991 (HCFA, 1991). Some parts of the rule-making process were not scheduled to be completed until spring 1992.

These regulatory changes resulted largely from a perception that the care for the nation's 1.5 million nursing home residents was inconsistent and often inadequate. Table 5.1 highlights some of the clinical problems (including those related to medical care) that the regulations were intended to address.

These revised regulations say very little about the medical director. Although original federal regulations required a medical director only in SNFs, the OBRA '87 regulations have mandated a medical director in all the nation's nursing homes (now referred to in the regulations as nursing facilities). The only explicit requirements are to oversee the medical care and to coordinate the facility's resident care policies. There are many implicit responsibilities, however, because of the many expectations for improved clinical care and oversight placed on facilities. The interpretive guidelines accompanying the regulations hold the medical director accountable for

TABLE 5.1 Clinical Issues Addressed in the OBRA '87 Regulations

---

More consistent access for nursing home residents to necessary medical care
More consistently adequate and accurate medical and nursing assessments
More services to maximize function and minimize side effects and complications of treatments
Improved mechanisms to enable nursing home residents to participate in their own care
Better evaluation of resident competence
More adequate medical coverage and information on discharge from facilities
More judicious use of restraints and psychotropic medications
Better continuity of care during resident transfers across the health care system
Greater consistency in nursing care plans to address residents' needs, condition, and wishes
More timely and pertinent physician evaluations after admission
More nursing, medical, and other services to maintain the highest possible levels of mental, physical, and functional well-being
More consistent creation and implementation of policies and programs to prevent and manage clinical problems
More timely physician response to changes in patient status
More consistent evaluation of rehabilitation potential
Maintenance of more complete, accurate, useful, and systematically organized medical records

---

helping ensure the application of appropriate professional standards and for taking action when clinical care is inconsistent with those standards.

Some people question whether these OBRA '87 regulations will help improve outcome among the elderly in nursing homes, or whether they will cost more money, demand more time, and simply shift from one set of rules to another. If they work as intended, the new nursing home regulations could help improve the professionalism and the care in many nursing homes nationwide. But their success will require the full collaboration of all concerned including physicians.

Optional and Mandatory Responsibilities

In 1988, a group of medical directors met under the auspices of Dr. James Pattee to develop a comprehensive list of roles, functions, and tasks for nursing home medical directors (Pattee, 1991). Table 5.2 list these major administrative functions.

Only the first three of these functions are mandated. The remainder represent a broader, more "activist" physician role that could help improve the quality of care in the nursing home. It remains for further studies to demonstrate to what extent that is true.

TABLE 5.2 Major Medical Director Functions

Participate in administrative decision making, and recommend and approve policies and procedures

Organize and coordinate physician's and other professional's services as they relate to patient care

Ensure the appropriateness and quality of medical and medically related care

Participate in the development and conduct of education programs

Help articulate the facility's mission to the community, and represent the facility in the community

Participate in the surveillance and promotion of the health, welfare, and safety of employees

Acquire, maintain, and apply knowledge of social, regulatory, political, and economic factors that relate to patient care services

Provide medical leadership for research and development activities in geriatrics and long-term care

Participate in establishing policies and procedures to assure that the rights of individuals are respected

---

PHYSICIAN'S ROLE

The need of nursing home residents for quality medical care is being recognized and the message disseminated. Though many of the problems of nursing home residents are more functional and psychosocial than medical, the increasing acuity of medical conditions in this population requires greater physician involvement. Indirectly, the OBRA '87 regulations hold physicians increasingly responsible for adequate assessments, better documentation, and justification of poor outcomes of care (Ouslander, 1989).

One likely reason for minimal physician participation in nursing home care is the relative lack of formal training and professional support for nursing home practice. Although there is more formal postgraduate training in geriatric medicine and the principles of nursing home care than in the past, and more graduates of geriatrics fellowship training programs, the statistics on physician participation in nursing homes are still not encouraging. Although primary care practitioners render most nursing home medical care, only a small minority of such physicians care for nursing home patients (Mitchell & Hewes, 1986). Some communities only have one or two physicians to provide such care. Only a few nursing homes retain any full- or part-time medical staff.

Like other practitioners, physicians find that providing good care to nursing home residents is emotionally and physically demanding and time consuming. There may be abundant external social, political, and regulatory pressures, but little concrete support. Often, reimbursement for individuals and facilities has not been commensurate with the time and effort spent to provide good quality care. Medicine's highest monetary and professional rewards have traditionally been reserved for physicians who deliver high-technology care or perform procedures, not for those who deliver care in such settings, or for those who spend time to solve complex problems. Reimbursement for nursing home visits has been among the lowest of all physician services.

A new "Relative Value Scale" system for reimbursing physicians, effective in 1992, is expected to increase reimbursement for primary care services and lower it for those who do procedures; allow practitioners to see more than one patient per visit without being penalized; and be reimbursed for time spent reviewing information with the staff, patient, and family, and for time spent to comply with the regulatory requirements intended to improve quality of care (Medicare Program Fee Schedule, 1991). It remains to be seen how much this will improve the reimbursement to physicians treating nursing home residents.

As in the past, nursing homes will likely continue to rely heavily on general internists and family physicians in private practice to provide most medical care to the residents. Thus, those physicians providing nursing home care need considerable support, including an effective, efficient system of care, to help them meet these clinical demands appropriately. The medical director is a key person to offer such support, and to integrate the medical care successfully with other services and programs for the facility residents.

INTERDISCIPLINARY CONCEPT

Consistent with the emphasis of contemporary geriatrics, physicians are appreciating more the interdisciplinary nature of nursing home care. The diverse nursing home population requires medical flexibility. The management of a short-stay rehabilitation patient differs significantly from that of a short-stay terminally ill person, or of a long-term ambulatory but cognitively and functionally impaired person. Many problems of nursing home residents are not medical symptoms. Only some of their medical problems may respond—often, only partially—to current medical treatments.

To meet residents' care needs and comply with regulations, attending physicians must collaborate with many others involved in that care including social workers, dietitians, nurses, nurse aides, and physical and occupational therapists. Others impacting care include families, administrators, regulators, ombudsmen, and lawyers. Also, there are greater expectations for the resident's participation in care decisions.

The new comprehensive assessment (the MDS), mandated by OBRA '87 regulations, expands the role of nonphysicians in doing systematic geriatric assessments. Attending physicians must make diagnoses and prescribe treatments, but other staff also must observe, monitor, document, and report information. Now, nursing staff may be able to provide attending physicians with better clinical information, or may be better informed about a medical diagnosis or treatment, or the possible complications of treatment (e.g., medications causing side effects or a plan of care that does not appear consistent with a resident's functional problems).

One significant medical director role is to encourage attending physicians to respect this interdisciplinary approach, and to pay more attention to the information provided by other staff. The medical director should help attending physicians understand the potential benefits of broader support for gathering information and making decisions. These benefits could include earlier detection of acute illness and its complications, better prevention of iatrogenic illness, greater family and resident satisfaction with care, and reduced legal liability.

CLINICAL SUPPORT OF LONG-TERM MEDICAL CARE

There is growing recognition of important distinctions between providing care in the acute and long-term care setting. Although acute care emphasizes treating a medical disease or condition, nursing home care emphasizes restoring and maintaining functional capabilities, supporting maximal autonomy and quality of life, and providing comfort and dignity for those who are dying. Nursing home medical interventions focus on managing chronic medical conditions and preventing and recognizing acute medical and iatrogenic illnesses (Ouslander, 1990).

Medical directors can help improve clinical care by helping attending physicians and other caregivers manage acute and chronic illness more effectively in the nursing home. Several studies have suggested a high incidence of potentially remediable medical conditions in the nursing home including malnutrition, dehydration, hyponatremia, depression, and infections. Apparently, many such problems could be treated successfully in their earlier stages in the nursing home, thus preventing costly and traumatic hospital admissions (American Medical Association Council on Scientific Affairs, 1991). Although some studies now offer useful data to support clinical decision making on nursing home patients, more information is needed about optimal management of chronic and intercurrent acute illnesses in this population.

Used appropriately, such information can help attending physicians give better advice and help enhance residents' quality of life through more rational care decisions. As Table 5.3 illustrates, however, the medical decision-making process in the nursing home is multifaceted. Many people, including physicians with nursing home practices, still seem not to recognize these

TABLE 5.3 Questions in Medical Decision Making in the Nursing Home

When is a symptom, change, or problem a *medical* problem?
If it is a medical problem, is it due to aging or disease, or both?
Is it at least somewhat treatable?
Can the patient give a useful medical history?
If not, what useful medical information do we have?
Is the problem due to existing treatments (medications)?
Would a test be helpful?
Is there a regulation?
What are we treating?
Is it a new illness or a complication of an existing one?
Should we be treating it at all?
What are the potential risks-benefits of the treatment?
How vigorously should it be treated and for how long?
What is the goal of treatment?
Who determines what the treatment should accomplish?
Does the patient know what he or she wants?
Can the patient participate in making decisions?
If not, did the patient complete an advance directive?
Does the family know what the patient wants?
Does the family agree on what the patient wants or should have?
Did the doctor explain all this, and did anyone listen?
Is there a regulation?
Does the staff understand what they are treating and why?
Is the staff giving the treatment consistently and correctly?
If not, will anyone inform the physician?
How will the doctor know if the treatment is working?
If a medication or treatment is not working, should we give more of it, less of it,
    something else, or nothing at all?
Do we need a consultant?
Is a consultant available?
Should the resident be sent to the acute hospital?
How will the tests and treatments be paid for?
Is there sufficient documentation to understand the reasons for these conclusions and
    decisions?
Did others document enough so the doctor knows what is going on, because the
    patient often cannot give this information?

complexities, or how they can affect the management of medical illness in nursing home residents.

The extent to which medical problems (e.g., fever, shortness of breath, aspiration pneumonia) of nursing home residents should be treated depends on available therapy, prognosis, and the wishes of the resident and family. An effective system to ascertain those wishes must be combined with good communications and policies and protocols for cooperative management between physicians and other caregivers.

The management of terminal illness deserves special consideration. Many elderly are now dying in nursing homes, instead of in acute hospitals or at home. They require measures for comfort and pain relief. Also, studies suggest that nursing home residents are interested in discussing limited treatment options, and that there is limited value in doing cardiopulmonary resuscitation in the nursing home (Gamble, McDonald, & Lichstein 1991; New law, 1990).

Thus, medical directors must have, and should promote, a broader understanding of the meaning and implications of clinical care in the nursing home beyond the medical management of acute and chronic illness. This implies helping both physicians and nonphysicians—facility staff, residents, administrators, families, regulatory agencies, and so on—appreciate the potential benefits and limits of medical intervention, and promoting an appropriate interdisciplinary care process. More than ever before, attending physicians in the nursing home must coordinate their management of diseases, including their orders, with the patients' wishes and the plans and activities of other caregivers.

ESTABLISHMENT OF MEDICAL DIRECTOR ROLE

Most medical directors serve part time, and cover one or two facilities. Most are either primary care internists or family physicians, who take care of at least some patients in their facilities. Currently, there are two groups of medical directors: one of physicians toward the end of their careers and the other of physicians recently out in practice. Older medical directors have a lot of experience, and younger ones tend to have more formal training in, or exposure to, geriatric medicine. Efforts are being made to reduce the gap between experience and training.

Both new and experienced medical directors are searching for tactics to help them fulfill their expanding responsibilities in a time- and cost-effective fashion. Table 5.4 lists the steps by which they may accomplish this objective. These steps are discussed in more detail later.

Understanding of Job

The first step is to try to understand a medical director's roles, and the required and optional functions of those roles. As noted, OBRA '87 regulations require a medical director to at least be responsible for the medical care in the facility and to implement resident care policies. The Interpretive Guidelines accompanying these regulations expand somewhat on these responsibilities, as follows (Interpretive Guidelines, 1991).

The medical director is specifically responsible for implementing resident care policies (regarding admissions, transfers, and discharges; infection con-

TABLE 5.4 Steps to Establishing the Medical Director Role

Understand the job
Assess the facility
Create a job description and medical director contract
Clarify legal liability
Establish and refine relationships and lines of communication with key people including committees
Organize the medical staff as needed
Create or refine bylaws or other practice guidelines as indicated
Create effective policies and procedures to guide physician practices and establish standards for care
Help create effective communications and information management systems
Oversee and evaluate the care
Review physician practices according to established standards
Provide feedback and education to the attending physicians and the other staff based on these and other assessments
Help the facility deal with regulatory and related issues
Advocate for change and improvement within the facility
Liaison with other physicians and medical directors locally and nationally
Arrange personal continuing medical education to keep abreast of relevant administrative and clinical issues

trol; physician privileges and practices, responsibilities of non-physician health care workers (e.g., nursing, rehabilitation therapies, and dietary services in resident care, emergency care, and resident assessment and care planning); accidents and incidents; ancillary services such as laboratory, radiology, and pharmacy; use of medications; use and release of clinical information; utilization review; and overall quality of care. The guidelines note, however, that a medical director who only approves resident care policies does not meet the requirement..

The regulations also require facilities to operate and provide services in compliance with federal, state, and local laws, *and* consistent with accepted professional standards and principles pertinent to professionals providing services in the facility. Thus, the medical director is also responsible for assuring that the facility is providing appropriate care in general, and that the care of individual residents is adequate. When inadequate or inappropriate care is identified, the medical director is responsible for taking action to try to correct the situation including consultation with the resident or the resident's physician. The medical director also must ensure timely visits and adequate medical coverage.

Few medical directors will have the same scope or priority of responsibilities. Many will focus primarily or exclusively on the mandatory functions, whereas others will also handle additional areas. How the medical director meets these and other responsibilities, and to what extent, depends substantially on an assessment of each facility compared with personal availability, knowledge, skills, and interests.

Assessment of Facility

Before accepting a position as medical director, and periodically thereafter, a physician should assess the job requirements and work circumstances.

To decide what is personally relevant, a medical director should assess the facility, and discuss with the administrator and director of nursing their priorities and other desired activities. This process includes (a) evaluating a facility's current and planned goals, programs, and services, and their pertinence to the needs of the population to be served; (b) assessing the commitment of the ownership and management to providing quality care, to giving the medical director essential support, and to being receptive to medical input; and (c) evaluating a facility's or organization's overall soundness (e.g., by reviewing representative financial statements).

The physician should then consider whether he has the time and willingness to commit to the relevant on-site and off-site activities. In doing this, he should distinguish the administrative responsibilities from the time spent on direct patient care, although both roles overlap somewhat.

Creation of Job Description and Contract

A physician's time commitment will vary with facility size, the medical complexity of the residents, and the expectations of the administrator and director of nursing. It also depends on the extent to which the medical director is new to the job or is organizing a new medical staff system, as opposed to improving or refining an existing system. Once a medical director establishes effective systems, ongoing management should take less time.

Every medical director should have a written job description. This is best done after first reviewing the requirements of medical direction, and then assessing the facility's desires and needs for additional roles and responsibilities.

A medical director's contract should specify responsibilities and approximate time expectations; terms of the relationship (employee, contractor, etc.); compensation and benefits; secretarial support; and any financial support for education, meetings, and acquiring pertinent reference materials. Also, it should ensure that the medical director will receive adequate support and authority to do the job properly.

With their expanded responsibilities under OBRA '87, medical directors may need at least 4 to 8 administrative hours a month per 100 beds to be effective. Less than an hour a week is almost certainly insufficient.

Clarification of Liabilities

Medical directors have certain legal liabilities separate from those related to direct patient care.

Medical directors must carry out their oversight functions appropriately and take effective action as needed. Under OBRA '87 regulations, medical directors are expected to oversee care, to look for certain high-risk or high-volume problems, to help institute preventive measures, and to *do something* or encourage the facility and its staff to do something when inadequate or inappropriate care is observed. Concurrently, they will be more liable than in the past for failing to oversee care and take effective action. The era of nominal medical direction, of merely signing orders or completing forms, is past.

Nationwide, lawyers have been taking more nursing home cases, and juries have been making more awards (Lawyers find gold, 1991). For instance, a Houston, Texas jury awarded $39.4 million to the family of an 84-year-old resident who died by strangulation from a vest restraint. A McComb, Mississippi, jury awarded $250,000 in compensatory and punitive damages to each of two families for generally negligent care in a nursing facility (Suits against nursing facilities, 1990).

Recognizing that basic preventive measures can reduce significantly risk to patients, facilities, and professionals, medical directors should support effective risk-management programs in their facilities. Many of these risk-reduction measures are discussed openly in the OBRA '87 regulations (e.g., comprehensive periodic assessments, careful use of medications, prompt communication of significant changes in condition, and effective communication with residents and families including more involvement in care planning).

The medical director also should clarify liability coverage, because a medical malpractice policy may not cover performance of administrative duties. Often, the medical director can be covered under a facility's blanket administrative liability policy.

Establishment of Relationships

A medical director should understand how the facility is organized. how the physicians fit in, to whom the medical director is responsible and who is responsible to him, and how best to communicate with the administrator, director of nursing, and other key staff.

In general, the nursing home medical director is the functional equivalent of the medical executive committee in the acute hospital. Representing both the physicians and the facility, the medical director has an essential role in coordinating medical services with other disciplines. Representing the physicians, the medical director's role is to handle many of the systems issues (such as committees, regulations, and creation of protocols for managing clinical problems) that affect medical care, freeing the attending physicians to provide the care as effectively and efficiently as possible. Representing the facility, the medical director must ensure adequate, appropriate, timely, and good quality medical coverage that meets the residents' health care needs and helps the facility fulfill its legal and regulatory obligations.

As a manager, the medical director arranges coverage, oversees performance, and gives information and performance feedback to physicians and nonphysicians. This also involves explaining rules to people, attaining their cooperation, and sometimes asking them to change their practices or patterns of care.

Attending physicians are generally independent minded, and often frustrated by the problems and limitations of nursing home care. The typical medical director is a primary care practitioner who may find it difficult to shift to a management mode, and to perform quality assurance activities on the patients of friends and colleagues. At times, nursing home medical directors may also be handicapped by limited authority and capacity to enforce change. For those medical directors who provide primary care to nursing home residents, oversight of such care may also become problematic.

Many medical directors have found it helpful to assess their personal styles of communication and management, and to understand how these may help or hinder their efforts to interact with many different physicians and nonmedical people, with their widely varying personalities and styles. These variations in personal management styles relate mostly to the degree of authority used by the manager and to the amount of freedom available to subordinates to participate in decisions (Pattee & Otteson, 1991, p. 81).

Committees

Under the OBRA '87 regulations, the medical director must oversee the resident care policies. Committees are an important part of interdisciplinary communication, and the backbone of policy formulation in the nursing home.

The medical director must work effectively with committees in the nursing home, so they will support the medical staff and the medical care. The OBRA '87 regulations require only a Quality Assurance (QA) committee. However, other common nursing home committees include pharmacy and therapeutics review, medical records, and infection control.

More medical directors are finding that they can be more effective by better understanding group dynamics, and the means to make committee meetings more effective. The medical director and other key staff should decide together on an efficient way to hold these meetings. Many facilities hold combined meetings, in which the same key staff participate in handling several functions (medical records, infection control, risk management, etc.) consecutively. Often, nursing home staffs are finding the QA committee to be a valuable focus for solving and preventing problems, and for obtaining critical interdisciplinary participation.

Organization of Medical Staff

The medical director must ensure adequate and timely medical coverage for the facility's residents. This may be accomplished in several ways.

Typically, nursing facilities have used any of several different physician staffing arrangements. Most still use open staffs of community-based attending physicians. Possible advantages of direct care provision by private attendings include having knowledge of and familiarity with patients; allowing residents more choice of physician; and avoiding conflict of interest of the medical director having to evaluate his or her own care.

Especially in larger nursing homes (more than 200 beds), some medical directors are turning to closed staffs, sometimes hiring full- or part-time salaried physicians. Possible advantages of closed staffs include more timely medical intervention, more control over staff performance, easier access to medical input for problem solving, better follow-up and continuity of care, loyalty to the facility and its goals and philosophy, better interactions with nursing home staff, and better compliance with regulations.

More medical directors are realizing the importance of organizing their attending physicians to some degree. They have found it difficult to exercise their responsibility without a system that enables them to assert some authority. Attending physicians must know the regulations, policies, and expectations underlying their performance. This is also critical if the medical director is to fulfill QA oversight functions.

More medical directors are using bylaws (also referred to as practice agreements) to organize attending physicians and to create a foundation for medical care. Bylaws describe the legal foundations and the structure and functions underlying medical staff activity, establish a broad general framework of expectations for physician performance, create a mechanism for enforcing responsibility, and establish ground rules for the medical staff to carry out its responsibilities to the residents and the facility. They establish the medical staff as a self-governing entity and define its relationship to the governing body, which is ultimately responsible for the care delivered in the facility. Sample bylaws are available from the American Medical Directors Association and elsewhere (Levenson, 1988; Pattee & Otteson, 1991).

Because the nursing home medical director typically serves the functions of the chief of staff and medical executive committee in the acute hospital, nursing home medical staff bylaws can be simpler than those for hospital medical staffs. At the least, these bylaws should have practitioners acknowledge that they understand the regulatory and clinical demands on contemporary nursing homes, are willing to cooperate with the medical director and facility staff to provide good geriatric medical care and help meet those requirements, and are receptive to suggestions from the medical director, based on medical QA activities, about ways to improve care.

Physician Assistants and Nurse Practitioners

Increasingly, physician assistants (PAs) and nurse practitioners (NPs) are being used in the nursing home in a new role at the interface between the physician, nurse, and social worker.

The few studies that have been done in the nursing home, usually focused on NPs, have shown clinical advantages (Kane, Kane, Garrard, et al., 1991). Nurse practitioners may be sponsored by physicians, the nursing home, or the medical director. For attending physicians, they can also provide acute and chronic assessment and in-service education. As nursing home representatives, they may conduct previsits and follow-up visits, perform acute evaluation and treatment, and coordinate rehabilitation care and family communication. Under medical director sponsorship, they can also perform QA and committee functions, assist with physician visits, perform employee health evaluations, and improve liaison with attending physicians.

Thus, with appropriate physician support, PAs and NPs can assume various clinical roles and administrative functions. Potential obstacles to their use include physician or nurse resistance, legal restrictions in some states, and limits on payment—although Medicare now pays for both PA and NP services.

Creation of Policies and Procedures, and Standards for Care

The medical director is responsible for implementing effective clinical policies and procedures. These will be both physician specific, and general clinical issues requiring physician participation and input.

In any complex system, such as the one delivering care to nursing home residents, policies and procedures are essential guides to performance. Effective policies and procedures are the "rules of the game" that guide collections of individuals of diverse experience and backgrounds toward common standards and expectations, and a common understanding of essential goals and objectives.

Policies may be defined as officially interpreted general goals, objectives, and expectations. Managers or directors of businesses, departments, facilities, or oganizations establish policies for those who work with or for them.

Procedures are the specific steps or mechanisms for achieving these goals or objectives.

Medical directors must not only create and help implement effective medical policies and procedures, but must also ensure that such policies and procedures are compatible with those of other disciplines, and reflect good care standards. Several references now exist to provide medical directors with comprehensive medical policies that can help them and their attending physicians fulfill their responsibilities under OBRA '87 (Levenson, 1990; Ouslander, Osterweil, & Morely, 1991).

For example, when, why, how, and how urgently should nurses notify physicians of changes in a resident's condition? This appears to be a common source of physician-nurse disagreement in many nursing homes nationwide. Nursing home staff need a timely physician response to notification of changes in condition, and physicians desire an effective system to distinguish emergencies and urgent problems from routine ones. Thus, protocols and policies for notification are important communications and clinical tools.

Policies and procedures should be reasonable, supportable by some objective information, based on widely accepted standards, and clear enough to be understood and followed. Selecting clinical information or principles to serve as practice standards depends on which services are offered at the facility, the availability of published studies to support the standard, other information in the geriatric literature, federal and state regulations, and facility, state, and local experience. To try to increase physician compliance, medical directors should include attending physicians in reviewing proposed policies and any pertinent medical literature. This allows physicians to have some input in the QA process and alerts them to applicable standards.

Evaluation of and Improvement of Systems for Communicating and Managing Information

The medical director should be concerned with evaluating and improving the quality and consistency of the clinical information available in the nursing home, and systems for collecting, storing, retrieving, analyzing, and reporting that information. Such systems are needed not only for individual patient encounters, but for management decisions and compliance with regulatory expectations.

Current medical records systems in health care are often inadequate for dealing effectively with complex patient care, especially with high volumes of regulations and standards, and where there is substantial variability in staff skills and performance. Poor quality, and inaccurate and inconsistent information should be considered a significant risk factor for the facility and its practitioners. They create and contribute to errors of omission and commission. The reliability of sources of clinical information in the nursing home is hampered by the many cognitively impaired residents with a limited ability to give an accurate history, and the often limited number of caregivers with adequate assessment skills to be helpful in gathering clinical data (Ouslander, 1989).

Partially because of pending requirements to record MDS information in a computer-usable format, many facilities are beginning to realize the potential value of computerizing clinical as well as financial information. The creative use of computers and other technologies may be necessary for the industry to meet growing expectations for quality care for a growing population. The OBRA '87 Interpretive Guidelines explicitly allow for computerized medical records, provided they meet certain safeguards.

Some developments in the computer field that will likely impact significantly on nursing home practice in the next 5 years include cheaper and more portable computers, declining cost of linking users in effective networks, growing interest by vendors in nursing home software, and voice and handwriting recognition capabilities. There are great possibilities for staff and patient education, communications, and the more efficient collection and use of information for multiple purposes, such as clinical care, quality assurance, and regulatory compliance (see chapter by Bock and Kane).

Medical directors should become more knowledgeable about information management and the potential uses for computerized information systems in long-term care. The needs of all caregivers, including the attending physicians, must be represented effectively as facilities consider and then reorient towards the creation, and then future automation, of effective clinical information systems.

Process of Overseeing and Evaluating Care

The OBRA '87 regulations mandate physician participation on a facility QA committee. Most likely, the medical director will serve in this role. To do so effectively, medical directors should have some role in setting up monitoring systems; deciding how to collect data; reviewing and analyzing those data; helping identify high-risk, high-volume, and problem-prone areas, and educating attending physicians based on analysis of this information.

The Joint Commission on Accreditation of Healthcare Organizations has recommended a so-called 10-step process for QA activities (Joint Commission on Accreditation of Healthcare Organizations, 1989). This includes (a) assigning responsibility, (b) defining the scope of care, (c) considering the important aspects of care, (d) developing key indicators, (e) creating evaluation thresholds, (f) collecting and organizing data, (g) evaluating care, (h) taking problem-solving actions, (i) assessing the results of those actions, and (j) communicating relevant information. In some form, these principles apply to all disciplines including the medical staff.

The goals of medical QA in the nursing home are to safeguard good care already being provided, recognize opportunities to improve care, and identify and resolve problems. Briefly, a successful medical QA program in the nursing home involves the following steps. The medical director and attending physicians identify important aspects of care and collaborate on establishing appropriate policies and medical care standards, and quality indicators (criteria for reviewing specific aspects of care). The medical director, perhaps assisted by other medical staff, then ensures a mechanism for collecting pertinent data, reviews the data when collected, assesses problems or seeks areas for possible quality improvement, provides feedback to attending physicians (both QA information and education), and follows up to see if education and policy making improve care and prevent subsequent problems.

Though responsible for evaluating data and taking follow-up actions, the medical director can rely mostly on data that others already collect or report for other purposes (e.g., incident and accident reports, pharmacist reports, and reviews of infections). Medical directors typcially evaluate care and identify care problems by reviewing accident and incident reports, reviewing pharmacist reports, reviewing infections, making observations while delivering care and on rounds, attending QA committee meetings, reviewing change of condition reports, and helping design special studies and ongoing audits.

Medical directors may respond to identified problems with care by communicating with individual physicians (orally or in writing), communicating with the medical staff about care problems in general (not pertaining to a specific resident), communicating with nonphysician staff regarding their clinical care, participating in facility inservices to correct general care problems, and preparing written reports of actions taken.

Also, organized QA programs and minor research activities such as medical care evaluation studies can help test hypotheses and provide data used to improve care. Medical care evaluation studies are somewhere between normal QA activities and formal research studies. Examples of questions examined in these studies are

- Is there value in treating asymptomatic bacteriuria in nursing home residents? (Elon 1991)
- Can we decrease morbidity or mortality by routinely irrigating indwelling Foley catheters? (Lefton, Ergun, and Jones 1991)
- Do nursing home residents with the diagnosis of "diabetes" really need calorie-restricted or diabetic diets? (Rosen, Gohr, & Smith, 1991)

Risk management (RM) may be defined as the preventive arm of QA programs. RM activities seek potential problems that may impact negatively on care, or on those providing care, and try to reduce or eliminate those risks. The medical director should play a role in the facility's RM program including reporting pertinent observations (e.g., about safety hazards, or potential sources of clinical errors or miscommunications) to the director of nursing and administrator; through a role in the employee health program; and by educating physicians to help reduce risks—for example, by timely response to nursing notification of changes in condition, assuring adequate alternate coverage in case of unavailability, and reducing the use of medications that may increase the risk of functional problems such as dizziness and falling.

To fulfill their required functions better, medical directors may need to spend more time on QA activities and critical follow-up and feedback to attending physicians. In some cases, they may need to adjust their total time commitment, or perhaps reduce somewhat the time spent in direct care to nursing home patients. Nursing homes should consider compensating their medical directors accordingly for this additional commitment.

OTHER POTENTIAL MEDICAL DIRECTOR ROLES

Because of the complexities of nursing home care, good clinical geriatric medical practice is essential, but not sufficient, to assure optimal outcomes and effective care overall. Besides having an important role in improving medical care, medical directors also can help influence other related processes within the facility, that may in turn affect care positively.

For example, the medical director can play a major role in helping *professionalize* the nursing home. Among other things, professionalization implies attitudes and methods of thinking, centering around a more systematic rational problem-solving process. These include

- Thoughtful, careful definition of objectives and standards
- Systematic data gathering and analysis
- Better understanding of methods used to evaluate information and draw conclusions
- Considering alternative explanations for events
- Systematic application of conclusions for problem solving
- Retesting conclusions based on new or changed information

In facilities, medical directors can make the care process more rational by supporting an appropriate problem-solving process in meetings, and by educating both physicians and nonphysicians. For example, the medical director can provide attending physicians with information about geriatric medicine, provide the facility staff with medical information in a form they can understand and use, and help to ensure that medical knowledge is translated into good care and desirable outcomes.

For instance, the OBRA '87 regulations emphasize the reduction of "unnecessary medications." The medical director can approach this issue in several ways: (a) provide the medical staff with articles from the geriatric literature about the prescribing of as-needed medications or the use of psychotropics; (b) provide other staff with guidelines for reducing medication use in the facility; (c) translate such knowledge into policies and procedures that facilitate appropriate physician actions, and (d) explain the benefits, risks, and limitations of medication use in the elderly.

Employee health is another important area that could benefit from more medical director attention. Appropriate physician input into the medical and psychological well-being of nursing home employees has the potential to improve care by creating a healthier, better trained, and more functional work force. Areas of possible medical director policy and procedure participation in employee health include the preemployment examination, screening for infections, vaccination, worker's compensation, and back-to-work evaluations.

Survey and Regulatory Issues

Medical directors can help facilities deal with regulatory issues and the actual survey process. Before the survey, medical directors can help improve overall physician compliance with physician-centered regulations such as visit requirements, and encourage attending physicians to support care by talking to staff and patients and coordinating their orders with staff care plans. They can also recommend to the facility's administration and staff ways of improving care in general, and help ensure good communications, information management, and documentation systems.

During and after the survey process, the medical director can help by answering general or case-specific questions on medical care, requesting clarification of citations regarding clinical care, helping to draft corrective action, and communicating with health department physicians who might understand better the nuances of disputed complex medical issues.

Because most medical directors with nursing home patients are also on the staffs of local hospitals, they also have an opportunity to try to improve hospital care of the elderly, which can in turn help the nursing home in its care responsibilities.

Many acute care hospitals and their medical staffs have yet to realize their potential role in helping nursing homes give better care. Some examples of areas for improvement include placement of indwelling urinary catheters in nursing home residents while in the hospital; development of pressure sores in nursing home residents while hospitalized; and incomplete documentation or inadequate instructions about ongoing care when hospital patients are transferred to the nursing home. Possible approaches to improving such support may include informal discussions and presentations at grand rounds or other medical meetings.

MEDICAL DIRECTOR'S IMPACT ON QUALITY CARE

Defining quality care in the nursing home is a complex issue, because nursing homes provide both personal and medical care (Levenson, 1989b). Demonstrating quality care is also difficult. Many negative outcomes (death, complications of treatment, worsening of condition) occur despite adequate and appropriate treatment. Without knowing the expected course for a given resident beset by a number of chronic conditions, it remains very difficult to define "quality care outcomes."

Regulatory and QA activities in the nursing home must consider not only the purpose of care in each individual, but must also differentiate unavoidable negative outcomes from those resulting from inadequate or indifferent care. It is hoped that the future regulatory role will continue to shift away from a traditional punitive structure and process orientation toward a more selective focus on outcome and constructive feedback as well as sanctions.

As a leader in the nursing home, the medical director should understand and advocate for tactics and systems that help both physicians and nonphysicians work more effectively. According to one perspective, professional and facility leaders must take the lead in seeking continuous quality improvement, promoting a vision of a health care system undergoing continuous improvement, and using modern technical, theoretically grounded tools to improve these processes. Also, individual physicians must join in the effort for continous improvement (Berwick, 1989).

Although the value of the "continuous quality improvement" in the nursing home remains to be proved fully, it appears that an effective system *is* critical to providing good care. The medical director should at least encourage and help attending physicians to understand their role in a common effort to improve care, instead of seeing themselves as isolated practitioners treating disease in individual patients.

RESOURCES FOR MEDICAL DIRECTOR

Many medical directors nationwide still seem to feel they are alone, with little effective support or information to help them do their job. As of 1991, however, any new or experienced medical director can have access to a variety of references and organizations to help do an effective job with much less effort. No medical director needs to "reinvent the wheel." There are other clinical and administrative references (Katz & Calkins, 1989, Levenson,

1989a) besides those already noted. Also, more education programs address these administrative functions specifically, review regulatory requirements, and explain how the medical director can influence medical and other professional care effectively.

The American Medical Directors Association is a growing nationwide organization dedicated to helping physicians serve effectively as long-term care medical directors. It offers a newsletter and journal, samples of useful documents and materials, an annual meeting, and various continuing medical education conferences and training programs.

A certification program has recently begun to encourage medical directors to learn more about medical direction and to help nursing homes choose better qualified medical directors. The goals of this certification process are to ensure that physicians serving as medical directors in the nation's nursing homes will possess the skills and knowledge necessary to fulfill their roles as medical directors, and that medical directors will get the respect and credibility they deserve.

The certification program was guided by the philosophy that medical direction in the nursing home requires a unique blend of clinical and administrative knowledge and skills, and that most medical directors will continue to be primary care practitioners. Facilities have various requirements, and the physicians coming to the medical director role have diverse interests, background, and experiences. The program was designed to accommodate both academicians and community practitioners of several different primary care specialties (e.g., general internal medicine, family physicians), and to use existing specialty certification programs rather than create new ones. It also requires physicians to maintain and improve skills in both medical direction and geriatric medicine.

Physicians considering medical direction, or medical directors interested in continuing education, training programs, and certification can obtain more information by contacting the American Medical Directors Association (10480 Little Patuxent Parkway, Columbia, MD 21044.

FUTURE OF MEDICAL DIRECTION

Twenty years after the nursing home medical director was conceived, the position is assuming greater importance and responsibility, fueled considerably by the OBRA '87 regulations effective in October, 1990. Also, the medical director's mandatory and optional roles and responsibilities are being clarified better.

The future of nursing home medical direction looks brighter than in the past. With current regulatory requirements, medical directors will have greater responsibility for organizing medical care and coordinating it with other programs and services, creating and refining policies and procedures, and overseeing medical and general clinical care. Undoubtedly, the extent of medical director participation and influence in individual facilities will vary widely. The full potential impact of the medical director on clinical care remains uncertain. It will be useful to study the effect on outcomes and quality of care of the time that medical directors spend on activities such as quality assurance, employee health, education and training, and research and development.

Some medical directors believe their efforts are handicapped by a shortage of attending physicians, the relative lack of cooperation or interest of some attending physicians, the relative lack of facility support, the quality and skills of nonphysician personnel working in nursing homes, regulations, and paper work. A substantial minority of medical directors, however, do not appear to face any significant impediments to improving physician or nonphysician care in their facilities. Currently, several nursing facilities have satisfied and effective attending physicians, because of effective collaboration between these physicians and their medical director, enhanced by effective collaboration between the medical director and the other facility staff and administration. They represent a useful model for the entire industry to observe and follow.

REFERENCES

American Medical Association. (1977). *The medical director in the long term care facility.* Chicago: Author.

American Medical Association Council on Scientific Affairs. (1990). American Medical Association white paper on elderly health. *Archives of Internal Medicine, 150,* 2459–2472.

Berwick, D. M. (1989). Sounding board: Continuous improvement as an ideal in health care. *New England Journal of Medicine, 320,* 53–56.

Elon, R. (1991). Urinary tract infections/asymptomatic bacteriuria: Treatment of the positive urine culture. *Annual of Medical Direction, 1,* 32–39.

Fanale, J. E. (1989). The nursing home medical director. *Journal of the American Geriatric Society, 37,* 369–375.

Gamble, E. R., McDonald, P. J., & Lichstein, P. R. (1991). Knowledge, attitudes, and behavior of elerly persons regarding living wills. *Archives of Internal Medicine, 151,* 277–280.

Garrard, J., Kane, R. L., Ratner, E. R., & Buchanan, J. L. (1991). The impact of nurse practitioners on the care of nursing home residents. In P. R. Katz, R. L. Kane, M. Mezey (Eds.), *Advances in Long-Term Care* (vol 1, pp. 169–185). New York: Springer.

Health Care Financing Administration. (1991, September 26). Part 483 — Requirements for long term care facilities, *Federal Register, 56,* 48867–48879.

Ingman, S. R., Lawson, I. R., & Carboni, D. (1978). Medical direction in long-term care. *Journal of the American Geriatric Society, 26,* 157–166.

Institute of Medicine. (1986). *Improving the quality of care in nursing homes.* Washington, DC: National Academy Press.

Interpretive Guidelines for Long-term Care Facilities (1991). Washington, DC: Health Care Financing Administration.

Joint Commission on Accreditation of Healthcare Organizations. (1989). *Quality assurance in long-term care.* Chicago: Author.

Kane, R. A., Kane, R. L., Garrard, J., et al. (1988). Geriatric nursing practitioner as nursing home employees: Implementing the role. *Gerontologist, 28,* 469–477.

Katz, P. R., & Calkins, E. (Eds.). (1989). *The principles and practice of nursing home care.* New York: Springer.

Lawyers find gold in nursing facilities. (1991, September). *McKnight's Long-Term Care news, 12,* 1.

Lefton, E., Ergun, C. Y., & Jones, L. (1991). Benefit or detriment of urethral catheter irrigation. *Annual of Medical Direction, 1,* 40–43.

Levenson, S. A. (1988). *Medical direction in long-term care.* Baltimore: National Health Publishing.

Levenson, S. A. (1989a, Spring). The nursing home medical director: A new era. *Journal of Long-Term Care Administration,* 6–9.

Levenson, S. A. (1989b). Quality care in the nursing home – defining and providing it in a new era. *Geriatric Medicine Today, 8,* 29–40.

Levenson, S. A. (1990). *Medical policies and procedures for long-term care.* Baltimore: National Health Publishing.

(1990, December). *McKnight's Long-Term Care News, 11,* 1.

Medicare program fee schedule for physicians' services: Proposed rule. (1991, June 5). *Federal Register,* 25792–25978.

Mitchell, J. B., & Hewes, H. T. (1986). Why won't physicians make nursing home visits? *Gerontologist, 26,* 650–654.

New law will require providers to inform patients of living wills. (1990, December 10). *Modern Healthcare, 20.*

Ouslander, J. G. (1989). Medical care in the nursing home. *Journal of the American Medical Association, 262,* 2582–2590.

Ouslander, J. G., Osterweil, D., & Morley, J. (1991). *Medical care in the nursing home.* New York: McGraw-Hill.

Pattee, J. J., & Otteson, O. J. (1991). *Medical direction in the nursing home.* Minneapolis: Northridge Press.

Reichel, W. (1983). Role of the medical director in the skilled nursing facility: Historical perspectives. In W. Reichel (Ed.), *Clinical aspects of aging* (2nd ed., pp. 570–579). Baltimore: Williams & Wilkins.

Rosen, W. K., Gohr, K. A., & Smith, C. N. (1991). The diabetic diet reconsidered. *Annual of Medical Direction, 1,* 44–47.

Solon, J., Roberts, D. W., et al. (1957). Nursing homes: Their patients and their care (Public Health Monograph No. 46). Washington, DC: U.S. Department of Health, Education and Welfare.

Staats, D. O. (1988). The role of the nursing home medical director. *Clinics in Geriatric Medicine, 4,* 493–506.

Suits against nursing facilities: Are they on the rise? (1990, June). *McKnight's Long-Term Care News,* 11.

6

Influence of the Environment on Falls in Nursing Homes: A Conceptual Model

Jeanie Schmit Kayser-Jones

Falls are one of the most serious problems encountered by the elderly in the community, acute care hospitals, and especially in nursing homes. Thirty percent to 50% of nursing home residents fall each year (Gryfe et al., 1977; Tinetti et al., 1986; Tinetti & Speechley, 1989). Many elderly people live in fear of falling, knowing that a fall may result in an injury that necessitates hospitalization or admission to a nursing home.

Although most older people who fall do not sustain serious physical injuries, falls among the elderly carry high social, psychological, and economic costs (Kellogg, 1987). Following a fall, an elderly person may lose confidence in his or her ability to walk independently and thus restrict physical and social activities. Families may feel guilty that they did not anticipate and prevent the fall and consequently impose further limitations on their activities and independence, resulting in social isolation, withdrawal, and depression (Kellogg, 1987). Although most falls do not result in a serious injury, the fear of suffering an injury such as a hip fracture is not unrealistic.

In the United States, there are 172,000 hip fractures annually among people 65 years of age and older (Baker & Harvey, 1985). The incidence of hip fracture increases sharply among the very old; 32% of women and 17% of men who live to the age of 90 will suffer a hip fracture (National Institutes of Health, 1984). The economic cost of hip fractures has been estimated at about $7 billion annually (Melton & Riggs, 1983). As more people live to very old age, falls will become an increasingly important problem in our society.

Most of the research on falls has attempted to identify people who are at a high risk of falling, looking primarily at intrinsic (host) factors such as age; mental, physiological, and functional status; diagnosis; muscle weakness;

sensory, gait, or balance impairment; and number and type of medications (Campbell et al., 1981; Granek et al., 1987; Nevitt et al., 1989; Robbins et al., 1989; Rubenstein et al., 1988). Many investigators, however, acknowledge that falls are the result of an interaction between host and environmental factors.

The purpose of this chapter is to discuss the influence of environment on falls in nursing homes. A brief review of the literature on environment and aging will first be presented to illustrate how this theoretical framework can be useful in the study of falls in institutional settings. Next, articles and research studies that have discussed environmental factors will be reviewed, and empirical findings from a qualitative study (conducted by the author) that investigated the environment in nursing homes will be described. Lastly, building on the work of theorists in the field of environment and aging, a conceptual model to guide practice and future research will be presented.

THEORETICAL FRAMEWORK: ENVIRONMENT AND AGING

Broadly speaking, the environment is defined as all that surrounds us and affects our lives. This includes the roads we drive on, the neighborhood we live in, the people with whom we interact, the air we breathe, the architectural design of a building, and the furnishings within. Several models have been developed in an attempt to understand and predict the effect of the environment on older people, and some investigators have attempted to define optimal environments (Kahana, 1974; Lawton, 1975; Lawton & Nahemow, 1973; and Moos & Lemke, 1985).

Grant (1989) has presented a review of three theoretical approaches to understanding how the institutional environment affects adaptation and patient (resident) outcome: (a) the transactional model, (b) the social-ecological model, and (c) the person-environment congruence perspective. Briefly, a transactional model predicts outcome by looking at the transaction between a person and the environment. The relationship between a person and the environment is seen as a dynamic process. Cognitive appraisal and coping mediate the transaction and determine how environmental stressors, for example, affect outcome.

Social-ecological models have been developed by Lawton and Nahemow (1973) and Moos (1980). These models view the person, the social environment, and the physical environment as interdependent parts of a general ecological system. These theorists differ from one another in terms of how the environment is thought to affect outcome. Moos (1980), drawing on the transactional model, emphasizes that cognitive processes of appraisal and coping determine the outcome. Lawton and Nahemow (1973) predict behavioral outcome by looking at a person's "competence" relative to "environmental press" (i.e., the demands of the environment on the person). Both models describe a potentially bidirectional or reciprocal interchange between the person and the environment (Grant, 1989).

The third model, the person-environment congruence perspective, examines the goodness of fit between a set of personality characteristics (i.e., personal needs or preferences) and a commensurate set of environmental demands (i.e., environmental press). This model differs from those previously discussed in that it focuses on the difference between specific dimensions of personality and environmental demands. When a discrepancy occurs, it is a potential source of stress. Some studies have found that congruence between personal needs or preferences and environmental press predict life satisfaction and morale among the institutionalized elderly (Kahana, Liang, & Felton, 1977; Kiyak, 1977).

These models have provided a theoretical framework for much of the research on environment and aging. Despite the importance of the environment in providing care, however, there has been relatively little research on how environmental factors influence quality of care in institutional settings. A few studies have examined the effects of noise levels in intensive care units, recovery rooms, and acute care wards (Aiken, 1982; Hilton, 1985; Minckley, 1968; Topf, 1984; Woods & Falk, 1974). There is a small body of research in long-term care focusing on the modification of the environment for the cognitively and chronically ill patient (Andreasen, 1985; El-Sherif, 1986; Hatton, 1977; Hayter, 1983; Ryden, 1985), the effects of white uniforms on visually and cognitively impaired older patients (Steffes & Thralow, 1985), patients' wishes regarding type of room accommodation (Kayser-Jones, 1986), and how the environment affects quality of life and quality of care (Kayser-Jones, 1989a, 1989b).

Most studies have focused on four major features of the environment: (a) the physical characteristics, (b) the organizational climate, (c) the personal and suprapersonal environment, and (d) the social-psychological milieu. The physical characteristics include, for example, architectural design, color, lighting, type of floor surface, and space. Organizational aspects include items such as policy, patient/staff ratio, financing, nursing and medical leadership and supervision, and knowledge level and training of staff. Lawton (1975) defines the personal environment as the significant other who constitute the major one-to-one relationships of an individual (e.g., family, friends, and work associates). In the nursing home setting, a patient's personal world is also made up of family and friends, but it is the nursing home staff who constitute a major part of his or her personal world.

The suprapersonal environment is defined as the modal characteristics of all the people in physical proximity to an individual (e.g., the predominant race or the mean age of others in a neighborhood). In the nursing home, the modal characteristics of patients in physical proximity to one another include the following: They are typically very old (85 years); many are physically, cognitively, and functionally impaired; and they have multiple pathologies such as cerebrovascular, Parkinson's, and Alzheimer's disease.

The social-psychological milieu refers to the norms, values, activities, the philosophy of the administration, the attitudes and beliefs of the caregivers, and the interactions of all who are a part of the institution (e.g., residents, staff, and visitors).

ENVIRONMENTAL FACTORS THAT CONTRIBUTE TO FALLS

There is a large body of literature that describes the numerous environmental factors that contribute to falls. Although it is often said that most falls are due to an interaction between multiple intrinsic (host) and extrinsic (environment) factors, few studies have systematically investigated the role of environmental hazards (Ashley, Gryfe, & Amies, 1977; Nelson & Amin, 1990). The significance of environmental factors is often mentioned, especially regarding the prevention of falls. Environmental hazards such as slippery floors, the absence of handrails in corridors, and inadequate lighting, for example, are more easily corrected than intrinsic factors such as instability, gait disorders, and drop attacks.

Most authors discuss the physical characteristics of the environment that contribute to falls such as dangerous furniture, slippery hard, wet, or shiny floors, throw rugs, the absence of grab bars near the toilet or bathtub, the lack of appropriate handrails in corridors and on stairways, and inadequate lighting (Duthie, 1989; Gray-Vickrey, 1984; Hogue, 1982; Maciorowski, 1988; Rodstein, 1964; Rubenstein, 1983; Sorock, 1988). Equipment, especially canes, walkers, and wheelchairs, has also been identified as hazardous (Duthie, 1989). Tinetti and Speechley (1989) illustrate how the combination of host and environmental factors may contribute to falls. A frail man, they emphasize, with a decreased step height, wearing ill-fitting shoes and trousers that are too long is at a particularly high risk of tripping and falling.

A few nursing studies have described how organizational factors such as inadequate staffing contribute to falls (Colling & Park, 1983; Feist, 1978; Gross et al., 1990); when staff are not readily accessible, patients who are unable to walk without assistance may go to the toilet or attempt to get out of a chair or bed unassisted and fall.

Barrowclough (1979) in a brief but comprehensive discussion of host and environmental factors notes that psychological causes such as depression, overdependency, grief, and anxiety also contribute to falls. For many elderly people who have multiple sensory and physical impairments, walking safely can only be accomplished by maximum conscious effort and mental concentration. This necessary concentration can be adversely affected by psychological problems. A depressed patient, for example, may have a lack of concern for personal safety and be less aware of environmental hazards (Barrowclough, 1979).

RESEARCH STUDIES INVESTIGATING ENVIRONMENTAL FACTORS

Despite an awareness of the importance of environmental factors, relatively few studies have investigated the influence of the environment on falls. In many of the early studies, investigators did not include environmental factors as variables in the research design but did discuss them in their findings.

Sheldon (1960) was one of the first investigators to discuss the significance of environmental factors. In an analysis of the natural history of falls among 500 elderly people, he found that accidental falls frequently occurred on staircases, most often because of missing the last step. He believed that handrails were often too broad or too close to the wall to allow a person to grasp them effectively. Furthermore, he stressed that handrails should extend beyond the last stair and should be especially shaped so that one would know when the end of the stairway had been reached.

Gryfe et al. (1977) conducted one of the earliest longitudinal (5 years) prospective studies of falls in a 200-bed residential unit in a Jewish Home for the Aged in Canada. In an attempt to decrease accidents, non-slip floor coverings; adequate illumination; and handrails in corridors, toilets, and elevators had been incorporated into the design of the building. Despite these safety features, an annual fall rate of 668 incidents per 1,000 residents was found.

Ashley, Gryfe, and Amies (1977) observed that although the literature frequently made reference to the importance of extrinsic factors in falls, there were no systematic analyses of the constituents of these factors. Using the data from the 5-year longitudinal study described earlier (Gryfe et al., 1977), they described some of the circumstances of falling. In this study, extrinsic factors were defined as the hour of the day, day of the week, where residents fell, and the activity associated with falls.

This analysis disclosed that falls occurred at all hours of the day and were quite evenly distributed over all days of the week. A slightly lower percentage of falls occurred on the Sabbath (Saturday). Most falls occurred in the resident's room and toilet (bathroom), and the activity most commonly associated with falling was going to or returning from the toilet (44%). Interestingly, nearly as many falls occurred while residents were sitting in chairs (18.3%) or lying in bed (18.3%) as when they were getting in and out of bed (19.3%). Observing that residents spend many hours in chairs and beds, they emphasized the need for furniture designed specifically for elderly people with functional limitations.

In a small nursing study, extrinsic factors were extended to include improper footwear and clothing such as long gowns and bathrobes (Feist, 1978). Although these items were cited as potential problems, no mention is made as to whether or not they contributed to falls. Data from incident reports were analyzed during a 3 ½-year period in a 42-bed home for the aged. The study disclosed that the peak time of falls was between 6 P.M. and 9 P.M.; 57% of the falls occurred among residents who were confused at the time of the fall, and 35% of the falls were from wheelchairs. The author notes that confused patients need close supervision and must be "protected physically by soft restraints and chemically by tranquilizers." Notably, 57% of the residents were on regular doses of tranquilizers, and 43% were on tranquilizers as needed. Only 21.5% of the residents who fell were *not* taking tranquilizers. It is noteworthy that the author first observed that confused patients must be protected with physical and chemical restraints, yet later states that 35% of the falls were from wheelchairs, "often documented as an attempt to escape from the confinement of soft restraints in the chair." This author was one of the first to mention adequate staffing as an extrinsic factor. Staff-patient ratios during the time of the study were noted, and in an attempt to decrease the number of falls, they increased the number of nurse aides during the peak danger time. Further, from 8 A.M. until 8 P.M. one nurse aide was assigned specifically to respond to calls for help and especially to help patients who needed assistance in going to the toilet.

This study provides some insight into how extensively restraints and tranquilizers were used and accepted as a standard of care. This philosophy of care, of course, has continued until recently when the use of restraints has come into question (Evans & Strumpf, 1989).

In a study conducted in a 400-bed Canadian geriatric hospital, it was also found that most of the falls (71.9%) occurred in the patient's room or in the toilet. The ambulatory status of the residents was recorded; most used wheelchairs. About half of the falls were associated with getting in and out of bed or a wheelchair, or getting on or off the toilet. The authors concluded that because most accident victims were in wheelchairs, they are potentially a hazard, and their indiscriminate use as a convenience for caretakers should be discouraged. The psychological and physiological consequences of enforced immobility in wheelchairs was also identified as an important factor to be avoided (Berry, Fisher, & Lang, 1981).

Although many studies mention environmental factors when analyzing data, few investigators have actually designed studies to examine the significance of environmental hazards. An exception is Tinetti's (1987) innovative study that evaluated the contribution of chronic conditions (e.g., visual problems, musculoskeletal disease, and dementia), acute processes (e.g., dys-rhythmias and pneumonia), and environmental factors that may contribute to serious injury during falls among ambulatory nursing home residents. Environmental hazards were defined as "obstacles that might cause some healthy, fit people to fall (e.g. broken chair, wet floor)" (p. 645). The inappropriate use of a walking aid (cane, walker, or wheelchair) was the most common extrinsic factor associated with falling. An association between environmental factors and serious injury during falls was not found. The author notes, however, that significant environmental hazards might have been missed because incident reports do not supply sufficient data. Major hazards were not missed, but less obvious obstacles such as poorly fitting shoes were missed (Tinetti, 1987).

In a unique study designed to examine organizational staff attitudes (components of the organizational environment) as determinants of falls, Harris (1989) found that variables such as leadership, work group cohesion, job involvement, and expectations and attidues toward the elderly were related to falls. Interestingly, no significant correlation between medical diagnoses, length of stay, mental status, and number of falls was found (Harris, 1989). This study, while broadening the scope of research, did not investigate other environmental variables that may contribute to falls.

In a carefully designed study in two long-term care facilities, which included recurrent fallers and nonfallers, Lipsitz et al. (1991) found that environmental hazards accounted for only 10% of the falls. The authors state their findings are in contrast to earlier studies reporting that environmental factors account for as many as one third of falls among elderly patients (Brocklehurst et al., 1968; Campbell, et al. 1981; Clark, 1968; Sheldon, 1960).

This investigation, however, was conducted in "two high-quality nursing facilities, and dependent wheelchair bound and uncooperative residents were excluded from the study." The term, uncooperative, is not defined. These two important variables (type of facility and functional status) may account for the low percentage of falls attributed to environmental hazards. First, the nursing and medical leadership and the philosophy of care in two high-quality facilities (one was a Hebrew Rehabilitation Center for the Aged) may have been instrumental in preventing falls. Second, wheelchairs have been seen by other investigators as a dangerous piece of equipment, and wheelchair patients are most likely to be impaired physiologically and functionally. The difference in patient population is especially important because numerous studies have found that a large proportion of falls occurred while patients were getting in and out of wheelchairs (Berry et al., 1981; Feist, 1978; Gross et al., 1990).

Although the investigators in the Lipsitz study (1991) are to be commended for the comprehensive clinical data they obtained and the thorough and elegant analysis of those data, the exploration of environmental factors appears to have been limited to physical factors such as cluttered rooms and unstable furniture.

PROSPECTIVE STUDY USING PARTICIPANT OBSERVATION

Most of the major studies of falls have been retrospective, using incident reports as the primary source of data. To augment these studies and to describe further how environmental factors contribute to falls, prospective studies are needed. Consistently, investigators have found that most falls occur in patients' rooms, and that many accidents occur while patients are going to and from the toilet, and while getting in and out of beds and wheelchairs. Yet, we know little about why accidents occur in these locations and during these activities. Further, numerous papers, for example, discuss the importance of handrails in corridors and patients wearing properly fitting shoes. None of the investigators, however, have reported if handrails are used, and if patients wear comfortable shoes with a broad low heel, and if not, why not.

Interviews with patients and their families to obtain personal and historical data, as well as their viewpoint of institutional life, may reveal important factors that contribute to falls.

In an attempt to answer some of these questions and to augment findings from retrospective studies that analyzed incident reports, a prospective observational study was designed to investigate environmental factors that may contribute to falls. The study was conducted in a 100-bed two-story proprietary nursing home over the course of 1 year. The data will be presented under the four categories of the environment discussed earlier: (a) the physical environment, (b) the personal and suprapersonal environment, (c) the social-psychological milieu, and (d) the organizational climate. Although each of these categories will be discussed independently, it must be emphasized that factors in one category may influence those in another. For example, a shortage of staff (organizational environment) may contribute to negative attitudes toward patients (social-psychological milieu) resulting in a nurse aide's refusing to answer a call light. Subsequently this behavior may contribute to a patient's fall.

Physical Characteristics

The nursing home was nicely decorated. The rooms (private, and two and three beds) all had large windows that provided ample natural light. The rooms and corridors were wallpapered in pleasant designs and warm colors. A pleasantly decorated outdoor patio, adjacent to the lounge on the second floor, was easily accessible through sliding glass doors. Grab bars in the toilets and handrails in the corridors had been installed.

Most of the literature discusses the importance of handrails in the corridors, and regulations require this feature. Our observations disclosed, however, that patients seldom used the handrails. The corridors were very crowded at all hours of the day. Medicine, laundry, and food carts, cleaning equipment, laundry hampers, wheelchairs, and bedside tables were placed along the side of the corridor, thus obstructing the handrails. Further, artificial plants in plastic containers had been hung on the wall at eye level. If patients wanted to use the handrail, the plants would hit them in the face (possibly in the eye) as they walked up and down the hallway.

Studies have disclosed that most falls occur in patients' rooms, and while the elderly are getting in and out of wheelchairs or bed. The bathrooms and bedrooms were small, crowded, and cluttered. Patients using wheelchairs and walkers complained that they could not move about without bumping into the doorway, walls, or furniture. There were no comfortable chairs in the patients' rooms; the small rooms would not accommodate additional furniture. When patients were out of bed, they had to sit in a wheelchair in their room, in the corridor, or in the patient lounge. This room served as the activity, dining, and television room, as well as a visitors' lounge; the television was playing from early morning until bedtime. Although some wheelchairs had padded cushions on the seat, others did not. The wheelchairs did not provide back support. Patients said they became very tired sitting in the wheelchair throughout most of the day. Typically, patients were seen restrained, slumped over in their wheelchairs, resting their head on their arms on the bedside stand, which stood in front of the wheelchair.

The gray tile floors in the corridors, although not highly polished, appeared shiny and slick. The overhead lights produced a glare that may cause blurring of vision similar to what one experiences while driving into the bright glare of the sun. Our observations suggest that certain characteristics of the physical environment may contribute to falls. Studies to indentify additional hazards and measures to correct environmental problems may help to prevent falls and other accidents. Staats (1984) has presented an excellent discussion on the subject of color, lighting, acoustics, graphics, and texture in environments for the elderly.

Social-Psychological and Personal-Suprapersonal Factors

The factors in these two categories are often interrelated; they will therefore be discussed together. The research on falls has given little attention to social-psychological factors and their potential relationship to falls. Berry, Fisher, and Lang (1981) described the psychological consequences of enforced immobility among patients who are confined to wheelchairs. Tinetti

(1986) in an article that discusses the limitation of a disease-oriented approach to immobility, describes how a patient's mental and emotional status may affect mobility and falling. Some studies have examined mental status, but other social and psychological factors have not been investigated. A patient's social, psychological, and emotional status (e.g., anxiety, loneliness, or depression) or past life experiences may predispose them to falls.

Visitors who fail to come, or the death of another patient may cause a psychological disruption in the life of a nursing home resident. A cognitively impaired man became very anxious on the death of a female resident. She had become an important part of his social life, and he had become very attached to her. They had lunch together daily and were often seen walking hand in hand in the corridor. After her death, he repeatedly attempted to leave the facility, paced up and down the hallways, and wandered in and out of other patients' rooms. While in another man's room, who was also cognitively impaired, he was pushed, fell, and fractured his hip. One can posit that this agitated patient's behavior in response to his friend's death (social-psychological factors) precipitated an aggressive behavior in another cognitively impaired resident (personal-suprapersonal factors) that contributed to his fall.

Knowledge of a patient's past may help to understand his or her current behavior. While talking with the son of an 81-year-old woman who had been admitted to the nursing home from an acute hospital following a major stroke, we learned that during her childhood, his mother had spent some time in an orphanage. She had told her son that while in the orphanage if they wet their bed, they were required to wear the wet sheets all day. This past history was interesting in view of the fact that in the nursing home, she had fallen twice while attempting to leave her wheelchair unassisted to use the toilet.

Organizational Environment

The organizational environment is pivotal and indeed perhaps the most critical element in maintaining a safe environment. Policy issues, patient-staff ratios, leadership (especially nursing and medical), and the philosophy of the nursing home influence every aspect of care. A nursing home, for example, may have all the modern safety features, but without strong professional leadership and adequate staffing, it may be an unsafe environment for the elderly.

Most of the environmental factors we observed that may contribute to falls fell into this category. Specifically, patients were found to be at risk because of a lack of nursing leadership and supervision, or because of a low patient-staff ratio.

To illustrate, one evening we observed a cognitively impaired man on the second floor open the door from the corridor that led onto the stairwell. Fortunately, the door was alarmed. A male orderly (one of three employees caring for 47 patients) ran full speed the length of the hallway to prevent this man from possibly falling down a flight of concrete stairs.

The literature on falls repeatedly emphasizes the importance of patients wearing well-fitting, comfortable low-heeled shoes. Our observations disclosed, however, that on any given day about 70% to 80% of the residents were not wearing shoes. Some wore only stockings or slippers, and others were barefoot. A few wore shoes without shoelaces. The lack of supportive footwear may contribute to falls, especially when patients wear synthetic stockings that provide no traction.

When we asked the staff why so many residents were not wearing shoes, they informed us that some do not have shoes because when they are incontinent, their shoes become soiled with urine and have to be discarded. Families are unwilling to buy shoes that may soon become soiled. Measures taken by the staff to prevent incontinent patients from soiling their shoes and advising families to buy tennis shoes that could be easily washed when soiled would alleviate this problem.

The literature also stresses the importance of patients wearing properly fitting personal clothing. About 50% of the patients were dressed in night clothes rather than in daytime clothing. Several residents were seen walking in the corridor with long robes and ill-fitting slippers. One woman was pacing rapidly up and down the corridor. The hem was out of her robe, and it was dragging on the floor, thus increasing the risk of her falling.

As mentioned earlier, investigators consistently found that most accidents occurred in patients' rooms while getting in and out of chairs and beds. Numerous residents were seen sitting at the bedside restrained in their wheelchairs for long periods, with their signal cord out of reach. A 93-year-old mentally alert man, terrified and crying, was attempting to get out of bed. He could not understand why he had to be restrained. "I took the nap they wanted me to take; I want to get up now," he said. "Why do I have to be tied down?"

A woman in a wheelchair called repeatedly for something to drink and attempted to reach the water on her bedside stand. Although secured with a vest-type restraint, she had slipped from the wheelchair to the floor. The nurse put her back into the chair, restrained her tightly, but did not offer her anything to drink.

On the evening shift, a low staff-patient ratio may have been a key organizational factor that contributed to accidents. On the second floor, for example, one attendant was responsible for 15 patients. Most were moderately to severely impaired mentally, and required much care and attention. When the nurse aides were in one room, others were left unattended for long periods. This was especially true during mealtime when the limited number of staff was feeding patients. On one occasion, a large woman who was wheelchair bound, had been waiting for an hour to go to the toilet. When no one came to assist her, she wheeled herself into the bathroom. Right before our eyes and before we could intervene, she quickly grasped the sink to obtain leverage and transferred independently from the wheelchair to the toilet. She was wearing nylon stockings; the tile floor was slippery, and the wheels on the wheelchair were unlocked. It was remarkable that the wheelchair did not slip from under her, thrusting her to the floor, or that she did not fall while transferring to the toilet.

We observed that patients were often left in a wheelchair at the side of the bed for long periods. One resident said that she had been sitting in a chair for more than 8 hours. Her water and call light were out of reach; she was thirsty, tired, and wanted to go to bed. She was found attempting to return to bed unassisted. The urine in the drainage tube from her foley catheter was cloudy and thick with sediment. "Look at my urine," she said. "I need to drink more water." Because most accidents occur in patients' rooms, close observation and a regular assessment of and attention to patients' needs would undoubtedly reduce the number of accidents. This is difficult, however, when staffing is low.

The findings of this research illustrate the need for additional qualitative studies that will extend our knowledge of falls and other accidents in nursing homes. The data presented here do not allow us to establish cause and effect, but such studies will generate research questions and hypotheses to explore further those environmental factors that may contribute to falls. For example, would increasing patient-staff ratios during the hours when accidents most frequently occur decrease the number of falls?

CONCEPTUAL MODEL

Rubenstein, Robbins, and Josephson (1991) discussed the importance of doing an environmental assessment to help in the prevention of falls. The assessment focused primarily on physical characteristics such as floor surface, bed height, and poor lighting. Although this type of assessment is important and valuable, a broader approach is needed.

Building on Moos's (1980) conceptual framework described elsewhere (Kayser-Jones, 1989b), I shall present a conceptual model that illustrates how multiple factors in the physical, organizational, psychosocial, and personal-suprapersonal environment may effect the elderly nursing home patient with functional, cognitive, physiological, and sensory-perceptual disabilities (see Figure 6.1).

The two-way arrows illustrate that factors in one component of the environment interact with elements in another and that singularly or cumula-

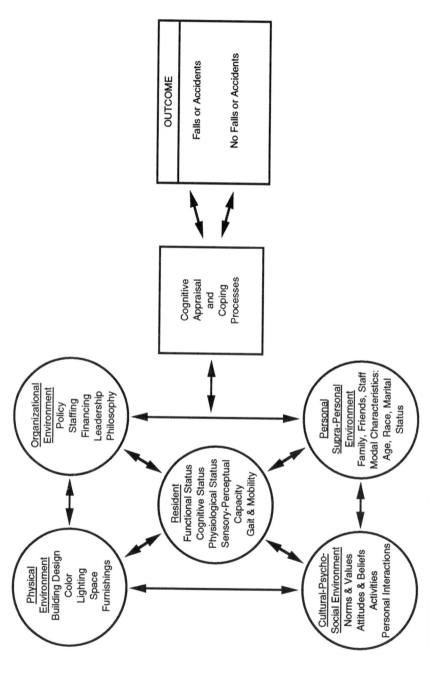

FIGURE 6.1 Conceptual Model for Study of Falls and Other Accidents in Nursing Homes

tively they may have an effect on the patient. If the philosophy of the nursing home, for example, is to use tranquilizers (organizational environment) and the rooms are crowded, poorly lighted, and the floors slippery (physical environment), the additive effect of these factors on a patient with gait and instability problems may or may not precipitate a fall, depending on the cognitive appraisal and coping ability of the patient. Moreover, financial considerations (the organizational environment) may determine the amount of space within patients' rooms as well as the number and size of communal spaces such as lounges and dining rooms (physical environment). If communal rooms are few and crowded and noise levels high, this may cause confusion, stress, and anxiety (psychosocial environment) that in turn contribute to falls. Furthermore, such an atmosphere may discourage friends and relatives from visiting (personal-suprapersonal environment), which may then cause the patient to be anxious, lonely, or depressed (psychosocial environment). One can hypothesize that the greater the depression, the higher the risk for accidents.

To illustrate further, policies regarding staff-patient ratio and staff salaries (organizational environment) may influence the attitudes and behavior of the caregivers (psychosocial environment), which may have a negative effect on patients. Allowing patients to sit restrained in chairs for hours is the norm in some nursing homes. Staff maintain that they do not have time to attend to their needs. As we observed, patients became restless, needed to use the toilet, or wanted a drink of water and fell while attempting to move unassisted. A change in one part of this complex network of variables can have an impact throughout the system. For example, a change in nursing leadership or the death of a patient can have wide-ranging consequences.

Furthermore, although the environment has an impact on the patient, the patient also has an effect on the environment (as indicated by the two-way arrows). A lonely, unhappy, or cognitively impaired patient may create an unpleasant atmosphere (psychosocial environment) that causes staff, other patients, and their visitors to be restless and upset (personal-suprapersonal environment).

Within this environmental system, elderly people, many with cognitive, functional, and sensory-perceptual impairment; gait and mobility problems; and multiple pathologies (for which they may be taking several medications) are placed. It is a new and strange environment, frequently devoid of friends, family, and personal belongings, such as a favorite chair that may help patients adapt to their new circumstances. It is not surprising that accidents occur. In fact, nursing homes can be a dangerous environment, and it is remarkable that even more falls and accidents do not occur.

An important component of this model is how each individual person responds to or copes with the environmental factors. Cognitive appraisal and coping processes (see Figure 6.1) mediate the person-environment transactions. These mediating factors emphasize the active participation of residents, even those who are cognitively impaired, in choosing those aspects of the environment to which they will respond (Moos & Lemke, 1985) and how they will respond. Two patients who need to use the toilet, for example, may respond differently to an unanswered call light. One may choose to remain in the chair and be incontinent, whereas another, such as the woman who was in an orphanage as a child, may independently attempt to go to the bathroom and fall.

This conceptual model illustrates that simple linear cause-and-effect relationships are not always easy to identify. More likely, a combination of multiple variables contributes to falls and other accidents. A cognitively impaired patient, for example, receiving psychotrophic drugs, who is trying to negotiate his or her way unassisted (because of a shortage of staff) down a crowded, poorly lighted corridor, is at a high risk of falling.

This conceptual model is not meant to be all-inclusive. Rather, it serves to illustrate how the dynamic interaction of multiple environmental factors contribute to falls and other accidents in nursing homes. The model is intended to be a conceptual framework to guide research and practice. It may be modified by practitioners and investigators involved in the care of the elderly.

PATIENT CARE AND PROFESSIONAL PRACTICE

An essential first step in preventing accidents is to assess the physical environment and plan interventions to eliminate factors that are potentially harmful (see Rubenstein et al., 1991), thus making the environment as safe as possible for elderly disabled people. In-service programs that focus on environmental factors that contribute to accidents and nursing care plans that emphasize their importance will also reduce the incidence of falls.

An organizational climate that fosters strong, consistent nursing and medical leadership, and professionals who take responsibility for individualized care will also reduce the number of falls. Nurses and physicians working together must try to identify patients who are at a high risk of falling and collaboratively plan interventions. Careful medical and nursing observation of and attention to any changes in physiological, cognitive, functional, or psychosocial status may prevent falls.

A psychosocial atmosphere that is attentive to individual needs, staff who philosophically believe in treating people with dignity and respect, and an environment that is peaceful, pleasant, and yet provides stimulating and meaningful activities is essential in preventing falls. When patients sit in wheelchairs for hours, day after day, this inevitably contributes to muscle weakness, anxiety, and frustration. Such patients will undoubtedly attempt to leave their wheelchairs and are at risk of falling.

Regular exercise programs, including taking patients outside for walks, will prevent muscle atrophy and may reduce restlessness and wandering that sometimes results in falls. Even patients who cannot walk should regularly be taken outside in their wheelchairs. This will reduce restlessness and boredom and help to keep people in touch with the world outside of the nursing home.

Although some nursing homes do make an effort to dress patients in their personal clothing, patients frequently are seen walking about poorly groomed in hospital gowns, bathrobes, and slippers. One woman insisted that she be dressed every day. "I feel like a patient when I am in my gown," she remarked. The lack of personal clothing and inattention to grooming deprives patients of their individuality, and contributes to low self-esteem, withdrawal from social interaction, and depression (Kayser-Jones, 1981). Depression may, in turn, contribute to falls. One could hypothesize, for example, that the greater the number of patients who are dressed in night clothes, the higher the number of falls.

SUGGESTIONS FOR FUTURE RESEARCH

Much research on falls has focused on identifying risk factors such as polypharmacy, gait and mobility problems (Wolfson, 1990), muscle weakness, dementia, and specific diagnoses such as arthritis, depression, and incontinence (Rubenstein et al., 1991). Such research needs to be continued. Far less attention, however, has been given to the environment and the interaction between host and environmental factors that may contribute to falls. Perhaps this is because it is difficult to design studies that will unravel and quantitatively measure the numerous intertwining factors and how they interact in causing falls. Furthermore, falls often occur unobserved in patients' rooms, and potential falls are prevented by staff intervention. Although some progress has been made, especially, for example, in documenting the role of medications in relationship to falls, continued progress will not occur until further attention is given to the environment.

Future research questions might include (a) Are patients who have frequent family visitors (e.g., daily) at a lower risk of falling than those who seldom have visitors? (b) Are patients who are dressed in their personal clothing and wearing properly fitting shoes less likely to fall than are those who are dressed in night clothes and slippers? (c) Would offering the bedpan or taking patients to the toilet on a regular 2- to 3-hour basis decrease the number of falls (see Kayser-Jones, 1981)? (d) Because most falls occur in the bedroom, if staff made rounds regularly attempting to identify and meet patients' needs, would the number of falls decrease? (e) How many falls are due to staff turnover and does high staff turnover and shortage of staff at certain hours of the day contribute to falls? (f) What type of inservice educational programs would effectively reduce the number of falls? (g) Would regular programs of indoor and outdoor exercise strengthen muscles, reduce restlessness, and thereby decrease the number of falls?

Although it has been fruitful to identify risk factors for falls and to delineate items associated with serious injury during falls (Tinetti, 1988), it is imperative that a more comprehensive approach including identification and analysis of environmental factors be a significant part of future research efforts.

To advance this area of research, a new conceptual framework, such as the one proposed here that views nursing home residents as an integral part of a complex environmental system is needed. This chapter presents a conceptual framework within which the current knowledge regarding falls can be examined, environmental variables identified, and further study of the etiology and prevention of falls be facilitated.

REFERENCES

Aiken, R. J. (1982). Quantitative noise analysis in a modern hospital. *Archives of Environmental Health, 37*, 361–364.

Andreasen, M. E. (1985). Make a safe environment by design. *Journal of Gerontological Nursing, 11*, 18–22.

Ashley, M. J., Gryfe, C. I., & Amies, A. (1977). A longitudinal study of falls in an elderly population: Some circumstances of falling. *Age and Ageing, 6*(Pt. 2), 211–220.

Baker, S. P., & Harvey, A. (1985). Fall injuries in the elderly. *Clinics in Geriatric Medicine, 1*, 501–508.

Barbieri, E. B. (1983). Patient falls are not patient accidents. *Journal of Gerontological Nursing, 9*, 165–173.

Barrowclough, F. (1979, June 14). Danger! Why old people fall. *Nursing Mirror.*

Berry, G., Fisher, R. H., & Lang, S. (1981). Detrimental incidents, including falls, in an elderly institutional population. *Journal of the American Geriatrics Society, 29*, 322–324.

Blake, C., & Morfitt, J. M. (1986). Falls and staffing in a residential home for elderly people. *Public Health, 100*, 385–391.

Brocklehurst, J. C., Exton-Smith, A. N., Lempert Barber, S. M., Hunt, L. P., Palmer, M. K. (1981). Fracture of the femur in old age: A two-centre study of associated clinical factors and the cause of the fall. *Age & Ageing, 10*, 264–270.

Campbell, A. J., Reinken, J., Allan, B. C., & Martinez, G. S. (1981). Falls in old age: A study of frequency and related clinical factors. *Age and Ageing, 10*, 264–270.

Clark, A. (1968). Factors in fracture of the female femur: Clinical study of the environmental, physical, medical, and preventive aspects of this injury. *Gerontologia Clinica, 10*, 257.

Colling, J., & Park, D. (1983). Home, safe home. *Journal of Gerontological Nursing, 9*, 175–192.

Dimant, J. (1985). Accidents in the skilled nursing facility. *New York State Journal of Medicine, 85,* 202–205.

Duthie, E. H. (1989). Falls. *Geriatric Medicine, 73,* 1321–1336.

El-Sherif, C. (1986, May–June). A unit for the acutely ill. *Geriatric Nursing,* 130–139.

Evans, L. K., & Strumpf, N. E. (1989). Tying down the elderly: A review of the literature on physical restraint. *Journal of American Geriatric Society, 37,* 65–74.

Feist, R. R. (1978). A survey of accidental falls in a small home for the aged. *Journal of Gerontological Nursing, 4,* 15–17.

Grant, L. A. (1989). Environment and quality of life: A reaction from the perspective of social science and environmental design. In *Indices of quality in long-term care: Research and practice* (Publication No. 20-2292). New York: National League for Nursing.

Granek, E., Baker, S. P., & Abbey, H. (1987). Medications and diagnoses in relation to falls in a long-term care facility. *Journal of American Geriatric Society, 35,* 503–511.

Gray-Vickrey, M. (1984, May-June). Education to prevent falls. *Geriatric Nursing,* 179–183.

Gross, Y. T., Shimamoto, Y., Rose, C. L., & Frank, B. (1990). Why do they fall? Monitoring risk factors in nursing homes. *Journal of Gerontological Nursing, 16,* 20–25.

Gryfe, C. I., Amies, A., & Ashley, M. J. (1983). A longitudinal study of falls in an elderly population: Incidence and morbidity. *Age and Ageing, 6*(Pt. 1), 201–210.

Harris, P. B. (1989). Organizational and staff attitudinal determinants of falls in nursing home residents. *Medical Care, 27,* 737–749.

Hatton, J. (1977). Aging and the glare problem. *Journal of Gerontological Nursing, 3,* 38–44.

Hayter, J. (1983). Modifying the environment to help older persons. *Nursing & Health Care, 4,* 265–269.

Hilton, B. A. (1985). Noise in acute patient care areas. *Research in Nursing and Health, 8,* 283–291.

Hogue, C. C. (1982). Injury in late life: 2. Prevention. *Journal of the American Geriatric Society, 30,* 276–280.

Kahana, E. (1974). Matching environments to needs of the aged: A conceptual scheme. In J. F. Gubrium (Ed.), *Late life: Communities and environmental policy.* Springfield, IL: Charles C Thomas.

Kahana, E., Liang, J., & Felton, B. (1977). *Alternative models of P-E fit and wellbeing of the aged.* Paper presented at the annual meeting of the Gerontological Society, San Francisco.

Kayser-Jones, J. (1981). A comparison of care in a Scottish and a United States facility. *Geriatric Nursing: American Journal of Care for the Aged, 2,* 44–50.

Kayser-Jones, J. S. (1986). Open-ward accommodations in a long-term care facility: The elderly's point of view. *The Gerontologist, 26,* 63–69.

Kayser-Jones, J. S. (1989a). The environment and quality of life in long-term care institutions. *Nursing and Health Care, 10,* 125–130.

Kayser-Jones, J. S. (1989b). The environment and quality of care in long-term care institutions. In *Indices of quality in long-term care: Research and practice* (Publication No. 20-2292). New York: National League for Nursing.

Kellogg International Work Group on Prevention of Falls in the Elderly. (1987). The prevention of falls in later. *Danish Medical Bulletin, 34*(Suppl. 4), 1–24.

Kiyak, A. (1977). *Person-environment congruence as a predictor of satisfaction and wellbeing among institutionalized elderly.* Unpublished doctoral dissertation, Wayne State University, Detroit.

Lawton, M. P. (1975). Competence, environmental press, and adaptation. In P. G. Windley, T. O. Byerts, & G. Ernst (Eds.), *Theory development in environment and aging*. Washington, DC: Gerontological Society.

Lawton, M. P., & Nahemow, L. (1973). Ecology and the aging process. In C. Eisdorfer & M. P. Lawton (Eds.), *The psychology of adult development and aging*. Washington, DC: American Psychological Association.

Lipsitz, L. A., Jonsson, P. V., Kelley, M. M., & Koestner, J. S. (1991). Causes and correlates of recurrent falls in ambulatory frail elderly. *Journal of Gerontology, 46,* M114–122.

Louis, M. (1983). Falls and their causes. *Journal of Gerontological Nursing, 9,* 142–149.

Maciorowski, L. F., Munro, B. H., Dietrick-Gallagher, M., McNew, C. D., Sheppard-Hinkel, E., Wanich, C., & Ragan, P. A. (1988). A review of the patient fall literature. *Journal of Nursing Quality Assurance, 3,* 18–27.

Margulec, I., Librach, G., & Schadel, M. (1970). Epidemiological study of accidents among residents of homes for the aged. *Journal of Gerontology, 25,* 342–346.

Melton, I. J., & Riggs, B. L. (1983). Epidemiology of age-related fractures. In I. V. Avioli (Ed.), *The osteoporosis syndrome* (pp. 45–72). Orlando: Grune & Stratton.

Minckley, B. B. (1968). The study of noise and its relationship to patient discomfort in the recovery room. *Nursing Research, 17,* 247–250.

Moos, R. (1980). Social-ecological perspectives on health. In G. Stone (Ed.), *Health psychology*. San Francisco: Jossey-Bass.

Moos, R. H. (1980). Specialized living environments for older people: A conceptual framework for evaluation. *Journal of Social Issues, 36,* 75–96.

Moos, R. H., & Lemke, S. (1985). Assessing and improving social-ecological settings. In E. Seidman (Ed.), *Handbook of social intervention*. Beverly Hills: Sage.

Nelson, R. C., & Murlidhar, A. A. (1990). Falls in the elderly. *Emergency Medicine Clinics of North America, 8,* 309–324.

Nevitt, M. C., Cummings, S. R., Kidd, S., & Black, D. (1989). Risk factors for recurrent nonsyncopal falls: A prospective study. *Journal of the American Medical Association, 261,* 2663–2668.

National Institute of Health. (1984). Consensus development conference on osteoporosis. *Osteoporosis, 5,*

Riffle, K. L. (1982). Kinds, causes, and prevention. *Geriatric Nursing, 3,* 165–169.

Robbins, L. J., Boyko, E., Lane, J., et al. (1987). Binding the elderly: A prospective study of the use of restraints in an acute care hospital. *Journal of American Geriatric Society, 35,* 290–296.

Robbins, A. S., Rubenstein, L. Z., Josephson, K. R., Schulman, B. L., Osterweil, D., & Fine, G. (1989). Predictors of falls among elderly people: Results of two population-based studies. *Archives of Internal Medicine, 149,* 1628–1633.

Rodstein, M. (1964). Accidents among the aged: Incidence, causes and prevention. *Journal of Chronic Diseases, 17,* 515–526.

Rubenstein, L. Z. (1983). Falls in the elderly: A clinical approach. *The Western Journal of Medicine, 138,* 273–275.

Rubenstein, L. Z., Robbins, A. S., Josephson, K. R., & Schulman, B. L. (1989). Benefits of a falls workup: A randomized clinical trial. *Clinical Residency, 37,* 324A.

Rubenstein, L. Z., Robbins, A. S., & Josephson, K. R. (1991). Falls in the nursing home setting. In P. R. Katz, R. L. Kane, and M. D. Mezey (Eds.), *Advances in long-term care* (Vol. 1, pp. 28–42). New York: Springer.

Rubenstein, L. Z., Robbins, A. S., Schulman, B. L., Rosado, J., Osterweil, D., & Josephson, K. R. (1988). Falls and instability in the elderly. *Journal of the American Geriatric Society, 36,* 266–278.

Sheldon, J. H. (1960). On the natural history of falls in old age. *British Medical Journal,* *10,* 1685–1690.

Sorock, G. S. (1988). Falls among the elderly: Epidemiology and prevention. *American Journal of Preventive Medicine, 4,* 282–288.

Staats, D. O. (1984). Physical environments. In *Geriatric medicine: Vol. 2. Fundaments of geriatric care* (pp. 436–477). New York: Springer-Verlag.

Tinetti, M. E. (1986). Performance-oriented assessment of mobility problems in elderly patients. *Journal of American Geriatric Society, 34,* 119–126.

Tinetti, M. E. (1987). Factors associated with serious injury during falls by ambulatory nursing home residents. *Journal of American Geriatric Society, 35,* 644–648.

Tinetti, M. E., & Speechley, M. (1989). Prevention of falls among the elderly. *The New England Journal of Medicine, 320,* 1055–1059.

Topf, M. (1984). A framework for research on aversive physical aspects of the environment. *Research in Nursing and Health, 7,* 35–42.

Woods, N. F., & Falk, S. A. (1974). Noise stimuli in the acute care area. *Nursing Research, 23,* 144–150.

7

Assisted Living: A Model of Supportive Housing

Keren Brown Wilson

Housing options in the United States have developed haphazardly without significant thought to the relationship between shelter and services. Combining services with housing options to support more independent living arrangements has become an issue of great interest during the past several years. To pursue this goal of meshing housing and services it is helpful to identify past practices and current trends in the development of supportive housing options.

In the United States, home is most often synonymous with home ownership. Redfoot and Gaberlavage (1991) note that the home ownership rate for those older than age 65 increased between 1980 and 1987, although home ownership rates decreased for those in younger categories. Overall, about 14 million or 75 percent of older heads of households own their own home.

The cultural preference to reside in single-family households is strong among older Americans. Hurd (1990) points out that research has consistently demonstrated a desire by older adults to live apart from their children. Further, regardless of health, or economic or social status both older homeowners and renters show an inclination to "age in place" (Struyk, Page, Newman, et al., 1989; Wilson & Hunt, 1990).

This phenomenon has created strong policy pressures to create more community-based care programs such as in-home services as well as a greater variety of supportive housing options. Baker and Prince (1990) suggest that there is no consensus about what to call supportive housing. It is called among other things: congregate, retirement, sheltered, foster group, protective, residential assisted, and enriched housing. The lack of uniformity also is evident in the variety of structural, programmatic, and regulatory environments associated with supportive housing (Heller Institute, 1991; Leak, 1991; Mor, Sherwood, & Gurkin, 1986).

In looking at structural environments, for example, supportive housing options range from shared sleeping space in a single-family home to totally self-contained apartments in a building with shared common and support service space. Some supportive housing options offer only limited access to staff and selected hotel-type services; others provide ongoing personal and nursing care. It is not regulated uniformly, although most forms of supportive housing that offer any type of hands-on care, either directly or by contract, are licensed by state governments (Leak, 1991).

Although this variety causes confusion, the lack of uniformity has fostered creative structural, programmatic, and regulatory models for supportive housing. One variation of these models, assisted living, offers great promise in meshing housing with service for the most vulnerable, frail individuals (Kane, Illston, Kane, & Nyman, 1990). This model defines assisted living as 24-hour care capability in congregate apartments. The care capability, illustrated in Table 7.1 ranges from traditional hotel-type services, such as housekeeping, linen laundry, and meals, to personal and routine nursing care.

Although every client does not necessarily need nor receive each of these

TABLE 7.1 Core Care Capability in Assisted Living

Capability of assessing, planning, implementing, and evaluating necessary support services of resident's choices and independence

Capability of providing or coordinating three meals daily, 7 days a week including diets and evening snacks appropriate to resident's needs and choices

Capability of providing or coordinating personal and linen laundry including incontinent laundry

Capability of providing or coordinating opportunities of individual and group socialization, and using community resources to normalize the environment for community interaction

Capability of providing or coordinating medical and social transportation

Capability of providing or coordinating personal care to assist the resident in performing all activities of daily living including bathing, eating, dressing, personal hygiene, grooming, toileting, and ambulation

Capability of providing or coordinating routine nursing care such as medication management, injections, nail and skin care, dressing changes, health monitoring, nonskilled catheter care, and other nursing tasks as might be delegated

Capability of providing or coordinating services for residents who have behavioral problems requiring ongoing staff support, intervention, and supervision

Capability of providing or coordinating the ancillary services of medically related care (e.g., physician, pharmacist, therapy, podiatry), banking, barber-beauty, social-recreational opportunities, hospice, and other services necessary to support the resident.

Capability of providing or coordinating the household services essential for health and comfort of residents (e.g., floor cleaning, dusting, bed making, etc.).

Source. From Wilson, K. B. (1990). *Assisted living: The merger of housing and long term care services.* Durham, NC: Duke University, Center for the Study of Aging and Human Development.

services, the provider must be able to ensure they are available when needed by each individual. Each client lives in a small private apartment; double occupancy is by personal choice. Further, the model embraces a mode of service delivery with emphasis on client empowerment through a shift in values orientation. The experience of one state, Oregon, in implementing this model provides an illuminating case study worthy of close examination. It is useful first, however, to examine conceptual underpinnings and policy decisions that influenced the development of the model.

CONCEPTUAL BASIS FOR ASSISTED LIVING

The conceptual basis for assisted living is rooted in environmental and client normalization. Alluded to previously is a cultural preference for adults to live independently in single-family households. These households are character- ized typically as habitable dwelling units with a private entrance for the family unit, cooking capacity, a separate bathroom, and a means to regulate room temperature, regardless of household size. A functional design that incorporates these features embraces a fundamental principle of environmen- tal normalization. Another aspect of this normalization is a residential, as opposed to an institutional, environment. A residential environment, in addition to the creation of a recognizable private household described earlier, uses materials in common or public spaces that are intended to replicate, as closely as possible, those used in private individual residences.

Finally, the emphasis placed on these structural elements overlaps with strong beliefs surrounding the emotional and social context of "home." Emphasis is placed, for example, on controlling access to the household and uniquely defining the life-style preferences of those in residence. Tully (1986) defined the elements of home to include security, small familial groups, control over the course of daily life, unity of purpose, and group identity. Taken together these reflect a minimum definition of "homelike" in the United States. Environmental normalization reflects the attempt to repli- cate functional, emotional, and social elements of "home" in nonfamilial group living situations (Landesman, 1988). These same elements are re- flected in the functional design and the values orientation of assisted living as it is being defined by many (Regnier, Hamilton, & Yatabe, 1991; Wilson, 1988).

However, environmental normalization also incorporates the principle of space adaptation to accommodate individual limitations. The assumption is made that appropriate design can facilitate individual functional ability. Lawton's (1980) suggestion of the relationship between individual com- petence and the physical environment is central to key aspects of functional design in assisted living. Spivak (1984) also ties the environment to functioning. He forcefully makes the case that negative consequences occur when institutional environments are incongruent with the desires or capabilities of those who live in them.

How to achieve environmental normalization in design is a matter of some debate. Countries such as Sweden and Denmark encourage universal design (Raschko, 1982). The United States has emphasized the adoption of standards to promote accessibility. Assisted living blends the two approaches to create a new concept of an adaptable environment. This adaptable environment uses both features of universal design (e.g., wider doorways) and specialized design for "handicap" use (e.g., voice-to-voice communication system). Using both approaches results in a setting that appears more home-like overall but has built-in design capacity needed to respond to common individual functional limitations.

Environmental normalization seeks to reduce the effect of individual impairment through manipulation of the physical setting. Client normalization involves systematic intervention that focuses on increasing individual competence (Manfredini & Smith, 1988). This systematic intervention is directed toward the development of personal skills needed to function independently. In assisted living the direct expression of this systematic intervention is the service available to support individual efforts to assume culturally normative social roles and responsibilities. This approach involves both individualization and flexibility of service.

Although client normalization traditionally has been used with other special-needs groups such as the developmentally disabled, services for older adults were patterned using a medical model of care. Focused on illness, a linear model depicting decreasing good health was developed. This model, the continuum of care, views service in terms of the setting in which it occurs. It links increasing dependency with a more bureaucratic, institutional model of service delivery. Concurrently, assumptions are made about the relationship between disease, dependency, and service need.

Subsequently, programmatic interventions have focused on bundles of service assumed generally to be appropriate in select settings. One significant consequence of this model of service delivery was the development of a bimodal system. This system focuses on "in-home" services delivered in single units by multiple providers and "institutional" services delivered in fixed packages by a single provider. Both approaches often result in a poor fit between available services and actual individual service need.

Improving this fit implies rethinking how service could be delivered to match more closely individual preferences as well as actual need. Conceptually this means coordinating unbundled services to generate more cost-effective, consumer-oriented packages focused on client normalization. One obvious programmatic approach is to expand the scope, range, and mix of services in settings where multiple clients live in close proximity who also have a high-probability service need that is likely to increase over a relatively fixed period. This, in effect, is the deliberate combining of housing and services.

Many types of supportive housing theoretically could support client normalization. Assisted living has the potential to respond to the most complex, enduring, and intense need for systematic intervention. Wilson (1991) illustrates this potential in a matrix that matches client service need across four settings (see Table 7.2). Although most services can be delivered in most settings, issues of access, cost, and consumer preference interact to create patterns of demand for services.

Table 7.2 uses four service criteria that help define a probable "goodness of fit" between service need and service settings. The first criterion, caregiver availability, is measured by the degree to which someone, apart from a paid provider, is able, willing, and capable of providing services needed in a timely and predictable manner.

Thus, someone who lives alone but who has a family member, neighbor, or friend who regularly assists with Instrumental Activities of Daily Living (IADLs) and ADLs may eliminate or postpone the need for supportive services. Conversely, living with someone does not necessarily mean that the person is available to give care. For example, the spouse may be too frail or the adult daughter may not be able to provide daytime care.

In assessing need, thus, we might assume a range of caregiver availability to be

0 = No availability of caregiver
1 = Nominal availability—limited by health, skill, lifestyle, etc.
2 = Intermittent availability—limited by type, timing, duration of need
3 = Routine availability—limited only occasionally by unique caregiver needs (e.g. respite, etc.)

More important than the level of assistance or number of impairments an individual has in determining need is the frequency and duration of service needs. Frequency is determined not only by the number of times a task must be performed, but by the scheduling of the task and the predictability of performance. Duration is measured by the length of time the service need is expected to continue.

In examining need for services, the more often, the more unpredictable, and the longer a task must be performed the greater the probability that traditional in-home support services may be too costly to provide, too difficult to coordinate, or too difficult to locate. The range for frequency and duration of need might be assumed as

TABLE 7.2 Client Distribution in Articulated Service System

Service Criterion	In-Home Services	"Retirement" Housing	Adult Foster Care Homes	Assisted Living
Caregiver availability	Caregiver adequately available, or lack of availability does not impact need significantly.	Caregiver adequately available, or lack of availability does not impact need significantly.	Caregiver not adequately available, and lack of availability may impact need.	Caregiver not adequately available, and lack of availability impacts need significantly.
Frequency and duration	May be frequent if time limited or may be infrequent if ongoing. Must typically be scheduled during normal weekday hours. Must be delivered in single unit.	May be frequent if time limited or must be infrequent if ongoing. May be scheduled during normal weekday hours. May be delivered in group.	May be frequent and ongoing. Must be scheduled during normal waking hours. May be delivered individually if planned.	May be frequent and ongoing. May be scheduled anytime. May be unscheduled routinely for individuals.
Skill level	May be any skill level, but cost eligibility and availability will act to restrict services severely.	May be any skill level, but cost eligibility and availability will act to restrict services severely.	May be similar to other non-health-related service industry, but special training is necessary for basic hands-on personal care.	May be similar to other non-health related service industry, but special training is necessary for basic hands-on personal care and nursing services.
Protective oversight	Protective oversight not necessary or caregiver available to provide.	Protective oversight not necessary or caregiver available to provide.	Limited protective oversight may be needed.	Full protective oversight may be needed.

Source: Adapted from Wilson, K. B. Report prepared for the state of Delaware.

0 = Daily, unscheduled, ongoing needs
1 = More than once a week, unscheduled, ongoing, or daily scheduled needs
2 = Weekly or less, scheduled or time limited (e.g., 30 days or fewer) needs
3 = Episodic, scheduled, or time-limited needs

Many IADL and ADL tasks can be performed without significant or special training. Clearly, some require more skill than others. Occasionally, this skill is related solely to the task to be performed—such as providing care to a brittle diabetic on sliding-scale insulin. Often it is related to the ability of the person receiving care to direct and participate in his or her own care.

When care needs are complex, health condition is medically unstable, or the individual is unable to participate actively in getting care needs met, more skill, judgment, and professional insight are required. Thus, the range of skill level might be assumed to be

0 = Complex care needs, unstable medically, nominal ability to direct care
1 = Routine care needs, stable medically, nominal ability to direct care
2 = Complex care needs, stable medically, able to participate in directing care needs
3 = Routine care needs, stable medically, able to participate in directing care needs

The need for ongoing supervision for some individuals with nominal IADL or ADL needs long has been recognized. Generally these individuals suffer from some intellectual, psychological, or social impairments that significantly impair their independent living skills.

Even when IADL or ADL skills remain somewhat intact the individual who is intellectually compromised, has psychopathology that disrupts and impairs daily living, or is unable to evaluate risk-taking behaviors adequately must have their activities monitored closely. In this context the range of protective oversight can be assumed as

0 = Significantly intellectually compromised, moderate to severe psychopathology, poor life-preserving skills
1 = Significantly to moderately intellectually compromised, mild to moderate psychopathology, poor life-preserving skills
2 = Moderately to nominally intellectually compromised, mild to moderate psychopathology, adequate life-preserving skills
3 = Nominally intellectually compromised, nominal psychopathology, adequate life-preserving skills

Taken together, these criteria provide a way of assessing criteria for programmatic parameters as shown in Table 7.2. Clearly in such a system the lower the score the higher the service need and the more complex the intervention. Yet in an articulated system the intervention can be introduced more incrementally.

Assisted living, as previously defined in Table 7.1, generally appears better suited than other supportive housing options to carry out a program of client normalization when caregiver availability is compromised; service need is frequent, unpredictable, and ongoing; one-on-one care is required; and significant protective oversight is needed. Having core capability to deliver consistently a wide range of unplanned services is a distinguishing characteristic of assisted living.

POLICY PARAMETERS OF ASSISTED LIVING

Despite the inherent logic of combining housing with services, supportive housing has not developed naturally or gracefully in the United States. In part this is the result of federal policy. Historically, a strong policy imperative to view housing independent of services exists. Federal policy traditionally has not linked housing with services for any age group.

Although the number of federally sponsored units for older adults is very small in comparison with the demand for such housing, the clear federal policy of separating shelter from services has had far-ranging consequences. One consequence was the mandate of the Older Americans Act to serve older adults in their "own" homes. Subsequently, for the past two decades, most program efforts of State Units on Aging and Area Agencies on Aging have been directed toward individuals living in scattered-site settings. As a matter of policy, those living in age-segregated housing often were systematically excluded from service. This exclusion often was based erroneously on the assumption that their service needs were already being met.

The artificial separation of housing and services was heightened in 1965 by Title XVIII of the Social Security Act. In addition, the Miller amendments, passed in 1967, provided the basis for current Medicaid programs for older persons. Essentially by adopting a medical model of long-term care requiring that most services be authorized and performed by specially trained individuals (e.g., physicians, nurses, and certified personnel) in designated institutions (hospitals and nursing homes), the final link was forged to ensure 25 years of separation between housing and services, policy, funding, and regulation.

During the 1970s the number of age-segregated elderly independent living units without services continued to increase. Growth in the number of nursing home beds per 1,000 for the 65-plus population also increased. By the mid-1970s, however, the concept of a continuum of care emerged (Regnier and Pynoos, 1987; Struyk, Page, Newman, et al., 1989; Tilson, 1990). The concept played out under the Miller amendments recognized two ends of a continuum of need — totally independent living and nursing home placement. It did not, however, recognize, let alone legitimize, the role cf supportive housing.

In the real world of practice, of course, additional service options were created (Newcomer & Stone, 1985). Supportive housing in the guise of "boarding"-type homes existed. Board and care came to be used by many states as housing of last resort for the very poor who could not qualify for nursing home placement under Medicaid criteria, the chronically mentally ill (swept up in the de-institutionalization movement of the late 1960s), the developmentally disabled, and transient populations. In practice this option often has been used by states to house persons who did not fit federal categorical programs and who were too poor to pay privately for services. Generally, policy has been to minimize the public cost of supportive housing to individual states and the federal government.

At the same time demand for supportive housing was growing rapidly in the private market. This growing demand has been documented extensively (Newman, 1985; Regnier et al., 1991; Barnes, Burt, McBride, & Meyer, Zedlewski, 1989). One of the supportive housing options created for the upper middle class was the continuing care retirement community (CCRC's). This option was created to cater to those older individuals with sufficient resources to buy guaranteed access to long term nursing care. While CCRC's existed prior to the 1960's, in the past twenty years they have become targeted toward selected retirement destinations with less direct religious or philanthropic participation. Interest continues today in this option (Frankel, 1978; Pynoos, 1985; Tilson, 1990).

Another form of supportive housing for the upper middle class appeared in the 1970s and was marketed as a life-style choice of the active, independent person who lacked the means or inclination to purchase "life or continuing" care. Often called congregate care, a package of non–health-related services on a month-to-month rental basis was offered. The services were similar to those provided in boarding homes, but shelter and amenities in congregate care were designed to appeal to private-paying older adults (Lawton & Weeden, 1985).

Thus, by the late 1970s the continuum of care for older persons in the United States actually consisted of independent living housing options with limited support services routinely available, various types of boarding homes and nursing home placement. Efforts to expand this continuum of care focused almost exclusively on community-based care options for individuals residing in their own homes. These early options included programs such as property tax–relief programs, home repair, nutrition site meals, and chore services. The continual increase in the cost of nursing home care, however, began to result in more emphasis on targeting services toward more vulnerable older adults in the early 1980s. Programs such as home care and adult day care were implemented to reduce the risk of institutionalization. Community-residing older persons living alone in their own homes became a primary target group for these services.

During this same period, major changes were occurring in the populations of older persons living in all types of age-segregated housing. They were getting older and more frail. By the mid-1980s, two phrases had been coined to describe these phenomena and the attendant problems: "aging in place" and "delayed entry." As in-home service options expanded and the personal income of older adults increased, older persons began to further delay moving into settings where services might be more readily available. The average age at entry for every setting, from the Department of Housing and Urban Development housing to nursing homes, began to climb. At the same time, those who had entered age-segregated settings without services at a younger age stayed longer. The net effect of these consumer behaviors was to increase the range, mix, and scope of support services needed by individuals in all settings.

The effect of these trends was exacerbated further by the implementation of diagnostic-related groups (DRGs) by the HCFA in 1983. DRGs were a mechanism designed to control Medicare costs related to hospitalization. Under DRGs hospitals implemented a vigorous compaign to reduce the length of stay of Medicare patients. One result has been earlier discharge of individuals and increased demand for services in all settings. At the same time, older consumers have become increasingly resistive to nursing home placement.

Consumer resistance to nursing facility placement led to expanded efforts to increase traditional scattered-site services such as in-home health, meals-on-wheels, and remote emergency care monitoring. Many efforts have been made to create programs designed to keep older adults in single-family homes including home sharing, reverse annuity programs, ECHO housing and managed care programs such as ONLOK. These efforts to date have yielded little relief to states with increasing numbers of frail older adults needing ongoing services. A new option was needed that would serve more impaired individuals, cost less than traditional nursing facility placement, and be more acceptable to consumers (Newman, 1990).

At the same time states have been hit by revelations surrounding the conditions of nonfederally regulated board and care homes (Bolda, 1991). Aging advocates are seeking to institute minimum national standards to improve quality of care. Ironically, these regulatory efforts have not been aimed at the reformulation of policy to provide additional funding or a more viable programmatic approach (Wilson, Ladd, & Saslow, 1988). Despite the lack of a cohesive, informed federal policy, states are moving ahead to explore the development and regulation of new forms of supportive housing (Leak, 1991). In particular, states have begun to explore how to define and regulate the newest form of supportive housing—assisted living.

It is in this context of growing concerns about increasing frailness, vulnerability, cost, and consumer preference that states have begun to examine the policy parameters of assisted living. For states, policy formulation has been focused on issues related to definitions, standards, integration into existing service delivery systems, and cost.

CREATION OF A PARADIGM FOR ASSISTED LIVING

Linking conceptual and policy issues forges a paradigm for assisted living. As a type of supportive housing assisted living offers great potential for enhancing independent living for frail vulnerable adults (Wilson & Rankos, 1991; Wilson et al, 1988). Assisted living enhances this through

1. Normalization of the environment
2. Proactive strategies to enhance client functioning
3. Responding to prevailing cultural values
4. Refining service management and practices

Normalization of Environment

Essentially, the normalization of the environment for assisted living has focused on how to create more functional designs. These designs must facilitate the personalization of space and mediate the effects of individual limitations (Butler & Bjaanes, 1983). The personalization of space must weigh the need to establish territorial boundaries against the realities of communal living. In mediating individual limitations, the environment must not be devoid of all stimuli, nor can "public" safety be ignored.

The balance between territorial prerogatives and community goodwill in assisted living is enhanced by expanding on the concept of a multiunit building functioning as a microcommunity. Within this context, the "householder" has a private dwelling in supportive housing, and the common spaces function as communal resources. A significant problem, particularly in supportive housing, has been the assumption that private space is secondary to public space.

This assumption is based, in part, on the perception that public space functions the same as private space and could, in effect, act as an extension of it. Clearly, experience in age-segregated settings of all types suggests this perception generally is not accurate. Further, in those instances when public space is treated as an extension of private space, it can create confict in the larger community. Finally, by ignoring the differences between private and public space, social structures may be damaged.

Encouraging individuals to expand on a regular basis activities outside of their private space invites them to exercise territorial prerogatives in common spaces that can lead to group conflict. In group living it is not uncommon to see fighting over seats in the dining room, reluctance to invite others to join an activity, and hostility over perceived violations of rules in this extended personal space. When there is no cooking capacity in individual units, individuals mark space in the dining room. When there is no private personal living space, family encounters become public, ritualized events.

To substitute effectively public for private space often it is necessary to depersonalize it to the degree that conflict is limited over the use of that area. Assisted living, by creating private, self-contained living units, reduces the tension between the individual and the larger social unit. The capacity to create within a private, controlled individual space those activities most closely associated with home reduces the need by individuals to lay exclusive claim to public space.

Normalization also encourages accommodation within private space to support individual functional levels. In practical terms this means a careful blend of nonintrusive supports with an ability to manipulate the level of environmental press. To illustrate, an example of nonintrusive support would be lever door handles. Manipulating the level of environmental press is illustrated by the optional installation of grab bars in the unit bathroom.

Functional design elements also contribute to the normalization of an institutional setting by creating private space that is residential in character. Residential character is defined by structural amenities, furnishings, and ability to express life-style choices. Structural amenities ideally involve the replication of a scaled-down single-family household with defined areas for eating, sleeping, and entertaining. It involves having a private bath and a locking door to control access to the space. Residential furnishings means the total personalization of private space and normally shuns the use of specialized geriatric furniture. Ability to express life-style choices involves setting household standards for space use.

Thus, apart from size and nonintrusive environmental supports such as roll-in showers, the private space in assisted living should reflect those features primarily associated with a household. The environment is more than the private space called home, however. It is neighborhood or community as well. Whether community is defined territorially or culturally, clearly age-segregated multiunit buildings also have the potential to engender emotional and social feelings. Those who live next door are neighbors, and public space reflects neighborhood resources available to everyone. Maintaining the balance between the expression of life-style and neighborhood covenants generalize the sense of community.

Public space in assisted living mimics community space. There are all the expected areas — the dining room or the neighborhood restaurant, the activity area or the community social club, the lobby or the town square, and the medication room or the health clinic. The halls become streets, and the exits signal leaving the neighborhood. Use of this public space, when sufficient private space is available to individuals, is predictable. Residents come out of their own home to use a community resource, to socialize with friends, to find out what is going on, to collect their mail, and to entertain themselves. This pattern of use is both culturally and individually defined.

Enhancement of Individual Functioning

In addition to cost, providing services is linked to problems with availability and acceptability. Availability implies that capability exists. Acceptability infers that the method used meets with consumer approval. Assisted living expands availability and enhances acceptability in a unique proactive fashion to enhance individual functional ability.

Problems with availability stem from internal and external constraints that act to limit service. Those frequently mentioned as internal constraints are reluctance to expand staff responsibilities, lack of appropriate staff skills, and insufficient supplemental resources. External constraints involve interagency conflict over standards, conflict with market competitors, and uninformed consumers. The internal constraints are reduced by expanding expectations for capability, while encouraging the individualization of service to target the use of resources more effectively. External constraints are reduced by clarifying the articulation of services within the existing delivery system.

Core care capability in assisted living includes access to a broad array of environmental, personal, and routine nursing services using a modified system of care management. Several key service factors set assisted living apart from other forms of supportive housing. Chief among these is 24-hour care capability, which means that assistance is readily available on-site for most nonphysician care needs. In this arrangement problems with unpredictable (e.g., sleep disorders), unscheduled (e.g., incontinence), and irregular (e.g., ambulation) needs can be managed on an ongoing basis even for those unable to communicate their service needs and preferences to the provider.

Another factor is the range and mix of services addressed in the core capability of assisted living. Attempts to restrict services or to segment this range of services artificially encourages denial, increased costs, and forced relocation. To the extent that range is expanded (e.g., from medication monitoring to administration of controlled substances) and mix is extended (e.g., special-diet meals, coordination of dialysis care, and counseling for situational depression), overall capacity is enhanced. Enhanced capacity facilitates the potential for responding to increasingly complex unscheduled or unpredictable service needs.

Implicit in this expansion is the provision of services typically called nursing care, although many are related to ADL functioning and the management of chronic conditions. The ability to provide routine nursing services and to accept care management responsibility in assisted living distinguishes it from other forms of supportive housing that rely on third-party providers to coordinate and perform these services.

Thus, the range of services in assisted living extends beyond the typical "hotel" services found in many forms of supportive housing. Meals, structured group socialization, linen laundry, housekeeping, and transportation by themselves do not meet, even at a minimum, core care capability requirements of assisted living.

Level of service in assisted living must involve the expectation of consumer need for, and the ability of the provider to respond appropriately to, a variety of conditions stemming from impaired physical, intellectual, social, and psychological functional ability. Incontinence, dementia-related disorders, behavioral problems, and chronic conditions requiring active health management are other services that should be available routinely, in addition to assistance with medication management and ADLs.

Use of Values Orientation to Improve Quality

In assisted living values orientation is focused on autonomy and how it is implemented. Although autonomy has multiple meanings, in service settings it has come to be characterized as empowerment of the client to direct his or her own care (Cohen, 1988). Empowerment is centered on respecting and responding to client preferences in a way that fosters a sense of personal dignity, independence, privacy, individuality, and choice.

Further, consumer empowerment in assisted living reflects new assumptions about vulnerable adults. These new assumptions accept the premise that empowerment can occur only if values are seen in the context of shared responsibility, bounded choices, and managed risk.*

In many service models, older consumers are cast as helpless and without responsibility to contribute to outcomes. Yet, healthy adult relationships, including that of caregiver and care recipient, involve balancing the degree of control over decision making (empowerment) and the level of responsibility taken for the outcome. Assisted living assumes that responsibility and control are shared by the caregiver, the consumer, and others who may be designated

*Expansion of work first presented by the author in a paper, "Beyond Loving Care," written in 1988 for the Oregon Gerontological Association.

to act as an advocate for the consumer. It assumes that they will work together to set expectations, identify roles and tasks associated with them, as well as do their part in achieving agreed-on goals.

Shared responsibility is based on the premise that competence is relative to the situation and varies from one domain of functioning to another. Clearly, even severely compromised adults can be actively involved at some level in managing to meet some of their own needs. In assisted living service is organized formally to facilitate this sharing by segmenting tasks for the care recipient according to interest and ability of those sharing responsibility.

Setting expectations and contributing to agreed on outcomes, reflects a willingness to accept boundaries in the exercise of personal choice. How free individuals are to make choices depends on personal capacity, societal limits, and situational circumstances. The assumption in assisted living is that all individuals live with limits, but choices that reflect individual values and preferences should be honored whenever possible.

The right to have a choice honored is limited also by society, ability, and the personal risk inherent in the enactment of the decision. Civilization requires rules, bringing order and preventing harm. Additional limits are imposed culturally to help make life more predictable and pleasant on a personal level. Individuals who make choices outside of these boundaries risk refusal, rejection, or punishment on some level.

Often, however, choice is limited unnecessarily. Assisted living assumes that even choices that involve risk for vulnerable adults can be negotiated. In those situations when a decision involves significant likelihood of imminent or probable harm to self or others, demonstrates disregard for the rights of others, or is likely to result in social ridicule or isolation for the decision maker, the choice made is subject to a formal process of managed risk.

Managed risk involves determining why the choice may be a poor decision, providing information about the likely consequences of various options, developing alternatives that reduce the risk associated with various options but are responsive to individual preferences, and recording the negotiation process regardless of the decision outcome. It assures risks are evaluated, values respected, and liability managed prudently through a process of informed decision making and shared responsibility.

Refinement of Service Management

The key to implementing these precepts in assisted living is good case management. Assisted living incorporates fundamental principles of case management—service assessment, planning, implementation, and evaluation. Formalized comprehensive case management also sets assisted living apart from other forms of supportive housing. Case management enhances the individualization of services and promotes the concept of managed care even when third-party providers are used.

Although the focus on service planning is not unknown in settings such as nursing facilities, the method used is distinct. It goes beyond passive participation of the individual in a multidisciplinary planning process. Assisted living refocuses the process on the enhancement of individual competence. Such a focus is in keeping with the tenets of client normalization. This focus on competence extends to the active involvement of the individual in setting priorities, proposing strategies to meet them, and agreeing to service parameters as a part of the individualization of the service plan. Negotiation of the plan requires the consumer, the provider, and, at times, an advocate reaching consensus surrounding expectations and strategies to implement the services.

Service management in assisted living involves tying assessed service need directly to a service plan. Need is defined incrementally in terms of the level of support required to complete a given task adequately. These needs reflect not only ADLs, but the ability of the individual to manage other relevant facets of their lives (e.g., familial relations, leisure time, environment in which they live, etc.).

The implementation of the service plan is contingent on the agreement of the consumer or the consumer's designated advocate. The consumer is empowered to refuse service without being labeled as incompetent. Change in condition or preference results in renegotiation of the plan. When service is organized so that tasks are incrementally defined and consumers are empowered to take risks, service use not only decreases overall but becomes highly individualized.

CASE STUDY: IMPLEMENTATION OF ASSISTED LIVING IN OREGON

Assisted living in Oregon grew out of prototype initially developed in 1983 as a private-pay option. By merging consumer preference (home care) with need (core care capability), a new type of supportive housing emerged. The model was influenced by three events. First was the mode of financing. Using bond financing provided through the State Housing Agency meant building to specifications for the more traditional congregate project to secure funding. A second determining event was the decision to license the project under existing state rules for residential care. This decision was based on existing market demand for more service in congregate-type projects. Finally, those involved in developing the prototype were new to the field of supportive housing. Having few preconceived ideas about how institutional services traditionally were delivered, they pursued a course that blended theoretical assumptions and personal experience to forge a new paradigm for implementing assisted living.

Starting with a building design for congregate housing had significant impact on the normalization of the environment. At no time, for example, was there an assumption of "double-bed occupancy" rooms. Each client had a private apartment. Space was to be shared only by personal choice. Private space was defined in the context of a household with those features dominating design. The only concession was to size of the unit that was made smaller. This reduction was based on higher construction costs associated with building-code requirements for a structure meeting more stringent life-safety requirements (e.g., fully automatic sprinkler system).

The functional design elements of public space also were impacted. One major feature was the incorporation of space in the "town square" by the front door. Recognizing that this area was a major focus in the community for informal socialization, it was expanded and designed to facilitate such activities. Another normalization factor was the aggressive integration of residential furnishings suitably modified for their use in the project. The major departure in functional design, however, was the development of support services space intended to facilitate delivery of services associated typically with nursing care facilities (e.g., medication management, whirlpool bathing, incontinence laundry, etc.)

Getting a license proved to be the more significant event. Existing residential care rules were vague about the scope, range, and mix of services that could be provided in a licensed facility. There were some limitations related to mobility, incontinence, and nursing care. More significant were the interpretative limitations historically imposed by the licensure agency and providers themselves. The decision was made to develop a service planning approach that emphasized the provider's pivotal role in managing care including that which had to be assessed through third-party providers. As residents aged in place, staff became more committed to pushing the outer boundaries of rule limitations for individuals through the innovative organization of services.

Aggressive care management illustrated that the issues related to the imposition of admission and retention criteria for residential care were not properly focused. Clearly, the problem revolved around the capability of the provider to respond uniquely to a given set of needs. Individualization of service required more interaction and more negotiation, but it also created the capacity to adjust services radically in response to personal competence central to client normalization.

Overlaying the entire development of this prototype was an underlying belief that theory could be brought to bear on practice in a systematic way. The reported lack of success in existing models was attributed to a faulty paradigm, the continuum of care, as well as a misguided values orientation. This assumption had interesting results.

One result was the approach to service that was visualized as being made up of interchangeable units combined and recombined in response to changing needs. This approach automatically resulted in an expansion of core care capability and ultimately fewer discharges to nursing facilities. Another result was less differentiation in traditional staff roles. Focusing service on individual consumer priorities meant more ability and flexibility on the part of staff to respond. Finally, rethinking who and what services were to be provided resulted in a more profound shift in values orientation from "best practice" to client empowerment.

From Prototype to State Policy

In 1987 the state of Oregon determined to support a pilot project for Medicaid clients in one of the two now existing assisted living projects. The Senior and Disabled Services Division (SDSD) based this decision on a long-standing commitment to community-based long-term care and the prospect of reducing Medicaid costs for nursing facility–eligible clients.

Since the first project's opening it had been recognized as a successful, innovative model. Its success led the developers to plan a second one. In conjunction with its opening an offer was made to SDSD to conduct a demonstration project with a limited number of Medicaid clients. The goal was to provide an incentive for the state to examine formally the model developed as a means of illustrating the extensive role supportive housing could play in long-term care.

Terms of the first Medicaid project were straight forward. The state would select clients who were eligible financially and by virtue of their impairment level. Criteria included eligibility for nursing facility placement. Medicaid clients were provided a private studio apartment and a package of services tied to their level of impairment.

Of the original 22 clients placed, more than one half (59.1%) were relocated from nursing facilities and psychiatric units. Overall, one third (36.5%) were dependent in at least one of the six critical ADLs, with the remaining needing assistance in at least two of the same activities. Twenty percent were dependent behaviorally, whereas 75% needed full protective oversight. In a comparison, the state found significant overlaps in impairment between the Medicaid clients in the assisted living project and nursing facility clients.

An evaluation of outcomes for the assisted living Medicaid clients was conducted after 1 year. The state found significant improvements in mobility and orientation. Discharge data indicated 50% was due to death in the project. Analysis, in 1988, indicated an actual average total cost of $1,255 per client per month compared with $1,647 in a nursing facility. In both settings these costs included the client's contribution. Although the costs included shelter and food, they do not include other care costs such as hospitalization, drug use, physician visits, and durable medical equipment. In tracking the use of these services, the state did not find that assisted living clients used these services more frequently than comparable nursing facility clients. Based on these results the SDSD determined to make assisted living a Medicaid reimbursable service under the state's Home and Community Based Care Waiver. This decision led to a year-long process of policy planning to implement the program. Central to this process was the development of rules for assisted living.

The rule-making process tackled head on the relationship between housing and services as well as the role of supportive housing in long-term care. Facility standards were written that reflected a focus on environmental normalization. Further, the standards were developed by a broad-based group representing a wide range of concerns—fire marshals, loan officers, architects, building-codes inspectors, licensure surveyors, advocates, and providers. Concerns about safety, cost, and values were addressed. The end result was a stated value to maintain a residential feeling, a requirement to incorporate numerous features to protect and support residents, and an effort to minimize the financial impact by allowing greater flexibility in interpreting the standards.

Service standards also were developed by a diverse task force. Its goal not only was to define the range, mix, and scope of services to be provided, but to legitimize the importance of using a client-focused, outcome-oriented system of service delivery. These standards literally eliminated admission and retention criteria for assisted living. This flexibility reduces the rejection of clients seeking to move in based on a specific impairment (e.g., insulin dependency, transfer assistance, incontinence, etc.). It also reduces the need to move out based on a change in service needs. At the same time standards for core care capability were expanded with emphasis on the role of case management. Core care capability was defined to include all of the services identified in Table 7.2 including routine nursing tasks and behavior management services.

The most radical departure in the rules was the forthright statement of purpose that reflected a shift in values orientation. This shift emphasized that service quality was linked not only to outcomes, but the degree to which the service approach upheld the individual's dignity, engendered independence, facilitated choice, fostered privacy, respected individuality, and created a more homelike environment.

Some called the new rules an attempt to regulate philosophy. Others said they were too vague and did not provide enough direction to providers. The state's position was that prescriptive rule writing generally had not resolved issues of quality care in other settings. Thus, the regulatory focus in assisted living was to be tied to the skill of the provider in responding to client needs in a way that reflected the new values orientation.

After 15 months of effort the new rules went into effect in October 1989. They were accompanied by a five-level rate structure that overlapped on the low end with adult foster care and on the upper end with intermediate-care nursing facility rates (approximately $800–$1,600 per month). Rates were tied to assessed impairment levels, with priority for placement to be given to those with moderately high levels of impairment. Focus for placement in assisted living was on those hospitalized awaiting nursing facility placement, those seeking relocation from a nursing facility, those facing eviction from an existing facility, and private-pay clients who have exhausted their financial resources.

Turnover is averaging 30% to 35% annually for all details. Of other move-outs, 30% go to a higher level of care and 20% go to a lower level of care. Fifty-nine percent of private-pay clients who move into assisted living come from nursing facilities or hospitals. They pay, at an average, $52 per day for an apartment and services. The average private-pay, nonskilled nursing facility rate is approximately $80 per day plus add-ons.

Some unexpected events also have occurred. Perhaps the most significant is the development of smaller size assisted living projects in communities outside of the major population centers in the states. Of 15 projects currently licensed, 7 (46.7%) are outside of the major metropolitan areas of the state with an average size of 34 units. Of the projects currently being planned only two are in the metropolitan area, and only four are 50 units or more.

This has at least three potential implications. First, the demand exists in smaller, more rural communities. Second, smaller size projects can be economically viable, even advantageous, under the right conditions. Perhaps most important, such projects reflect a better understanding of the impact of size on client and environmental normalization.

A second impact has been revitalized attention to training of providers and of state surveyors particularly on values orientation. A consultative model has been used by the state to provide technical assistance to newly developed assisted living facilities that need more training in operationalizing the model. A key result of this is heightened cooperation between the state and providers in focusing efforts on upholding the philosophy of client empowerment using managed-risk techniques.

Not all of the news has been good. Perhaps the most serious is the problem of unlicensed assisted living. Some providers, unwilling or unable to meet facility or care standards to be licensed as assisted living, attempt to portray themselves as such to consumers. This is creating confusion among consumers as well as many professionals and legislators. Licensed assisted living providers themselves, in response, have bonded together to undertake a program of public education.

A second problem has been slower than hoped for development. Largely this has been due to the general slow-down of the economy and the difficulty in securing long-term financing for all types of projects. This is evident in the large number of projects still in planning after 2 years. Also disappointing is the interest shown by existing nursing facilities in conversion. Although four (26.7%) of the existing projects are residential-congregate care conversion, only one nursing facility conversion is even being planned.

By December 1991, 748 apartments in 15 buildings had been licensed for assisted living. With actual licensed capacity of 891 units, 216 (24.2%) house Medicaid clients of which 19 (08.8%) are younger or disabled adults. The sites range in size from 12 to 112 units, averaging 50 units. Each project has Medicaid clients with the percentage varying from 13% to 62%. Another 702 units are in some stage of development. Their additions would increase licensed capacity to serve an estimated 1,555 individuals.

Reflecting policy the majority of individuals placed by the state show moderate to high levels of impairment. Clients are significantly impaired. Thirty-four percent are older than age 85. ADL dependencies are high with 89% needing help with bathing, 84% being mobility impaired, 59% having behavioral problems, 52% needing assistance with toileting, and 34% unable to perform tasks associated with grooming or personal hygiene. Eighty percent need assistance with medication management, and 60% have a level of dementia that requires significant protective oversight. Clients average 3.4 dependencies in ADLs.

Average state payment is $891.00 per month, with clients contributing an additional average of $533.00 per month, for an average daily rate of $46.71. This compares to $75.00 per day for nonskilled Medicaid nursing facility care with clients contributing $405.65 per month. Private-pay rates range from approximately $1,049.00 to $2,800.00, with an average of $1,650.00 per month, while nursing facilities average $2,440.00 per month. This results in an average cost that is 65% to 70% of non–heavy care nursing facility rates.

Somewhat puzzling is the general lack of participation by nonprofits in the development of assisted living. Only two not-for-profit conversions are even in the planning stage. Some nonprofits, notably Continuing Care Retirement Communities (CCRCs), have created unlicensed assisted living units as a part of their campus.

The state, after 4 year's experience, remains convinced that assisted living is the type of supportive housing that is likely to become the predominate mode of custodial care in the future. Its own studies indicate that, despite an aggressive 10-year effort to use community-based care using foster care and in-home services, fully 40% of existing clients could be supported appropriately in assisted living. Thus, after 8 years of development, assisted living has evolved as a model of supportive housing for frail, vulnerable adults in need of substantial levels of ongoing personal and nursing care services.

ACKNOWLEDGMENTS

Assistance was provided by Richard Ladd, Janet Sehon, and Doug Stone, Senior and Disabled Services Division, state of Oregon, in preparing the section on the implementation of assisted living in Oregon.

REFERENCES

Baker, P., & Prince, M. (1990). Supportive housing preferences among the elderly. In L. A. Pastalan (Ed.), *Optimizing housing for the elderly.* New York: The Haworth Press.
Bolda, E. (1991). *Initial report on North Carolina domiciliary care policy.* Prepared for inclusion in the North Carolina Long Term Care Bibliographic Database, The Long Term Care Resources Program, Duke University Center for the Study of Aging and Human Development.
Butler, E., & Bjaanes, A. (1983). Deinstitutionalization, environmental normalization and client normalization. In K. Kernan, M. Begals, & R. Edgerton (Eds.), *The adaptation of mentally retarded persons.* Baltimore: University Park Press.
Cohen, E. (1988). The elderly mystique: Constraints on the autonomy of the elderly with disabilities. *The Gerontologist, 28,* 24–31.
Frankel, F. (1978). Health and social needs of the aged related to housing as provided by a life care community. *Long Term Care and Health Services Administration Quarterly, 21,* 245–249.
Hurd, M. (1990). Research on the elderly: Status, retirement and consumption and saving. *Journal of Economic Literature, 28,* 565–637.
Kane, R., Illston, L., Kane, R., & Nyman, J. (1990). Meshing services with housing: Lessons from adult foster care and assisted living in Oregon. University of Minnesota Care Decisions Resource Center, Minneapolis.
Landesman, S. (1988). Preventing "institutionalization" in the community. In M. Janicki, M. Krauss, & M. Seltzer (Eds.), *Community residence for persons with developmental disabilities: Here to stay.* Baltimore: Brooks.
Lawton, P. (1980). *Environment and Aging.* Monterey, CA: Brooks/Cole.
Lawton, P., & Weeden, J. (1985). Introduction. *Generations, 9,* 4–8.
Leak, S. (1991). State housing with services programs: New initiatives, striking diversity. *Lont Term Care Advances, 3,* 2–7.
Manfredini, D., & Smith, W. (1988). The concept and implementation of active treatment. In M. Janicki, M. Krauss, & M. Seltzer (Eds.). *Community residence for persons with developmental disabilities: Here to stay.* Baltimore: Brooks.
Merill, J., & Hunt, M. (1990). Aging in place: A dilemma for retirement housing administrators. *The Journal of Applied Gerontology, 9,* 60–76.
Mor, V., Sherwood, S., & Gurkin, C. (1986). A national study of residential care for the aged. *The Gerontologist, 26,* 405–414.
Newcomer, R., & Stone, R. (1985). Board and care housing. *Generations, 9,* 39–41.
Newman, S. (1985). The Shape of things to come. *Generations, 9,* 24–27.
Newman, S. (1990). The frail elderly in the community: An overview of characteristics. In D. Tilson (Ed.), *Aging in place.* Glenview, IL: Scott, Foresman.
Pynoos, J. (1985). Options for mid-upper income elders. *Generations, 9,* 31–33.
Raschko, B. (1982). *Housing interiors for the disabled and elderly.* New York: Van Nostrand Reinhold.

Redfoot, D., & Gaberlavage, R. (1991). Housing for older Americans: Sustaining the dream. *Generations, 15,* 35–38.

Regnier, V., Hamilton, J., & Yatabe, S. (1991). *Best practices in assisted living.* Long Term Care National Resource Center at UCLA/USC, Los Angeles.

Spivack, M. (1984). *Institutional settings: An environmental design approach.* New York: Human Sciences Press.

Struyk, R., Page, D., Newman, S., et al. (1989). *Providing supportive services to the frail elderly in federally assisted housing.* Washington, DC: Urban Institute Press.

Tilson, D. (Ed.). (1990). *Aging in place.* Glenview, IL: Scott, Foresman.

Tully, K. (1986). *Improving residential life for disabled people.* New York: Churchill Livingstone.

Wilson, K. (1988). *Beyond Loving Care.* Paper prepared for the Oregon Gerontological Society, Portland.

Wilson, K. B. (1990). Assisted living: The merger of housing and long term care services. *Long Term Care Advances, 1,* 208.

Wilson, K. (1991). Expanding residential options in Delaware. Report prepared for the Delaware Department of Health and Social Services, Dover.

Wilson, K., Ladd, R., & Saslow, M. (1988, November). Paper presented at the 41st Annual Scientific Meeting of the Gerontological Society of America, San Francisco.

Wilson, K., & Rankos, D. (1991). *Assisted living: New hope for long term care?* Paper presented at the Gerontological Society of America, San Francisco.

Zedlewski, S., Barnes, R., Burt, M., McBride, T. & Meyer, J. (1989). *The needs of the elderly in the 21st century.* The Urban Institute: DC: Washington.

Zedlewski, S., Barnes, R., Burt, M., McBride, T., & Meyer, J. (1991). *Supportive services in senior housing: Lessons from the Robert Wood Johnson Foundation demonstration paper prepared by The Policy Center on Aging.* The Heller School, Brandeis University, Waltham, MA.

8
Health Promotion and Health Maintenance for the Chronically Disabled

Kyle R. Allen
Gregg A. Warshaw

Among the very old chronic health problems are common. Eighty-six percent of persons older than age 65 have at least one chronic condition, and 52% of those older than age 75 have some limitation in their daily abilities (Federal Council on Aging, 1981). Common chronic conditions in older people include osteoarthritis, hypertension, hearing impairment, heart disease, cataracts, and diabetes (Fowks, 1990). The highest percentage of disabled persons are in the "old-old" age group (> 75 years) (Wedgewood, 1985). At first glance, it seems incongruent to discuss health promotion and preventive strategies for chronically disabled and frail older adults. The traditional goal of preventive medicine is to improve and maintain *health*, with a focus on primary and secondary prevention. For the chronically disabled and frail elderly, the goal is to improve and maintain function and quality of life – not necessarily to prevent or eliminate disease. In this way we can achieve some of the secondary goals of conventional health maintenance (i.e., to reduce the economic, social, personal, and political burden of disease and disability).

Health maintenance for the elderly is a complex and emotional topic (Kennie, 1988). Recommended guidelines are as varied as the number of professional organizations promoting them. The data available to support specific health promotion recommendations in the older population is limited. No wonder there is such frustration and confusion over implementing a health maintenance plan for older individuals. Furthermore, given such scant research data on the older population, it is even more difficult to discuss health maintenance for the chronically disabled and frail older adult.

The key to success is to use an approach that is specific for the individual, keeping in mind that person's medical history, degree of disability, life expectancy, resources, family support, quality of life, personal feelings, and goals. It is necessary to pay attention to the risk versus benefit of an intervention, burden of suffering, iatrogenic complications, and possible adverse effects. This will provide a framework for organizing an effective health maintenance plan with the ultimate goal of preventing further disability, maximizing function, and improving quality of life.

This chapter discusses general aspects of health maintenance and how they apply to chronically disabled and frail older adults. This information is directed primarily toward health care professionals in the long-term care sector: home care, nursing home, and long-term rehabilitation.

DEFINITIONS
Prevention

There are three basic preventive strategies: primary, secondary, and tertiary. Primary prevention is targeted toward identifying risk factors or environmental conditions that predispose persons to develop disease or injury. Examples include nutrition assessment and education, accident awareness and prevention, immunizations, and exercise programs. Secondary prevention is aimed at the preclinical or asymptomatic period of a disease. Most familiar screening strategies (e.g., mammograms, monitoring cholesterol, and fecal occult blood testing), are examples of secondary prevention.

Screening programs that uncover symptomatic but undetected disease are also important; this is known as case finding. It is a form of tertiary prevention. Though the chances of "curing" problems are limited, identifying symptomatic but unreported disease can have a dramatic impact on limiting the progression of disability and functional impairment, thereby helping the patient maintain independence. This is a valuable approach for promoting function in the chronically disabled and frail elderly (Kennie, 1988). The elderly tend to underreport disease and present late in the disease process. Williamson et al. (1964) reported the number of disabilities detected by screening persons age 65 or older living in the community in Scotland. They found that the men had a mean of 3.26 disabilities of which 1.87 were unknown to their physician, and women had a mean of 3.42 disabilities and 2.03 were unknown to the doctor (Williamson et al., 1964). A heightened clinical awareness and an index of suspicion can identify important clinical problems. In the aged this type of screening becomes as important if not more important than primary and secondary preventive strategies.

Disability

Most agree that disability means a loss of ability, be it physical, psychological, or functional. Disability can also be defined from different perspectives:

impairment—organ level, disability—personal level, and handicapped—society level. How the disability affects the patient's independence is more important than the disability per se. Furthermore, the patient's adaptation to loss and change predicts the actual long-term outcome. Age alone does not determine how a person manages a disability; it is rather a complex function of support, emotion, personality, experiences, resources, location, and other factors.

TASK OF HEALTH MAINTENANCE

An effective preventive approach to the chronically disabled, frail older adult requires that different sectors of society perform certain tasks. These include individuals, families, health care teams, long-term care institutions, and the health care system, working alone and collectively (Warshaw, 1988).

Individuals

Successful aging requires adaptation to loss. It is important to avoid becoming fatalistic and giving up adopting a healthier life-style or habits just because one is "disabled" or "frail." Prevention of further disability and functional loss by a willingness to change is important to maintain and improve quality of life. The emphasis on quality rather than the conventional quantity of life becomes the benchmark.

Families

Despite beliefs to the contrary, families provide approximately 75% to 85% of the care to the dependent elderly in the community (Stone, Cafferata, & Sangl, 1987). Their assistance is essential in promoting "health." Presently, the long-term care system is economically strained; therefore, the family is called on to play a greater role in supporting the ever-growing older segment of the population.

Health Care Teams

The health care team must also conduct certain tasks. There must be a reevaluation of traditional strategies and methodologies (i.e., screening versus case finding and an emphasis on functional outcome versus disease prevention). Teams need to provide an individual approach to health maintenance plans, bearing in mind issues of ethical concern, patient's beliefs, autonomy, caregiver support, convenience, and cost). Not only should teams assess frail older adults for support but make sure that it is adequate, not supplied inappropriately too early, or oversupplied. Furthermore, the team needs to be sensitive to the needs of family caregivers to prevent burnout and fatigue. Finally, the health care team must minimize iatrogenic insult, always keeping in mind "primum no nocere."

Long-Term Care

The long-term care institution must recognize how it homogenizes individuals. Older persons are diverse and have as much individuality as younger persons. In institutions, however, people can lose their uniqueness. Institutions need to be sensitive to this flaw and continue to consider health maintenance needs individually. They must carefully balance the risks, benefits, and costs in each situation. Admission policies should address health maintenance goals, ensuring a more effective outcome. Terminal care and advanced directives are of paramount importance.

Health Care System

Tasks of the health care system are multiple. Foremost, it must recognize its bias against prevention (e.g., the fact that less than 4% of current health care expenditures are spent on disease prevention) (Rogers, Eaton, & Bruhn, 1981; Sheffler & Parenger, 1980). Selective funding of preventive interventions for the elderly may represent effective "cost-control" strategies, though more data are needed to support this approach (Collen et al., 1970; Somers, 1984). There should be consideration of implementing financial disincentives for consumption of toxic products (e.g., alcohol or tobacco), or widespread use and easily accessed and administered subsidized funding for the poor elderly to guard against environmental hazards, such as hyperthermia or hypothermia. This would include widespread use of heating-cooling subsidies and insulation incentives.

Collectively there needs to be more education to dispel the myth and prejudice of ageism, involving individuals, families, government, and institutions. There should be increased efforts toward patient education about personal health, aging, disease, life changes with aging (e.g., retirement counseling), and risk assessment.

BARRIERS TO PREVENTIVE CARE

There are many barriers to adapting and implementing health maintenance in all age groups. Special circumstances further prohibit effective health maintenance in the frail older adult and chronically disabled.

The health care team itself poses specific barriers to a workable health maintenance system. Time is a precious resource, and it takes considerable time to discuss, implement, and plan effective health maintenance schedules for older adults. Regarding specific formal recommendations, target populations, target diseases, locations for screening, and intervals of screening there is little agreement; for the chronically disabled and frail elderly there is even less agreement (American Cancer Society, 1980; Breslow & Somers, 1977; Canadian Task Force, 1979; Frame & Carlson, 1975; U.S. Preventive Services Task Force, 1989). Despite the prevalence of ageism among all sectors, older adults are actually more amenable to life-style changes than younger persons and may be "more" successful with primary and secondary preventive recommendations. (National Center for Health Statistics, 1979a, 1979b; Harris, Louis, et al., 1986). For example, studies have shown that persons older than age 65 smoke less, drink alcohol and coffee less often, sleep 7 to 8 hours a night, eat breakfast, and maintain proper weight more than any other age segment of the population (Belloc & Breslow, 1972; Breslow & Enstrom, 1984; Harris & Guten, 1979; Steel & Brown, 1972). Most health care systems have inadequate reminder programs to prompt specific health maintenance activities (e.g., checklists for accepted health maintenance maneuvers, or postcard mailings to remind patients they are due for mammograms or Pap smears). Furthermore, teams have been trained under the disease-cure model, not a chronic disease management model. Under the conventional idea of health maintenance the functional perspective is lacking. Finally, reimbursement is a major obstacle because many preventive services are not covered by third-party payers, and health care providers are thus reluctant to order specific tests or provide health maintenance services.

Patients, too, present barriers to health maintenance (Black & Kapoor, 1990). They are generally undereducated about health practices or specific health maintenance recommendations. They may be fearful, angry, modest, or shameful in response to disease and therefore be reluctant to participate in any preventive health care. They may have denial, dislike the tests, or have irregular or infrequent doctor visits. They may dislike the amount of time involved or not be able to afford the care. Furthermore, older patients are also oriented toward a disease-cure model and sometimes self-fulfill the societal prejudice of ageism (e.g., "I'm old, I'm supposed to be incontinent"). Transportation and support resources can also be problems for the chronically disabled frail older adult.

The health care system has its own inherent barriers to effective health maintenance. The system is pluralistic, has no mechanism for coordination of care, and has not generated firm data on which to base sound guidelines. There is a lack of a well-grounded philosophy in long-term care, which only further obscures the implementation of health maintenance in the institutional setting.

Finally, in addition to barriers, ethical issues must be taken into account when considering a health maintenance plan for the chronically disabled. One must be certain each test or intervention meets the guidelines of prevention and screening (U.S. Preventive Services Task Force, 1989). Is the target problem sufficiently common to justify the investment of diagnosis, treatment, and follow-up care? Is the sensitivity or specificity of the proposed maneuvers acceptable enough to justify the use of resources? Unfortunately data are lacking on the "old-old" population.

The patient's autonomy and choice, based on cultural, religious, or personal belief systems, should be considered. Determining decision-making capacity must not be overlooked when caring for the frail elderly. This population has a high prevalence of dementia and cognitive impairment that can make obtaining informed consent difficult.

PRINCIPLES OF HEALTH MAINTENANCE

The first task, that of ensuring a sound scientific basis for any intervention strategy, has been addressed in recent years initially by the Canadian Task Force and, more recently, by the United States Task Force on the Periodic Health Examination. This task has been essential to protect the healthy population from iatrogenic insult, to prevent unnecessary costs both to the individual and to society, and to maintain the "scientific integrity" of the professionals concerned. It has led to careful study of the impact of disease, the efficacy of detection maneuvers, and the quality of evidence supporting the effectiveness of intervention strategies.

Yet, the relevance of this work to the elderly is somewhat limited, for it has focused on primary and secondary prevention strategies that address biomedical disorders in young populations. This is important, for old age is not a separate period of life but is part of a continuum, and, for full effectiveness, preventive measures need to start in childhood and continue throughout adult life. Nevertheless it does not provide the practicing physician with the details of what he or she should do or how to do it when confronted with frail elderly patients (Kennie & Warshaw, 1989).

SPECIAL ISSUES OF HEALTH PROMOTION IN THE LONG-TERM CARE INSTITUTION

Health maintenance and prevention strategies and goals for institutionalized elderly differ from those for elderly living in the community. Several investigators have looked at focused screening tests and health maintenance in the nursing home (Allen, Becker, McVey, et al., 1986; Israel, Kozarevis, & Satorius, 1984; Magenheim, 1989; Rubenstein, Josephson, Wieland, et al.,

1984; Teasdale, Schuman, Snow, et al., 1983). Overall, health screening and promotion may have important roles to play in the institutionalized, disabled elderly and that establishing routine schedules will provide a valuable contribution to overall well-being and health for chronic care patients.

Health maintenance in the institutionalized population should be individualized, respecting that long-term care patients are a heterogeneous group. Use a team approach. This should involve the family, nurses, nurses aides, physicians, social workers, and administration. This will facilitate the decision-making process in generating an individual health maintenance plan and lead to a more successful outcome. For each patient, the "team" must consider the already significant burden of chronic disease and whether detection and treatment of new problems will add or subtract from this burden. For example, should all 80-year-old women with no prior history of gynecological problems have routine yearly Pap smears? This group is particularly vulnerable to iatrogenic problems, and strict attention should be paid to not increasing the risk or burden to the patient, family, institution, and system.

There are special ethical concerns related to health maintenance procedures in the long-term care setting. Nursing home residents represent a captive audience (e.g., an individual's diet becomes a mixture of what the physician orders and what the institution is willing to provide). Smoking is usually prohibited or restricted. Caution and respect for a patient's autonomy and individuality should take priority. The health care team must be a patient advocate at all times. This may become difficult if there is a disagreement among team members (e.g., if a family member requests that tube feedings of their severely demented loved one be stopped and there is no clear evidence of what the patient would desire). Sometimes one must ask if prescribed maneuvers such as immunizations prolong the burden of suffering (e.g., "pneumonia can be the old man's friend") (Kennie, 1988). A high priority must be placed on gaining informed consent, though cognitive impairment may make direct patient consent unreliable. Teams may need to rely on surrogate decision makers and family.

Numerous specific health maintenance suggestions for long-term care have been made (Kane, Ouslander, & Abrass, 1989; Kennie, 1988; Magenheim, 1989). Though conclusive evidence is lacking, numerous clinical problems have been identified as possible areas of health maintenance and promotion in the chronically disabled and institutionalized elderly (Magenheim, 1989). These recommendations can be implemented by the health care team. It is important to individualize any plan. Table 8.1 may be used as a general guideline for specific health maintenance procedures. Data in many areas is weak and inconclusive. These recommendations are derived from available data, as well as the opinions of the authors. A practical point is to use flow charts and systematic checklists routinely. After contracting with

TABLE 8.1 Health Maintenance for Chronically Disabled and Frail Elderly

Target Area	Frequency	Comments or suggestions
Accident prevention	Ongoing	No unattended smoking for cognitively or physically impaired; limit restraint use; ensure correct footwear; avoid sedative medications; ensure adequate supervision; ensure proper use of assistive devices (e.g., walker, wheelchair when indicated); employ staff education and awareness programs; accept some risk that frail elderly may fall. Adjust lighting to reduce glare; employ gait-balance risk assessment to target high-risk individuals; use assessment instruments to uncover potential problems.
Advanced care issues	Ongoing as clinical course changes	Have policies that address these issues (e.g., literature, videovignettes); resolve issues of "resuscitate," "do not resuscitate," "transfer to hospital," "do not transfer to hospital," "tube feedings," "hydration." Educate families and patients about realistic goals; respect autonomy; respect cultural and personal differences; emphasis that "do not resuscitate" does not mean abandonment. Comfort care policies should be individualized according to need.
Alcohol	As needed depending on potential access	Caution; monitor for withdrawal symptoms; nutrition assessment; use vitamins, especially thiamine when indicated.
Audiological	Yearly	Check for cerumen impaction; assess for assistive devices and correctable problems.
Breast cancer	Yearly or per individualized assessment	Clinical exam yearly all ages and mammography based on individual case and circumstances.
Colerectal cancer	Yearly	Assess each case individually. Hemoccults, colonoscopy, and sigmoidoscopy as indicated.

Constipation	Ongoing	Hydration; review medications; use bowel agents when appropriate; maximize mobility; adequate fiber content; toileting schedules.
Dehydration	Ongoing	Facilitate access to fluids; target high-risk patients and make necessary interventions (e.g., adequate patient support for the most immobile and disabled).
Dementia	Yearly	Use screening instruments to provide objective data; minimize use of physical and chemical restraints.
Dental	Admission, yearly, and as needed	Oral and dental hygiene; oral cancer screening; denture fit and repair.
Depression	Ongoing, target those with recent or remote loss, bereavement, anniversary dates, medication changes, or past history	Formal screening instruments; use psychological services.
Diabetes	For those diagnosed monitor monthly For those undiagnosed, test if symptomatic	Blood sugar Hemoglobin A_1 C
Falls	Ongoing, after any fall	Formal assessment instruments; avoid sedative medication, must balance restraint or restrictions of patient against acceptable risks; target or identify high-risk patient and make necessary intervention to reduce potential injury. See "accidents."
Foot care	Yearly More frequently for diabetics and patients with peripheral vascular disease (PVD)	Podiatry treatment for nails, calluses, bunions, ulcerations, etc. Monitor for infection in diabetics and PVD.
Functional status testing	Yearly and with reported changes	Obtain baseline from which to measure changes. Standard instruments are available.

TABLE 8.1 Continued

Target Area	Frequency	Comments or suggestions
Gynecological/bimanual pelvic/Pap smear	Annually (each case must be individualized)	Pap smear may be omitted after two negative results in past 5 years and no prior history of cervical disease. Assessment for prolapse, atrophy, and incontinence.
Hypertension	Yearly	Individualize treatment according to degree, risks vs. benefit, medications, outcome, life expectancy, etc.; generally, advocate treatment of systolic blood pressure (BP) > 180 mm Hg and diastolic BP > 90 mm Hg.
Hyperthermia/hypothermia	During environmental extremes and per clinical changes	Prevention measures—keep thermostat at 70°F or greater. Ensure adequate fluids and nutrition as well as access. Appropriate clothing. Maintain index of suspicion.
Hypothyroidism/hyperthyroidism	Every 1 to 2 years and per clinical changes	Prevalence in the elderly may justify screening. Obtain thyroid-stimulating hormone and thyroxine.
Iatrogenic insult	Ongoing	Use principle of minimal interference; scrupulous use and review of medications. Respect patient autonomy. Informed consent, use forethought about results of tests and possible treatments.
Immunizations Influenza	Yearly	Use amantadine hydrochloride 100 mg/day within 24–48 hours of suspected outbreak of influenza A if not immunized. Need further reduction of dose if renal impairment present. In the nursing home unvaccinated residents and staff treated throughout outbreak; vaccinated persons until symptoms resolve.
Pneumococcal vaccine	Once	Efficacy debated
Tetanus	Every 10 years, or every 5 years with tetanus prone wounds	If unvaccinated, need tetanus series; when treating a wound use tetanus immune globulin and tetanus series or booster.

Tuberculosis screening	Admission to nursing home; aggressive control measures if active case develops	Two-step Protein Purified Derivative (PPD) Isoniazid 300 mg/d for 6–12 months for skin test conversions especially those with diabetes, end-stage renal disease, hematological malignancy, steroid or immunosuppressive therapy, and malnutrition. Must monitor for liver toxicity.
Immobility	Ongoing	Functional assessment all individuals; practice functional-oriented care; identify and treat any potential problem affecting or contributing to immobility; maximize function. Use appropriate assistive devices when indicated; reduce use of restraints; allow for an acceptable risk of falling.
Incontinence	Yearly and per episode	Incontinence warrants full diagnostic investigation. Improve mobility; use assistive devices as indicated after complete workup. Avoid indwelling catheterization except when absolutely indicated (e.g., persistent sacral decubitus, pain management in terminal illness).
Loss and bereavement	Yearly and per incident	Recognize not only personal but economic, sociologic, and physical losses. Provide supports and psychological services. Medical treatment for clinical depression.
Medications	Monthly and ongoing with any changes	Minimize use when feasibly and practically possible. Evaluate efficacy; review for adverse effects or interactions; monitor for drug-nutrient interactions.
Nutrition	Ongoing	Use formal assessment; dietitian to monitor; appropriate diet for clinical situation (i.e., obesity-weight reduction, diabetes-American Diabetes Association, etc.). Evaluate and treat unintentional weight reduction greater than 10% body weight. Ensure adequate staff-patient ratios to allow for adequate time to mouth-feed dependent individuals. Ensure hydration. Monitor for potential drug-nutrient interactions.
Ophthalmological	Yearly in diabetics; otherwise every 2–3 yr or per clinical changes	Maximize visual acuity. Use assistive devices and low vision aides when appropriate. Decrease glare.

TABLE 8.1 Continued

Target Area	Frequency	Comments or suggestions
Pain	Ongoing	Treat appropriately; must balance treatment against iatrogenesis.
Skin	Yearly, ongoing for patients at high risk for pressure sores	Screen for cancer. Screen for decubitus-pressure ulcers. Routinely employ prognostic rating scale for patients having a likelihood of developing pressure sores. Use appropriate preventive measures and devices when indicated. Vitamin and nutrition assessment.
Smoking	Individualize	Persons with cognitive impairment need supervision. Advocate smoking cessation based on quality of life and individual issues. Education of benefits of cessation can be worthwhile.
Stress/mental health	Ongoing	
Family	Ongoing	Counseling and education to help families cope with guilt of institutionalizing family members. Help resolve unresolved conflicts. Discuss openly prognosis and advanced care directives. Involve in "team" as much as they are willing to participate.
Staff	Ongoing	Open and clear communication. Education about prescribed treatments maneuvers and expectations. Provide support for those experiencing burnout or grief.

Source: Adapted from Kennie (1988); Lavizzo-Mourey et al. (1989); Magenheim (1989); and Warshaw (1988).

the patient and family about a specific health maintenance plan these charts can be used as reminders to facilitate and assure compliance.

One issue that needs further comment is advanced care directives. It is imperative that institutions and health care teams not ignore this important aspect of health promotion. People need to reflect and decide on the manner in which they wish to die and recognize that it can be a legitimate endpoint (Kennie, 1988). The new Patient Self-Determination Act requires institutions to introduce information on admission about advanced directives. This may be accomplished gracefully by using written materials or video vignettes the patient and family can review, followed by a visit to discuss options with the team. The patient and family should understand that deciding on "do not resuscitate" orders or "no gastrostomy tube" does not mean the patient will be abandoned.

SPECIAL ISSUES IN CHRONICALLY DISABLED AT HOME
General

For every disabled elderly person in the nursing home there are approximately one to three equally impaired and disabled elderly individuals living in the community (Kane, Ouslander, & Abrass, 1989). These patients usually see the physician only for acute medical problems. This population of frail and chronically disabled are at a high risk of not being screened or introduced to any form of health maintenance or preventive services. Chronically disabled and frail older adults at home, many of whom have a combination of physical, psychological, social, environmental, and economic factors that can affect their health, should be targeted for health maintenance procedures. An example is the frail 75-year-old widow who lives alone on a limited income and continually turns down the thermostat to save money, falls, and cannot reach the telephone, and dies of hypothermia. Another example is the disabled 80-year-old farmer who lives alone in the country, does not cook, and eats once a day to save money and conserve food because he can go shopping only once a month when a distant neighbor goes to town.

There are two groups of chronically disabled, frail older adults at home: those who are strictly home bound and cannot feasibly come to the doctor's office, and those who can, with assistance, make it to the physician's office — the "mobile home bound." These two groups have specialized needs for health maintenance and promotion that reflect issues such as caregiver burden, supports, transportation, compliance with visits, bureaucracy, and acceptability to the patient.

Home Bound

The proportion of noninstitutionalized persons aged 65 years or older who require assistance in basic and instrumental ADLs is substantial, and after age 85, the proportion needing this assistance increases dramatically. Among people who are 85 or older, the proportion who are dependent is double to triple those who are dependent among persons 75 to 84 years of age. For example, it is estimated that for individuals older than age 85 living at home nearly 30% need assistance with bathing, more than 20% need help with transferring, and 30% need help preparing meals (Leon & Lair, 1990).

For the home bound, as for those in the institution, a successful health maintenance plan requires an individual schedule using a team approach. The team consists of the patient, the family or caregivers, a nurse, social worker, and physician. The approach must be interdisciplinary to define deficits in physical, mental, or functional status as well as to address socioeconomic issues. One type of team intervention that may benefit the frail home-bound patient is comprehensive geriatric assessment. The settings in which effectiveness have been established is the combined geriatric assessment and rehabilitation unit and the inpatient geriatric assessment unit (Rubenstein, Josephson, Wieland, et al., 1984; Teasdale et al., 1983). There is less convincing evidence regarding comprehensive geriatric assessment in the home or ambulatory setting (Cohen & Feussner, 1989). The home-bound elderly may be a particularly successful group to target for comprehensive assessment because of the high likelihood of identifying reversible disabilities (National Institute of Health Consensus Conference, 1988).

The emphasis should be on case finding or detecting symptomatic but yet unreported disease (tertiary prevention). All patients need baseline functional and mental status assessment to understand initial needs as well as for future reference. Health maintenance recommendations for this group are as outlined in Table 7.1. Some issues warrant special attention. The team can help the caregiver and patient with planning for the future and for caregiver alternatives (e.g., respite and short-term placement). The team can help them prepare for the unexpected, such as caregiver illness or death, possible further loss of function, or financial losses. Social isolation and depression are common in this group, and the health maintenance schedule should include routine screening for depression, alcohol abuse, elder abuse, self-neglect, and weight loss. Assessment of each case for potential informal supports such as "adopt a grandparent program," visiting friends, or church member visitation is valuable. Environmental assessment is extremely valuable to guard against accidents or injury that could further reduce functional status, or lead to premature death. Educating patients and caregivers about heat stroke or exhaustion, and hypothermia is vital. Routine home visits using a standardized approach can often uncover potential problems (Currie et al., 1981).

The health maintenance plan can be carried out for the most part by the nonphysician (i.e., caregiver, nurse practitioner, or home health aide). The physician, however, needs to be readily accessible, either in the office by telephone or for home visits. Routine follow-up by different members of the team is important. Clinical assessment instruments that can be administered in the home may facilitate implementation and increase success of a health maintenance program. These instruments are readily available (Israel, Kozarevis, & Satorius, 1984; Lavizzo-Mourey et al., 1989).

Mobile Home Bound

The last group of chronically disabled and frail older adults is the home bound who are capable of coming to the office. These individuals are disabled but may not meet the criteria for Medicare reimbursement for long-term care resources.

In the traditional ambulatory care office this type of patient is not targeted or screened closely for early or as yet undetected problems. Moreover, sufficient time is not allowed for screening or discussing health maintenance recommendations. Though specific recommendations are similar to those for the other two groups, several areas deserve special comment.

Current Medicare reimbursement does not adequately reflect the cognitive skill or time it requires to provide comprehensive care to the frail elderly and chronically disabled older adult. Thus, there is an ever-present time-reimbursement constraint inherent in ambulatory care of this population. The primary care office can take practical steps to ease this pressure, however. More time should be allowed for the office visit, but nonphysician personnel should gather pertinent information or administer screening instruments. The "team approach" is a practical way to provide greater comprehensive care (Lavizzo-Mourey, 1989). The Folstein Mental Status Questionnaire (Folstein et al., 1975), Beck's Depression Scale (Beck & Beanesdenfer, 1974), or Physical Self Maintenance Scales (ADLs) (Katz, Ford, Moskowitz, et al., 1963), Instrumental Activities of Daily Living Scales (Casanasos, Stewart, & Cluff, 1974), and similar scales are relatively quick to administer and can be used as tools for case finding.

Iatrogenic problems secondary to medications are common in the geriatric population (Brennan, Leape, Laird, et al., 1991). In fact, one sixth of all hospital admissions for people older than age 70 are secondary to adverse drug reactions, and 25% of elderly admissions are related to medication noncompliance (Perspectives on Aging, 1990). The mobile home-bound elderly are particularly susceptible to these problems. A means of minimizing polypharmacy and adverse drug effects is to ask the patient or caregiver to bring in both prescription and over-the-counter medications at each office visit (i.e., the "brown paper bag" technique). Printed cards with dosages, frequency, and purpose of the medication can help the physician as well as other health care providers, caregivers, and patient. For persons with numerous medications or mild cognitive impairment, medi-planner pill boxes are extremely helpful. Additional priority areas for this population include alcohol abuse, falls, urine or fecal incontinence, depression, and self-neglect and abuse. Routine 3 to 4-month visits are advisable. Immunization recommendations and mammography are health maintenance procedures underused in this group. Because this group may not be as eligible for certain Medicare in-home resources or "skilled services," it is essential to evaluate in-home supports and caregivers to assure that they are adequate. Minimizing caregiver burden is essential. One means of accomplishing this in the office is to interview the patient and caregiver separately as well as together. This often reveals family dynamics, or stress and potential problems.

CONCLUSION

If we are to improve the application of health promotion interventions with the frail elderly more scientific data will be required. These studies should specifically address the improvement of function and the avoidance of dependency. In addition, a shift in health policy toward health promotion and prevention is required.

To be effective in promoting health or a health maintenance plan for the chronically disabled and frail elderly, one should be cognizant of how conventional methodologies and attitudes may interfere with an effective outcome. It is also important to implement an individualized approach, keeping in mind that optimizing function is the ultimate goal. Quality of life, quantity of life, iatrogenic problems, patients' personal attitudes and beliefs, convenience, and proof of effectiveness of a particular preventive method or procedure must all be scaled against optimizing function. The institutionalized, home-bound, and mobile home-bound frail elderly each have special prevention needs. This "holistic" approach with the emphasis on function is the cornerstone of geriatrics, and the use of the *health care team* is a key to success of any "geriatric" program. This is especially true for health promotion for the frail and chronically disabled older patient.

REFERENCES

Allen, C. M., Becker, P. M., McVey, L. J., et al. (1986). A randomized controlled clinical trial of a geriatric consultation team: Compliance with recommendations. *Journal of the American Medical Association, 255,* 2617–2621.
American Cancer Society. (1980). American Cancer Society report on the cancer related checkup. *Cancer, 30,* 194–232.

Beck, A. T., & Beanesdenfer, A. (1974). Assessment of depression: The Depression Inventory. In P. Pichot (Ed.), *Psychological measurements in psycho-pharmacology* (Vol. 7, pp. 151–169). Basel, Switzerland: Karger.

Belloc, N. B., & Breslow, L. (1972). Relationship of physical health status and health practices. *Preventive Medicine, 1,* 409–421.

Black, J. S., & Kapoor, W. (1990). Health promotion and disease prevention in older people: Our current state of ignorance. *Journal of American Geriatric Society, 38,* 168–172.

Brennan, T. A., Leape, L. L., Laird, N. M., et al. (1991). Incidence of adverse events and negligence in hospitalized patients. *New England Journal of Medicine, 324,* 370–376.

Breslow, L., & Enstrom, J. E. (1984). Persistance of health habits and their relationship to mortality. *Preventive Medicine, 9,* 469–483.

Breslow, L., & Somers, A. R. (1977). The life time health-monitoring program. *New England Journal of Medicine, 296,* 601–608.

Canadian Task Force. (1979). The periodic health examination. *Canadian Medical Association Journal, 121,* 1193–1254.

Casanasos, C. J., Stewart, R. B. & Cluff, L. E. (1974). Drug-induced illness leading to hospitalization. *Journal of the American Medical Association, 228,* 713–717.

Cohen, H. J., & Feussner, J. R. (1989). Comprehensive geriatric assessment: Mission not yet accomplished. *Journal of Gerontology, 44,* M185–M188.

Collen, M. F., Feldman, R., Siegelaub, A. B., & Crawford, D. (1970). Dollar cost per positive test for automated multiphasic screening. *New England Journal of Medicine, 283,* 459–463.

Currie, C. T., et al. (1981). Assessment of the elderly patients at home: A report of fifty cases. *Journal of the American Geriatric Society, 29,* 398–401.

Department of Health and Human Services. (1989). *U.S. Preventive Services Task Force: Guide to clinical preventive services.* Baltimore: Williams & Wilkins.

Federal Council on Aging. (1981). *The need for long-term care: A chartbook of the Federal Council on Aging* (Publication No. [OHDS] 81-20704, 29). Washington, DC: U.S. Department of Health and Human Services, Government Printing Office.

Folstein, M. F., et al. (1975). Mini-Mental State: A practical method of grading the cognitive state of the patient for the physician. *Journal of Psychiatric Resident, 12,* 189.

Fowles, D. G. (1990). *A profile of older Americans.* Washington, DC: American Association of Retired Persons.

Frame, P. J., & Carlson, S. J. (1975). A critical review of periodic health screening using specific screening criteria. *Journal of Family Practice, 2,* 29–35, 123–129, 189–194.

Harris, D. M., & Guten, S. (1979). Health protection behavior: An exploratory study. *Journal of Health and Social Behavior, 20,* 17–29.

Harris, L., et al. (1986, November). *Prevention Index '87: A report card on the nation's health. Summary Report: Consumer's survey.* Emmaus, PA: Rodale Press.

Israel, L., Kozarevis, O., & Satorius, N. (1984). *Source book of geriatric assessment.* Basil, Switzerland: Karger.

Kane, R. L., Ouslander, J. G., & Abrass, I. B. (1989). *Essentials of clinical geriatrics* (2nd ed.). New York: McGraw-Hill.

Katz, S., Ford, A. B., Moskowitz, R. W., Jackson, B. A., & Jaffee, M. W. (1963). Studies of illness in the aged: The Index of ADL: A standardized measure of biological and psychosocial function. *Journal of the American Medical Association, 185,* 94.

Kennie, D. C. (1988). Health maintenance of the elderly. *Clinics of Geriatric Medicine*, 2, 53–83.

Kennie, D., Warshaw, G. (1989). Health maintenance and health screening in the elderly. In W. Reichel (Ed.), *Clinics aspects of aging* (3rd ed.) Baltimore: Williams & Wilkins.

Lavizzo-Mourey, R. (1989). The home team. In R. Lavizzo-Mourey et al. (Eds.), *Practicing prevention for the elderly*. Philadelphia: Hanley & Belfus.

Leon, J., & Lair, T. (1990). *Functional status of the noninstitutionalized elderly: estimates of ADL and IADL difficulties* (DHHS Publication No. [PHS] 90-3462). National Medical Expenditure Survey Research Findings. Rockville, MD: Agency for Health Care Policy and Research, Public Health Service.

Lavizzo-Mourey, R., Day, S. C., Diserens, D., & Grisso, J. A. (1989). *Practicing prevention for the elderly*. Philadelphia: Hanley & Belfus.

Magenheim, M. S. (1989). Health maintenance in long-term care. In P. Katz & E. Calkins (Eds.), Principals and practice of nursing home care. New York: Springer.

National Center for Health Statistics. (1979a). *Acute conditions: Incidence and associated disability, United States, July 1977–June 1978* (Public Health Services Series 10-No. 123). Washington, DC: U.S. Government Printing Office.

National Center for Health Statistics. (1979b). Physician visits: Volume and interval since last visit, United States, 1975. (Public Health Services Series 10-No. 132). Washington DC: U.S. Government Printing Office.

National Institute of Health Consensus Development Conference Statement. (1988). Geriatric assessment methods for clinical decision-making. *Journal of American Geriatric Society*, 36, 342–347.

Perspective on Aging. (1990, July-August). Elders and their medications.

Rogers, P. J., Eaton, E. K., & Bruhn, J. G. (1981). Is health promotion cost effective? *Preventive Medicine*, 10, 324–339.

Rubenstein, L. Z., Josephson, K. R., Wieland, G. D., et al. (1984). Effectiveness of a geriatric evaluation unit: A randomized clinical trial. *New England Journal of Medicine*, 311, 1664–1670.

Sheffler, R. M., & Parenger, L. (1980). A review of the economic evidence on prevention. *Medical Care*, 18, 473–484.

Somers, A. (1984). Why not try preventing illness as a way of controlling Medicare costs? *New England Journal of Medicine*, 311, 853–856.

Steel, J. L., & Broom, W. H. (1972). Conceptual and empirical dimensions of health behavior. *Journal of Health and Social Behavior*, 13, 382–392.

Stone, R., Cafferata, G. L., & Sangl, J. (1987). Caregivers of the frail elderly: A national profile. *The Gerontologist*, 27, 616–626.

Teasdale, T. A., Schuman, L., Snow, E., et al. (1983). A comparison of outcomes of geriatric cohorts receiving care in a geriatric assessment unit and on general medicine floors. *Journal of the American Geriatrics Society*, 31, 529–534.

U.S. Pteventive Services Task Force. (1989). *Guide to clinical preventive services: An assessment of the effectiveness of 169 interventions*. Baltimore: Williams & Wilkins.

Warshaw, G. A. (1988). *Surgeon general's workshop: Health promotion and aging*. Washington DC: U.S. Department of Health and Human Services.

Wedgewood, J. (1985). The place of rehabilitation in geriatric medicine. *Rehabilitation Medicine*, 7, 107.

Williamson, J., et al. (1964). Old people at home: Their unreported needs. *Lancet*, 1, 1117–1120.

Williamson, J., & Chopin, J. M. (1980). Adverse reactions to prescribed drugs in the elderly: A multicenter investigation. *Age Aging*, 9, 73–80.

9
Information Systems in Long-Term Care

Warren H. Bock
Robert L. Kane

Information is the stuff of decisions. In long-term care settings, decisions affect the lives of dependent people who are extremely sensitive to their environment. The quality of those decisions depends on the amount, quality, usefulness, and organization of the information. The structure of information can influence the approach to care. Too often long-term care is viewed as a cross-sectional snapshot, with little appreciation for the dynamics of change that are occurring, albeit sometimes slowly. In a setting where further deterioration in physical and functional status of patients is common, it is especially important to provide some sort of yardstick against which the differences attributable to good care can be measured. Such comparisons are as important to the internal management of long-term care agencies as they are to external groups that monitor them. This chapter discusses the issues surrounding the acquisition, management, and use of information, and points to the role that modern information technology can play in helping long-term care move toward an era of more dynamic management.

ACQUISITION OF INFORMATION

Although the importance of conducting comprehensive assessments of persons *before* the design and implementation of a plan of care seems obvious, Congress, in 1987, legislated this process for nursing home care. The Omnibus Budget Reconciliation Act of 1987, (OBRA '87) contains specific language regarding not only the importance of assessments, but the uses to which they must be put in the care planning process. The way information is acquired will depend on the relationship between the findings of the assessment and the care planning and subsequent delivery of that care.

In its 1986 publication, *Improving the Quality of Care in Nursing Homes*, the Institute of Medicine's Committee on Nursing Home Regulation stressed the important effect initial and ongoing assessments had on the quality of care and the quality of life of persons living in nursing homes (Institute of Medicine, 1986). Relying heavily on this report, Congress mandated (in OBRA) the design, testing, and national implementation of a single, standardized geriatric assessment instrument. That instrument, the Minimum Data Set (MDS), is now in use throughout the country. Preliminary results from field trials suggest that this instrument, in its current pencil-and-paper format, will consume nearly 2 hours of nursing time for each resident (Morris et al., 1990).

To ensure accurate assessments, the Health Care Financing Administration (HCFA) has also contracted for the design of a survey protocol that will focus on the timeliness and accuracy of the assessments. The protocol will also measure the relationship between the care goals and the problems revealed in the assessment.

Apart from the need to acquire functional information on residents to develop relevant care plans, the increasingly complex regulatory and reimbursement practices are making demands for information that the typical administrator would not ordinarily collect. Case-mix reimbursement systems are being introduced more widely. The elimination of the distinction between intermediate and skilled levels of care may well be the harbinger of a national mandate to fund all long-term care using some form of severity or case-mix index. Case-mix systems require accurate and up-to-date information if facilities and agencies expect to receive the level of funds to which they are entitled.

Impending regulations will require the capture and storage of other group statistics such as incidence of decubiti, incontinence, use of medications, and many other group status indicators. As the inevitable shift of focus from input and process indicators to outcomes of care emerges, it will be important to maintain historical data to chart the impact of the facility's programs on its residents. Systematic gathering of these data must become routine, with virtually all staff of the facility participating in the process.

In summary, the acquisition of information is a large task that is likely to increase over the next few years. Agencies and facilities that expect to remain in compliance with these new demands will need to streamline its information-gathering practices to accommodate new regulatory standards on the immediate horizon. The forces behind this new emphasis are concerns for both quality care and fiscal accountability. Not only is the volume of the information needed increasing, the importance of the accuracy of the information will increase as data are used to plot trends.

In addition to the press of external forces, there are other reasons to reassess the way information is collected and handled. For example, nursing home personnel need some sense of accomplishment if they are to derive satisfaction from their work. The current approach to personal care is to view it as a task to be engaged in one day at a time. Each day brings a new set of problems and a group of patients that is gradually deteriorating. The result can often be a sense of futility and discouragement in a field that does not enjoy much prestige initally. Changing that mind-set requires moving from a static to a dynamic mode of practice. It means recognizing the positive effects care has made for patients including an appreciation that slowing the rate of decline is a positive and important function of care in nursing homes. Accomplishing this transformation in staff goals requires a dramatic change in the way we acquire and use information. The era of modern information technology makes feasible the graphic display of summarized information that can be understood and used by health workers at all levels.

MANAGEMENT OF INFORMATION

Long-term care settings face an ever-increasing need to gather information on their residents and on the programs and services they provide to those residents. The careful handling, manipulation, and storage of those data can become burdensome. The volume of information is now measured by bits. It is safe to assume that literally millions of bits of information need to be gathered, organized, and stored and, more important, be immediately available to a wide variety of users.

Traditional pencil-and-paper systems no longer suffice, especially if they must meet the "readily available" criterion. The volume of paper alone consumes more storage space than most nursing homes have available. A second problem with traditional systems is the inability to obtain the analytic power needed to look for patterns among individuals (e.g., rapidly sort across several persons on one or more bits of information, a requirement in the new conditions of participation in the Medicaid and Medicare programs) or to display longitudinal data on an individual. Third, traditional systems do not support the decision-making processes necessary for clinical and administrative functions. Finally, as the need to share information among various disciplines increases, the likelihood of losing information increases as does the frustration with never having all the information one needs when one wants it because someone else has it.

Undoubtedly many facilities will try to meet their information needs using the same methods they have always used. Some may even get by. Many will lose money if they are in a case-mix state or will receive deficiencies from the survey process without the documentation to argue their case with surveyors. Eventually, most will recognize the need for computerization.

Goals of Information Management System

Historically, most of the information systems developed for the long-term care setting managed financial data. In fact, most of the early vendors of software systems began as accountants; few vendors set out to develop clinical systems exclusively.

The reasons for the emphasis on financial status are obvious: Administrators and owners make the purchasing decisions, and their primary concerns are predictably financial management. Second, clinicians for the most part were not trained to use computers. Finally, and probably most significant, knowledge-based clinical systems are very difficult and costly to develop. The advent of OBRA '87, which mandates the Minimum Data Set (MDS) and the attendant Resident Assessment Protocols (RAPs), has shifted the focus from financial to clinical systems and has resulted in a flurry of software development activities.

The RAPs use a branching logic that is particularly well suited to computerization. The volume of information and the need to use that information both longitudinally and cross-sectionally argue for a strong role for computers.

The importance of good financial management systems to the efficient and profitable operation of nursing facilities is assumed. However, it is not the intent of this chapter to discuss financial systems. Rather, we will explore the goals, uses, attributes, and issues surrounding those less common systems that guide and record clinical functions.

The overarching goal of a clinical information management system (CIMS) should be to improve clinical decision making.

A well-designed information system should be capable of producing data for both individual clinical care and for aggregation for purposes of review and regulation. The current need to treat both the chart and the client should give way to a single information approach. Data that does not have clinical meaning is probably not worth collecting. The great advantage of computerization is the ability to use data, once collected, in a variety of ways.

Not only can a CIMS manage the sutstantial amount of information required to monitor change, it can facilitate the rapid recording of the information itself. However, the CIMS should not decide what care is given or how; that is, the role of the clinician. Rather, the CIMS should guide the decision-making process by prompting, reminding, and tracking decisions.

Improved decision making should result in improved care as evidenced by resident outcomes. The initial comprehensive assessment of a resident's status serves as a baseline against which all subsequent reassessments can be compared. Each of these reassessments can be likened to snapshots in time, which when strung together produces a motion picture of the resident's course of treatment. Thus, when the clinician is able to monitor change over time reliably and rapidly, she will be able to adjust the care by modifying or changing approaches.

Assessing the effects of care requires more than just longitudinal information. Some point of comparison is needed. This can be an internal standard of what should happen, or it can be a more empirically based expectation derived from analyzing data banks that store information on previous cases from a variety of facilities. The potential for this sort of organized analysis of clinical experience offers a means to improve the practice of long-term care and to base future practice decisions on established patterns of expected benefits.

Through its ability to aggregate data across residents and by monitoring change over time for client groups that share common problems and characteristics, the CIMS provides the clinician with the tools to evaluate the effectiveness of the decisions the CIMS helped shape. With this new ability, clinicians can now begin to predict outcomes of care and to compare the actual outcomes to the predicted ones. Individual levels of comparison can be further aggregated to establish the basis for program evaluations that reflect the extent that achievable goals were attained.

By extension, facilities can now be compared with other facilities (assuming all are using the same CIMS) to isolate exemplary practices, and approaches that show the best results (outcomes). Further, once the indices of status (MDS) are standardized nationally, groups of facilities (e.g., states) can be compared with other groups.

In the real world of long-term care, however, a CIMS that only meets the goal discussed previously will probably not be widely purchased given the limited resources available to facilities. Therefore, the CIMS must meet other goals albeit less noble than improved care.

Regulations

In addition to mandating comprehensive functional assessments using a minimum data set, OBRA '87 further requires that detailed attention be given to a wide range of quality-of-care and quality-of-life issues. No longer will paper trails and documentation necessarily suffice. The CIMS of the 1990s must play a central role in all aspects of monitoring the extent to which each of these new requirements are being met. Beyond the monitoring function, the CIMS should help manage the facility's operations by prompts, reminders, and "tickler" systems. It should further allow the facility to track both deficiencies and corrections over time because repeat deficiencies often trigger federal "look-behind" surveys. The CIMS should allow a facility to "self-survey" itself functionally on a continuous basis to assure full compliance with state and federal regulations.

Efficiency

The management of information currently generated in today's nursing facility often falls to the director or assistant director of nursing. Unfortunately, registered nursing personnel are typically in short supply throughout the long-term care industry. The burden of "paperwork," which is expected to increase, on these valuable clinical resources diverts scarce professional time away from patient care. To reduce the clinician's time spent in nondirect contact activities while simultaneously meeting the enhanced documentation requirements of OBRA '87, the CIMS must be sufficiently "user friendly" to allow aides, clerks, and computer-nonliterate persons to use it. More time can be saved by eliminating all redundant data-recording tasks.

Reimbursement

As stated earlier, more and more states are moving toward severity-based reimbursement models. Central to all severity-based, or "case-mix" systems, is the need to monitor changing client conditions accurately and efficiently. The CIMS should automatically compute and report each resident's functional status as it changes over time. If a given state permits electronic billing, the CIMS should contain this feature. In states with case-mix systems, nursing homes can forego payments if they fail to monitor and document clients' changing status accurately.

Uses of Information System

The number of uses to which a CIMS can be put are currently limited only by the imagination and creativity of the users and the creators of the system. As clinicians become more familiar and comfortable with computers, they will demand new and more complex functions of the CIMS. The list of uses discussed subsequently are only the beginning of what could become commonplace over the next several years.

At the center of any CIMS to be used in the era of OBRA must be the ability to capture the MDS. Some assessment tools have been designed to facilitate scoring. Computerization has the advantage of allowing an orderly collection of information in a clinically logical sequence and then permitting that data to be reformatted to yield scores of other aggregations as needed.

A great challenge to assessment is how to be both comprehensive and sensitive. One seeks a measure that will cover the full performance spectrum and at the same time provide sufficient distinction at each point along the way to detect meaningful clinical change. These two goals have the potential to produce a cumbersome measure whose items are inappropriate for any single client. One answer to the dilemma lies in branching formats. Aided by the computer, an assessor can identify the general level of performance in a domain and then move on to a more detailed examination of that level. Comparability is assured because the same set of general questions is used for all clients, but more discriminating levels of change can also be detected. The same branching approach can be used to collect more detailed clinical data to help identify the client's needs in specific areas of dysfunction. This logic underlies the RAPs in the MDS.

A well-conceived structured assessment system can also provide a better way to integrate client preferences into the routine assessment. Rather than setting them aside as a separate component, client preferences can be collected within their appropriate domains. For example, in the section on nutrition preference about foods, mealtimes and dining situation can be collected. Items like privacy, activities, smoking, and sleeping patterns can be collected as routine evaluation topics and hence given greater credibility and importance as issues around which to shape care plans. At the same time a separate report can be created on client preferences as a basis for evaluation.

Diagnostic information is primarily useful for its contribution to a plan of action. Although there is a role for prognosis, even in the absence of any specific treatment, most diagnostic or assessment information should be evaluated in terms of its contribution to a care plan. Indeed, the best assessments may be arrived at by working backward, starting from a determination as to what interventions are feasible and then identifying what information is critical to deciding among treatment options. However, such an approach runs the risk of limiting one's perspective. New ideas are less likely when the system is heavily structured and frustrating data is censored. A combination of inductive and deductive approaches is probably best.

To be effective, assessment data must be linked to a decision-making system that translates the findings of the assessment into a plan of action. Such planning requires a structure. In long-term care, while care needs are primarily driven by the residents functional status, other factors are important. The care plan must take cognizance of clinical information, especially as it pertains to etiology of illness and implied prognosis. Impaired mobility from congestive heart failure has a very different course from that owing to a fractured hip. The care plan should identify the full scope of clinical problems, their modifying factors, and the alternative treatments available. The decision about which treatments to use should be based on a combination of professional judgment and client preferences, once the risks and benefits are clear. Once a decision has been made, responsibility for carrying out the treatment should be clearly fixed.

An important component of information is feedback. In long-term care, feedback takes on a special meaning. Because many long-term care clients are chronically impaired, the normal course is for decline. The feedback provided by routine care thus runs the risk of promoting a sense of futility if the observed changes are in the direction of deterioration. The same principle of learned helplessness that Seligman has described for long-term care clients can affect the staff with consequent burn out (Seligman, 1976). Structured clinical feedback, which displays for staff the difference their care has made, can provide one means to counteract this tendency. Such feedback needs to compare the results obtained to what would be expected under conditions of good care. At a minimum, it should contrast the results to those for similar clients in comparable and other settings.

The same feedback approach can form the heart of a meaningful regulatory system. Rather than emphasizing adherence to preordained criteria for how things should be done, regulations can examine actual outcomes achieved. Of course, any use of outcomes must recognize at the outset the importance of comparing actual outcomes to expectations based on case-mix elements. The ratio of observed to expected becomes the basis for judging good results and hence good care. The same ratios are used to compare individual care for clinical feedback and aggregated care for regulatory purposes. Hence, the caregivers and the regulators are working toward a common goal of improving care. The same information is used for both purposes. Moreover, it is the same information used to develop and evaluate care plans. This technique is not only harmonious, it is efficient.

Information is also needed at the programmatic level. The discrepancy between services needed and those provided defines the agenda for program development. Well-documented evidence of deficiencies is critical to obtaining additional programmatic support. The CIMS should be capable of profiling the gaps in services and ideally indicating some of their consequences.

An information system should also be capable of producing administrative reports including summary data on important operational indices. It is useful, for example, to understand what services were used by which clients and what were the reasons for termination of care. Clearly, any information to be summarized must first be built into the basic design of the information system. Because it is not always possible to anticipate all the information one wants to analyze, the system should be flexibly designed to allow for modifications. Individual components should be able to be added and changed without having to alter the fundamental architecture.

The centrality of outcomes data in long-term care has already been emphasized. Especially when the relationship between the processes and outcomes of care are not well understood or causal pathways are poorly developed, an emphasis on outcomes seems like the best way to avoid the trap of premature orthodoxy. The same outcomes information, with appropriate adjustments for client characteristics, can be used on at least two different levels for monitoring purposes beyond direct feedback to the individual care provider. A large clinical data base of consistently collected information on clients' progress and the services they received forms the substrate for useful clinical epidemiological analysis. Outcomes can be thought of as the result of two forces: client characteristics and care. The effectiveness of the latter can be inferred by analyzing sufficient samples that provide enough information on the former to determine the relationship between the type of care rendered and the clients' characteristics. In other words, one can deduce what kinds of care work best for what kinds of clients. Thus, epidemiological analysis can help to ascertain the state of the art of care.

However, doing the right thing may not be enough (nor is there necessarily only one right thing to do). The skill of an individual practitioner can be inferred from comparing the adjusted outcomes for a given caregiver who did the appropriate things to the adjusted outcomes for the same problems achieved by others.

Attributes of an Information System

A good CIMS should be efficient; that is, it should eliminate all unnecessary redundancy. At present, nursing home recording is plagued with duplicated effort. Each discipline collects information, much of which is common to several disciplines. In an era when time spent on charting seems to be time not spent with clients, this unneeded duplication drains scarce resources. Computerization makes information available in multiple places with no added cost. Thus, information collected by one discipline can automatically be displayed in the forms used by another. Opportunities can be provided to allow the second professional to differ with the findings of the first and to highlight these discrepancies for reconciliation at team meetings. Likewise, multidisciplinary participation does not mean that a representation of every discipline has to see each client. The costs of assessment can be greatly reduced if disciplinary expertise is used to identify the information that should be collected while the actual collection of at least the basic data set is accomplished by a single professional. Specific expertise can be called in if the need for more detailed data is identified by the basic screening questions.

Computerized information is also portable. It can be transferred by telephone. Copying it does not diminish its availability centrally. Especially in situations like home care, or sending patients to an emergency department, this means that one can access information from the main data source and still maintain the integrity of the original record.

The CIMS should make inputting data easy. One of the frustrating problems with computerized systems can be the failure to discriminate among various levels of familiarity with the operations of the system. New users need a lot of instructions, which are unduly cumbersome to those already familiar with the details. A well-designed system provides different levels of assistance through devices like pop-up help screens that can be called on as needed.

A critical feature of any information approach is consistency. Entries must mean the same thing to different users. Terms must be carefully defined. Here again, help screens can provide definitions for those not familiar with the system. Internal logic programs can avoid inappropriate responses and make necessary calculations that might otherwise create errors.

In addition to consistency, accuracy is vital. One of the most frustrating problems with most forms is the inability to distinguish between missing information and negative values. A structured approach to data collection will specify the component data elements and avoid general (and meaningless) summary comments like "normal." Programming can require an answer when an answer is appropriate before the user can go on to the next item.

Because the data is designed to be used, it must be complete. Using branching logic, as discussed earlier, provides a means to cover the performance spectrum and still assure comparability and individual information. Structured data, including reminders and stimuli to consider specific issues, can enhance completeness.

Structured data entry will also minimize entry effort. Computerization means that a user need enter only a short answer perhaps not more than a letter, but the report produced will come out as full narrative test. The structured format should not preclude narrative commentary, however. Often the items themselves will not tell the full story. Clinicians need to be able to explain their answers, if they are expected to be willing to adhere to a fixed format. The CIMS should accept narrative comments, which can be printed at the end as part of the report in the appropriate places.

It is essential that the information system be viewed as supplementing and enhancing professional practice rather than supplanting it. Too much structure may rankle clinicians and give them a sense of using a cookbook. The system should structure decision making by providing a way to review all of the relevant information, but the professionals should make the choices about the priorities. It is very useful to stimulate memory and even to offer suggestions, but it is dangerous to offer overt algorithms.

A strong advantage of computerized information is the ability to display it in multiple modes. Once recorded, the same data can be transformed into flow sheets, summary tables, narrative text, and graphs. Modern long-term care practice requires a longitudinal perspective. Change over time is the key to understanding progress in LTC. Graphic presentation can display at a glance the changes in a client's status for designated parameters and can contrast that course with what might be expected from ordinary care. As noted earlier, much of the positive feedback and job satisfaction for providers will come from this contrast. Moreover, many of the front-line workers in LTC have minimal training and may even have problems with literacy. Graphic presentations can make vivid the accomplishments for such workers. Simple entry systems can likewise make it possible to engage many of these front-line workers in active data use and thus remind them of tasks to be accomplished and point to progress being made. The very act of displaying data in terms of changes over time encourages all users to think in these terms.

Practical Issues

One of the considerations in introducing computerized record keeping is how to assure access to users. The logistics will depend in part on the type of care provided. For home care, where workers are rarely at a base station, each worker will need some means of entering data and maintaining updated files. Lap-top computers are now becoming affordable and can be linked by modems to base stations to both transmit and receive data. In nursing homes, different strategies may pertain. It is feasible to use lap-tops at the clients' bedsides. Although some people fear the anonymity implied by these machines, experience suggests that clients actually become fascinated with them and see such care as being more professional. Alternatively, one can collect the information in more traditional ways and enter it at a terminal at the nurses' station. It is important that there be adequate access to terminals. When professionals are forced to wait to use the machine, they will see this as a major impediment and will be reluctant to use them. Moreover, the quality of the data will deteriorate if too much time elapses between gathering and entering it. Usually notes are just stimuli to memory. The next generation of machines will see even greater portability with new lines of hand-held devices that can be used for modest data-entry tasks. These machines can be pre-programmed to create stimuli for entry and then be downloaded into more powerful machines for analysis.

Typing skills should not be an issue. Well-designed CIMSs will demand short answers at most, although there will be the opportunity for narrative text. Bar codes, light pens, and touch screens can each be used to make the data-entry process even faster and easier.

Bar coding has a great potential in long-term care. It is already widely used in inventory control and is familiar to most shoppers at the checkout counters of today's supermarkets. It is easy to imagine its extension into nursing homes. Medication errors can be virtually eliminated by a system that pre-programs medications schedules, including dosages, and compares the information to the patient's bar-coded identification tag. By reading both the caregiver's and the patient's tag the internal clock on the bar-code reader can maintain a tamper-proof record; by comparing the medication code and the patient code, the system will beep when a potential error is committed.

Bar coding can also be used for behavioral programs. Aides can be readily trained to use a simple instruction card to go through a standardized routine for such things as toileting. For example, a system already developed to manage incontinence has each aide approach a patient, read the patient's bar code and her own (which logs the time of the contact), and then record the answers to a series of questions listed on a laminated bar coded card. For instance, is the patient wet? If so, how much? If not, was the patient toileted? Was urine passed? This is accomplished using a small hand-held bar-code reader no larger than a credit card. The reader is recharged at the end of each shift, while the data is downloaded simultaneously into a larger machine, which prints a summary of the shift's activities. Aides are given immediate feedback (including graphs) of their performance (in terms of toileting frequencies, percentage of time patients were wet, etc.) and are compared with other aides on the same and different shifts, and to their own prior performance. This system has been well received by aides, who seem to respond well to the instant feedback offered by an analysis of data at the end of each shift.

Indeed, in a low-technology environment like long-term care, computerized information seems to have a better chance of acceptance than in more complex environments like hospitals. Technology is viewed as a means of increasing the prestige of the job, and the feedback, if well presented, is seen as an important source of positive supervision. Busy nurses have remarked that they are now able to gain a perspective about the work of the aides they supervise.

Twenty Criteria for Judging a CIMS

Clearly, electronic data management is likely to be a major clinical and fiscal tool in the future of many long-term care facilities and agencies. Only the very largest facility systems can afford the time and cost of developing such information management themselves. Therefore consideration must be given to the criteria that are appropriate to selecting an externally developed system and the consulting organization that will provide, install, and support it.

A CIMS must be chosen carefully. Generally speaking, they are not available "off the shelf," ready to be purchased and installed by the facility staff. This means that the choice must be made of the system itself, and equally importantly of the organization that will provide and service it. Twenty salient criteria to use in making these selections follow. The list does not start with technical details of the system itself, but with broader and more critical considerations. Regardless of the techincal excellence of a CIMS, if it is not actually used and depended on it is a lost investment.

Training and Support

The quality and availability of the training programs in the use of the CIMS, and the ongoing support of the system once it is in place, will often determine whether the system is used and whether it is used to maximum benefit. Most of the people who will personally use the CIMS will have had little or no prior experience with computers. Many will actually fear what they see as a new-fangled technology and will resist it initially. This resistance will increase over time if the initial experience is not positive.

Not only must the CIMS have sound, easy-to-comprehend training packages provided during installation, but the ongoing support must be responsive and available on nearly a 24-hour basis via an 800 telephone number. While all software companies advertise support, it must be recognized that the support required by the typical nursing facility will be extraordinary in comparison with that needed by the user of a standard application software package. Further, the personnel who provide the support should have a working knowledge of nursing practices carried out in facilities to deal with the issues that will arise.

The quality of the support to be expected of a company can be judged by requesting copies of logs of support requests that have been dealt with, as well as the results of customer satisfaction surveys. These records should reveal the prevalence of both problems encountered owing to software bugs, those resulting from clinical issues, and those incidental to problems encountered by the novice user.

Development Team Credentials

Technical competence in computerization is not the only consideration in a system vendor. The development team that created and supports the software program should have had hands-on experience in long-term care facilities, especially experience in actual nursing activities.

Software programs that manage the finances of a nursing facility and software systems that guide and monitor nursing functions are necessarily different. The latter systems must have a look and feel that is characteristic of the way things are typically done in the facility. Nurses have developed and perfected the ways they plan and deliver care in an environment that is often understaffed, crisis driven, and short of resources. The CIMS that requires major changes in standard operating procedures will not fare well.

The unique clinical information needs of the nursing facility in the 1990s are complex, substantial in scope, and critical to maintaining compliance with regulation. To ensure that this information is gathered, managed, and used to the betterment of care delivery, the CIMS must make sense to the nursing personnel. It must fit into the way they carry out their daily activities so that time is saved, care is improved, and regulatory compliance is achieved.

Decisions: Supplemented or Supplanted

Central to the spirit of OBRA is the role of the interdisciplinary team. This concept holds that the best care decisions are reached through the consensus of a group of professionals representing the disciplines of nursing, social work, dietetics, activities (occupational therapy, physical therapy, etc.), and medicine. In addition, the lawmakers recognized the importance of the participation of the resident or the resident's representative.

The CIMS must not only accommodate each of these disciplines through discipline-specific content to the assessment, but it should facilitate communication among and between disciplines. The process through which clinical decisions are made, both individually and collectively, can be guided by the CIMS, but they must not be made by the CIMS. In other words, the CIMS should supplement the decision process by offering products, reminders, and clues that follow best practice and structure to the process. The CIMS that supplants the decision process by offering canned solutions to standard problems or diagnoses is not acceptable.

The key concept in the new regulations and in contemporary understanding of best practice is individualization of the care plan. No two plans of care should be the same, even when two residents appear on the surface to present identical problems. Individual differences always exist in terms of preferences, past histories leading to placement, severity of the conditions, and best approaches to addressing problems in individual circumstances. To ensure individualization of care plans, the CIMS must present multiple options to the team members as they select and prioritize problems, goals, approaches, and criterion levels of goal attainment according to the assessed needs of each individual resident.

Resident Assessment

The resident assessment instrument (RAI), selected by each state to comply with the OBRA requirement that each resident be assessed using a uniform data set, is the core element of a CIMS. For a CIMS to be even considered by a facility, it must incorporate the RAI as its central feature. The HCFA-designated MDS has been published in draft form and is accompanied by a set of RAPs that are triggered during assessment. The MDS, RAPs, and triggers, and the instructions for using each of these elements, combine to form the RAI. The RAPs "trigger" clues to the nurse assessor about what additional assessment data should be gathered, what factors related to an identified problem should be considered, and in some cases suggestions for care planning activities.

Most experts agree that the MDS alone does not meet the OBRA requirement for a comprehensive assessment. A minimum set is only a minimum set. Consequently, the extent to which the CIMS's assessment module goes beyond the MDS will prove to be an important evaluative criterion in choosing the right computer system. Several expanded versions of the MDS already exist (e.g., the MDS plus) and several more are being developed. The ideal CIMS should be capable of expansion to accommodate these developments.

Time

Reports of assessment findings output by the CIMS must follow the federal and state requirements and should also contribute directly to the care planning process for which the assessment was done (see next criterion). The forms on which the reports appear should be legible and of a size that fits into standard medical records. Graphics are a highly desirable feature that enhances the multiple uses of reports.

Another evaluative criterion is the time required to use the CIMS. This is not merely an incidental consideration. Assessment using the CIMS should take no more time than assessment using the pencil-and-paper medium and preferably should take less time. The ease and speed of assessment will be largely determined by the competence of the software program. Items must be presented in the correct order; selection sets should be displayed in a manner that allows single-key selection; resident preference items should be paired with required items (e.g., preferred type and time of day of bath with the bathing activities-of-daily-living item); contingent items should have built-in skips (e.g., if "no behavior exhibited" is selected, the screen should automatically clear to the next section).

Care Planning

The main purpose of conducting a comprehensive assessment is to develop a care plan that directly addresses, in priority, the problems and needs of the resident. This relationship between the assessment findings and the care of the resident is not only of paramount importance to the well-being of the resident; it is also the central criterion of the entire assessment planning function that OBRA emphasizes. By extension, the next important criterion that will be used in judging the quality of care delivered by the facility is the relationship between the plan of care and the actual care that is delivered. In other words, do the problems identified in assessment have corresponding goals and approaches in the care plan, and are these approaches being followed in the daily care that is being delivered?

Most CIMSs will have a care planning module. The feature that will distinguish one CIMS from another is the extent to which the assessment and care planning modules are integrated. Do they operate in the same file and talk to each other? Functionally, does practice move smoothly between the two? In practical terms, the problems identified in assessment should generate a plan unique to the individual and the plan should not be merely selected by the team from a standard library of options in the planning module. An advantage of an integrated system is that no single problem of the resident will be overlooked in the plan. Other advantages, besides accuracy of description itself, is that a properly integrated system will be faster in that only problems relevant to an individual resident will be displayed; the direct relationship between assessment and care is assured; and each care plan will be individualized so that no two care plans will be the same.

There are care planning modules, and there are care planning modules. It is essential to distinguish those that operate dynamically from those that simply call up fixed response screens triggered by a problem. The desired module is one that will allow an individualized care plan to be developed from the several elements that distinguish and describe the full extent of the client's problem. The care plan should contain specific actions to be taken and a clear assignment of responsibility for carrying them out.

The incorporation of resident preferences as part of a comprehensive plan of care directly contributes to a measure of the quality of life a person experiences in a care facility. If preferences are addressed in the assessment module as stated earlier, they should be incorporated into planning for care. As with individual problems, an integrated CIMS will assure that these important findings will not be overlooked in the care planning process.

Clinical Base of the CIMS

OBRA's legitimate emphasis on the quality of care and its focus on outcomes dictate that the clinical logic must meet the tests of "best practice." It follows that any CIMS that purports to reflect best practice should truly do just that. The obvious questions then are: What constitutes best practice, and what criteria can be used to judge a given CIMS's clinical base against the standards of best practice?

Fortunately, a set of criteria do now exist in a recent publication of the American Nurses Association. Standards and Scope of Gerontological Nursing Practice (American Nurses Association), offers the most current set of criteria that can be used in the evaluation of a CIMS's clinical base. The criteria will not be repeated here. Despite the fact that these standards place a higher value on the nursing diagnosis approach than the authors of this chapter would, it does represent an excellent source of evaluative criteria.

User-Defined Capability

Although a well-developed CIMS will deal adequately with the external and regulatory standards that now require a RAI, it is not necessarily true that "one size fits all." The facility may well have good reason for making the CIMS serve related or even unique purposes in addition. The flexibility of the CIMS to provide capabilities that are defined by the user facility is a proper evaluative criterion.

Caution is advised here, not to discourage dialogue with a potential vendor but to recognize the closed-end nature of some (but not all) available CIMS packages. It is also necessary to resist the urge to use the CIMS as the vehicle for all the facility's computerization. Moderation is the key. A well-designed CIMS will have the flexibility necessary to add a moderate amount of user-defined capability and link it to the existing modules without either overwhelming the CIMS or costing an inordinate amount of adjustment at installation.

It is by definition impossible to list all the user-defined capabilities that might be wanted, ranging from generating reports on a nonstandard schedule to adding an item to a problem checklist in the assessment module. Questions that clarify the flexibility of a CIMS include: Does this system permit content editing by the user, and can this feature be installed at all? What will be the added cost of programming, modifying manuals, and training? Will it be integrated in the same way as other features in the CIMS? How long will it take to make the modification? How much space remains in the recommended or furnished hardware configuration, and how much of that will this use? Will it affect the speed at which the program will run? Will it be covered by the same performance guarantee as the rest of the CIMS?

Guarantees of Changing Regulatory Compliance

Regulations governing long-term care facilities will continue to change. As they do, a well-designed and well-maintained CIMS will be able to adapt with minimum fuss.

Unlike user-defined capabilities, the flexibility demanded by changes in regulation cannot be defined and questioned in detail in advance. The pertinent questions are whether the vendor guarantees that changes will be made, what is the maximum time the changes will take, and what are the limits of the changes that will be accommodated without extra cost in the regular updates of the system (see next criterion). During this discussion it should be possible to estimate what planning the vendor has given to these contingencies; this is a consideration in vendor competence. Because the matter is technical, it will not always be possible to clarify directly just how the changes will be programmed, but the contract should deal with performance in regard to this kind of flexibility.

Frequency, Content, Cost, and Ease of Upgrades and Enhancements

The CIMS should have a stated policy of upgrades and enhancements as part of its offer. There may be a schedule. For that matter, a completely designed CIMS will probably have a built-in date on which it will become inoperative without intervention by the vendor (a "drop-dead" date), to prevent use beyond the contracted or otherwise proper time.

The basic architecture of the CIMS, if it has been well tested in the field, will not likely need upgrade. No upgrade should make previous files unusable, of course, and this is not likely and should be covered in the contract. But other changes of a less drastic nature and improvements will inevitably be found, in addition to the changes that are impelled by changes in regulations. These are the subjects of upgrades and enhancements, most of which should be a part of the normal contracted cost of CIMS maintenance and support.

Some enhancements will be optional, being essentially additions to the things that the CIMS will do for the facility. Additional cost should be expected for them. There may be upgrading cost associated with what are in effect new versions of the CIMS.

Source Code Escrow

Vendors of CIMS are like other businesses in not being immortal. They can, for example, go out of business through bankruptcy. An important criterion thus is the existence of an escrow of the CIMS source code. This is an archive of the source code and the means for regenerating the entire CIMS in the event that the vendor cannot continue to service the CIMS and its user facilities. Provision should be made in the escrow for some other entity to be authorized to service the CIMS in the event of the vendor's demise.

The escrow has the additional advantage of serving as a secure backup in case of physical loss of the vendor's working master copy. The physical location of the escrow archive should minimize simultaneous loss in a common disaster. A prudent vendor will have made this provision and can describe it.

The user facility should know how to access the escrow if the vendor goes out of business, and how to resume service or stand it down with the preservation of its contents in commonly usable form. There should be assurance that all versions and upgrades of the CIMS are escrowed.

User Friendliness

The much-used term, "user friendly," should simply mean that a nontechnical user will readily learn the system and easily use it. The dimensions of friendliness include considerations of hardware, ease of putting in and getting out information, intuitiveness of look and feel, minimal distraction from professional duties while using it, and in this context compatibility with good practice above all.

The part of the CIMS that the user deals with should be clearly in the format that the actual user is accustomed to using, disregarding for the moment that the computer itself may be novel. The actual user is often not a highly trained professional person (this is, among other things, a cost consideration) nor is he or she necessarily a typist. The features of user friendliness are too lengthy to cite here in detail, but it is worth repeating that matters should be simplified and made as essential, intuitive, and comfortable as possible for the user, considering the skills typically brought to the task. The training program and pop-up help screens that accompany the system can make a critical difference here.

An often overlooked friendliness feature is the need for the person who puts in the information to get personal benefit from the system. There are many ways to provide this, once the need is recognized. For example, it may reward the person to see, after entering data, a summary of what has been put in, perhaps personalized with the person's name credited. Some users, of course, will be best rewarded with the CIMS's standard reports. The criterion here is to determine what direct satisfaction this particular CIMS provides to the person who is operating it.

Standardized Screens

Each CIMS has a particular look and feel. The criterion at issue is that the look and feel should not be chaotic nor disruptive. Standardization of screens — the displays that the person looks at when interacting with the system — can provide a familiarity with where and how pertinent information and questions will appear. This standardization should be unobtrusive and as compatible with human visual perception as possible.

At some points in operating the CIMS, the user is variously presented with the need to select among listed choices, to enter something from a keyboard, or even just to look at and understand a statement of information before continuing. The CIMS may use a single style of presentation for all these things, or it may present each required interaction in a different way. In general, it has been found that a uniform style of presentation or standardized screens will function best if the format gives clear clues as to what the user should do with it.

Operating Systems

Modern computers found in business each use one of a limited number of operating systems: MS/PC-DOS (the "IBM" system), OS-2, Unix, Xenix, or the Macintosh system; or a network variation. Software, including CIMSs, is written in one or another of these fundamental languages and in general will not work on a computer that uses a different one. A few CIMSs may have versions in more than one operating system.

Security, Backup, and Storage Capabilities

The data in a CIMS are valuable and perhaps irreplaceable. Data must be protected from damage and loss.

A CIMS vendor will be able to state clearly what provisions have been made to protect the data from unauthorized or accidental alteration or loss, and may speak of error traps, redundancy, automatic backup, and password levels. To apply the criteria in this set of considerations, the facility needs to have these and similar terms replaced with plain English descriptions of the features so that their meaning in this particular CIMS is clear.

The facility should have its own local backup of current data, and the system manual can describe how this is managed with this CIMS. Some systems are more convenient in this than are others. In addition, if the CIMS entails transmittal of data to the vendor for processing, the facility should determine whether the data set can be reconstructed from the vendor's files if local recovery from disaster is not possible.

Data management is not a snapshot; as an ongoing process, the data of days, months, and even years past are pertinent and must be stored. The criterion here has to do with whether the data are stored as part of a single file that is always active, how the historical data interact with current data, how often and in what manner archive copies of the data set are made, and how they are stored. Both convenience and security should be considered.

Quality Assurance Features

The facility has obvious interest in the quality of the CIMS's performance and usage. The vendor also has a large and legitimate interest in this, with reputation and proprietary control at stake.

The training and support programs are major quality assurance features, effective in proportion to their thoroughness and vigilance. If the CIMS package entails transfer of data to the vendor for processing, it should be determined whether any quality assurance evaluation is made of that data. Management oversight by the facility's administration is the first line of quality assurance, though reliance on the vendor may be necessary for some technical aspects.

The ultimate issue in quality assurance, once accuracy of the data is assured, has to do with the use of data. Quality assurance checks should be made at this point not only on the accuracy and clarity of the application of the information but also on the regularity with which use is invoked, and the attention to and the consequences of the use of information.

Hardware and Compatibility Requirements

Electronic management of information requires hardware. Operating systems are one aspect of this (see earlier discussion on operating systems), and once that is dealt with other considerations come into play. Required and recommended minimum memory, size, and type of storage; graphics systems; display; portability; and keyboard features should be explicitly determined.

The criterion, by now a familiar one to those who deal with any computerized operation, is whether the CIMS will run on the facility's existing computers; if not, what it will take in cost, time, enhancement, or replacement of equipment or translation to either adapt or replace the existing equipment. Some CIMSs will come with their own hardware, such as a set of portable computers, as part of the total CIMS package. In that case the issue will be the compatibility of the new configuration with the existing facility system (to the extent, if any, to which the existing system will be involved).

Therefore a facility considering a CIMS should know the characteristics of its present system and should determine the exact requirements or furnished hardware of the CIMS. A competent vendor will be able to state just what are the minimum and recommended hardware and operating system requirements of the CIMS under consideration. The offer should be explicit on this and on what is included in the cost of the CIMS package.

Modularity

Though on the surface it must operate as a seamless system, a full-featured CIMS is likely to be made up of modules. This is a convenience in development and an efficiency in updating and modifying.

Typical modules include assessment with data input and editing, data sorting and transformation, retrieval and lookup functions, storage and file management, facilitation of planning and plan recording, report generating, and various utilities. A CIMS may be available as a basic system and with enhancing modules that will expand its capabilities, or it may be available only as a complete package.

Some features may be available only at extra cost. The offer should be clear as to what is included, and what if anything can be added. In any event, the facility considering a CIMS should determine from the vendor the characteristics of this system's modularity.

Trial and Pilot Permission

A CIMS offer should come with provision for a risk-free or low-cost "test drive," the opportunity to try it for a period to determine whether in the real situation it serves the purposes at reasonable cost and effort.

A reasonable time for trial application is 30 days, or for a full cycle that samples the output (reports, and data retrieval and application) of the system. The time to discover problems is before extensive investment has been made in data entry and in the revision of the facility's operating procedures and before the full cost of purchase has been committed. It is unavoidable that cost will have been incurred for some of the training, because the system cannot be tested without some trained users.

The offer and the contract should be clear on this criterion. The facility should also consider whether it is making a psychological commitment, in contrast to the formality of signing a contract, prematurely.

Cost

The cost of acquiring and operating a CIMS is an obvious criterion. It is approached in the same way as is the cost of any other business decision.

The offer will be clear as to up-front cost and as to what is included in this cost, or it should be clarified. Cost will be judged in relation to the necessity for and the capability of the CIMS, and alternatives to it. A reminder is in order that the facility should determine whether the training and installation are included in the quoted initial cost. If hardware is part of the CIMS package, its cost must also be considered.

The ongoing costs of operating the CIMS are more complicated. Criteria include the following: What fee, if any, is charged periodically for the continued use of the system? What is the cost, if any, of vendor support and help during the life of the system? Is this cost on a per-month basis or on the basis of hours of help used? Is there any guarantee that this cost will not be raised or any limits to what the raises will be? Will there be any required or recommended training refreshers offered and if so at what cost? If there is an upgrade in the system, what is it likely to cost? If there is a new version of the system, will the vendor continue to support the old version at presently quoted cost? Will there be any end-of-contract closure cost or a required notice period?

The indirect cost of having personnel trained and the cost of assigning personnel to operate the system must also be considered. This cost will be offset, to an extent that should be determined, by the cost of using an alternative system including the cost of a pencil-and-paper system, or the financial and other cost of not having a competent RAI.

CONCLUSION

There currently exists information technology to support and encourage better long-term care. Many vendors offer information systems. Some are quite good; others are not. Organizations interested in improving their approach to managing information must take the time to examine their options including testing the most likely systems. Decisions about which system to adopt should be made by both clinicians and administrators.

The potential benefits from and feasibility of computerization of long-term care would seem to argue inexorably for such a transition, but the response, even in the face of the new demands of OBRA, have been much less intense than one might expect. It is difficult to explain just why the moment has not been seized. A cynic might suggest that the long-term care industry has a history of not moving until pushed. For the moment at least, HCFA has not provided any inducements to computerize nursing home information systems, leaving the decision to the marketplace. Computerization does involve cost. Nursing home operators who feel themselves financially pressed will be less willing to spend money for an improvement that affects only quality than for one that can enhance revenue. At present, there is no evidence that having a computerized information system confers any direct market advantage.

If it is the case that nursing homes will not computerize until they are told to, then it falls to the government to provide some incentive to do so. HCFA's enthusiasm will be tempered by their conviction that computerization does indeed lead to better quality. At present, HCFA seems more content to leave that decision up to the industry, especially because such a step leaves them less responsible for paying for the cost of acquiring the technology.

It is frustrating to have reached a point where one can see the future, especially the potential of improved information management to transform the nature of long-term care services, and face so many reluctant participants. It appears that neither the government nor the long-term care industry is as yet prepared to initiate decisive action. At a minimum, one might hope to see at least more demonstrations of the possibilities to be achieved by changing our approach to information management.

REFERENCES

American Nurses Association Task Force to Revise a Statement on the Scope and Standards of Gerontological Nursing Practice. (1987). *Standards and Scope of Gerontological Nursing Practice.* Kansas City, MO: American Nurses Association.

Institute of Medicine. (1986). *Improving the quality of care in nursing homes.* Washington, DC: National Academy Press.

Morris, J. N., Hawes, C., Fries, B. E., Phillips, C. D., Mor, V., Katz, S., Murphy, K., Drugovich, M. L., & Friedlob, A. S. (1990). Designing the national resident assessment instrument for nursing homes. *The Gerontologist, 30,* 293–307.

Seligman, M. E. P. (1976). *Learned helplessness and depression in animals and men.* Morristown, NJ: General Learning Press.

Index

NOTES

NOTES

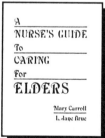

Managing Urinary Incontinence in the Elderly

John F. Schnelle, PhD

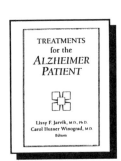

This unique new work takes a wholly different approach to the problem of incontinence in the elderly. Rather than treating it as an inevitable part of the aging process, Dr. Schnelle outlines a complete set of proven strategies for alleviating and even solving the problem for many elders.

Contents: The Problem of Urinary Incontinence. Starting a Program. Basic Incontinence Management. Assessment. Program Implementation. Quality Control. Night Incontinence Care. Incontinence Management at Home.

1991   144pp   0-8261-7360-8   hardcover

Treatments for the Alzheimer Patient

Lissy F. Jarvik, MD, PhD
Carol H. Winograd, MD, Editors

"...offering readers multiple strategies for treating the disease...emphasizes that Alzheimer's disease affects not only the patient but also the family and caretakers. Perspectives from physicians, family members and sociologists are well documented, and practical advice on handling difficult conditions commonly associated with Alzheimer's disease is provided...I recommend it to anyone involved in the care of elderly persons."

—American Family Physician

1988   288pp   0-8261-6000-X   hardcover

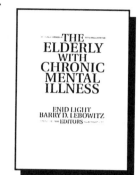
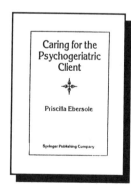